D0908869

Instructional Course Lectures

Volume XXXVII 1988

American Academy
of Orthopaedic Surgeons

Instructional Course Lectures

Volume XXXVII 1988

Edited by
Frank H. Bassett III, MD
Professor, Orthopaedic Surgery
Department of Surgery
Assistant Professor
Department of Anatomy
Chief, Sports Medicine Section
Division of Orthopaedic Surgery
Duke University Medical Center
Durham, North Carolina

With 397 illustrations

American Academy
of Orthopaedic Surgeons

American Academy of Orthopaedic Surgeons

Instructional Course Lectures
Volume XXXVII

Assistant Director, Scientific Publications: Marilyn L. Fox, PhD
Director of Communications and Publications: Mark W. Wieting
Editor: Wendy O. Schmidt
Editorial Assistant: Alice A. Michaels

Design: James Buddenbaum Design, Wilmette, Illinois
Typesetting: Impressions, Inc., Madison, Wisconsin
Printing: Malloy Lithographing, Inc., Ann Arbor, Michigan

The material presented in this volume has been made available by the American Academy of Orthopaedic Surgeons for educational purposes only. This material is not intended to represent the only, or necessarily best, methods or procedures for the medical situations discussed, but rather is intended to present an approach, view, statement, or opinion of the author(s) or producer(s), which may be helpful to others who face similar situations.

Contributors

Lewis D. Anderson, MD, Professor and Chairman, Department of Orthopaedic Surgery, Vice President for Medical Affairs, University of South Alabama, College of Medicine, Mobile, Alabama

Yoram Ben-Menachem, MD, Professor of Radiology, Baylor College of Medicine, Attending Radiologist, Ben Taub and V.A.M.C. Hospitals, Houston, Texas

Bruce D. Browner, MD, Associate Professor and Director, Division of Orthopaedic Surgery, The University of Texas, Health Science Center at Houston, Houston, Texas

Robert W. Bucholz, MD, Associate Professor of Orthopaedic Surgery, The University of Texas Southwestern Medical School, Dallas, Texas

Charles P. Capito, MD, Pelvic and Acetabular Fellow, Department of Orthopaedic Surgery, University of Pittsburgh, School of Medicine, Pittsburgh, Pennsylvania

Peter G. Carnesale, MD, Clinical Associate Professor, Department of Orthopaedics, University of Tennessee, The Campbell Clinic, Memphis, Tennessee

Norris C. Carroll, MD, FRCS(C), Head, Division of Orthopedics, The Children's Memorial Hospital, Chicago, Illinois

William G. Carson, Jr., MD, Assistant Clinical Professor of Orthopaedics, University of South Florida, Tampa, Florida

Frank M. Chang, MD, Director of Orthopaedics, The Denver Children's Hospital, Denver, Colorado

Sara C. Charles, MD, Associate Professor of Clinical Psychiatry, University of Illinois at Chicago, Chicago, Illinois

J. Roger Clark, MD, Southern Orthopaedic and Sports Medicine Center, Nashville, Tennessee

J. Dean Cole, MD, Assistant Professor, Division of Orthopaedics, The University of Texas, Health Science Center at Houston, Houston, Texas

Charles N. Cornell, MD, Associate Professor of Orthopaedic Surgery, Cornell University Medical College, Attending Orthopaedic Surgeon, The Hospital for Special Surgery, New York, New York

Andrei A. Czitrom, MD, FRCS(C), PhD, Associate Professor, University of Toronto, Toronto General Hospital, Mount Sinai Hospital, Toronto, Ontario, Canada

Henry Deleeuw, MD, Resident Fellow, Department of Orthopaedic Surgery, University of Pittsburgh, School of Medicine, Pittsburgh, Pennsylvania

Charles C. Edwards, MD, Associate Professor, Division of Orthopaedic Surgery, University of Maryland, Baltimore, Maryland

William F. Enneking, MD, Distinguished Service Professor, Eugene L. Jewett Professor of Orthopaedic Surgery, Department of Orthopaedics, University of Florida, Gainesville, Florida

Charles H. Epps, Jr., MD, Professor and Chief, Division of Orthopaedic Surgery, Howard University Hospital, Washington, DC

William E. Garrett, Jr., MD, PhD, Assistant Professor, Division of Orthopaedic Surgery, Duke University Medical Center, Durham, North Carolina

Gerard L. Glancy, MD, Director of Medical Education, Department of Orthopaedic Surgery, The Children's Hospital, Denver, Colorado

James M. Glick, MD, Associate Clinical Professor, Department of Orthopaedic Surgery, University of California Medical Center, San Francisco, Chief, Department of Orthopaedic Surgery, Mt. Zion Hospital and Medical Center, Team Physician and Associate Professor of Physical Education, San Francisco State University, San Francisco, California

Allan E. Gross, MD, FRCS(C), PhD, Professor and Head, Division of Orthopaedics, University of Toronto, Toronto General Hospital, Mount Sinai Hospital, Toronto, Ontario, Canada

Wm. Douglas Gurley, MD, Orthopaedic surgeon, Denver, Colorado

Charles E. Henning, MD, Clinical Assistant Professor, University of Kansas School of Medicine, Mid-America Center for Sports Medicine, Wichita, Kansas

Thomas A. Lange, MD, Associate Professor, Head of Orthopaedic Oncology, University of Arkansas for Medical Sciences, Little Rock, Arkansas

Fred Langer, MD, FRCS(C), PhD, Associate Professor, University of Toronto, Toronto General Hospital, Mount Sinai Hospital, Toronto, Ontario, Canada

Mary A. Lynch, MD, Mid-America Center for Sports Medicine, Wichita, Kansas

Richard E. McCarthy, MD, Associate Professor, University of Arkansas for Medical Sciences, Head, Section of Pediatric Orthopaedics, Arkansas Children's Hospital, Little Rock, Arkansas

Douglas W. McKay, MD, Chairman, Department of Pediatric Orthopaedic Surgery, Children's Hospital National Medical Center, Professor, Department of Child Health and Development, George Washington University Medical Center, Washington, DC

Dana C. Mears, MD, PhD, Associate Professor, Department of Orthopaedic Surgery, University of Pittsburgh, School of Medicine, Pittsburgh, Pennsylvania

Robert W. Metcalf, MD, Professor of Orthopaedic Surgery, University of Utah School of Medicine, Salt Lake City, Utah

Frederick N. Meyer, MD, Associate Professor, Department of Orthopaedic Surgery, Chief, Division of Hand Surgery, University of South Alabama, College of Medicine, Mobile, Alabama

Carl L. Nelson, MD, Professor and Chairman, Department of Orthopaedic Surgery, University of Arkansas for Medical Sciences, Little Rock, Arkansas

Sir Dennis Paterson, MD, FRCS, FRACS, Director and Chief Orthopaedic Surgeon, Department of Orthopaedic Surgery, Adelaide Children's Hospital, Adelaide, Australia

Paul Peters, MD, Chief Resident, Division of Orthopaedic Surgery, University of Texas Southwestern Medical School, Dallas, Texas

Gary G. Poehling, MD, Associate Professor, Bowman-Gray School of Medicine, Winston-Salem, North Carolina

Michael C. Reineck, MD, Orthopaedic surgeon, West Bend, Wisconsin

Thomas D. Rosenberg, MD, Assistant Clinical Professor of Orthopaedic Surgery, University of Utah School of Medicine, Salt Lake City, Utah

James H. Roth, MD, FRCS(C), Clinical Associate Professor, University of Western Ontario, London, Ontario, Canada

Eduardo A. Salvati, MD, Chief of Hip Clinic, Associate Attending Orthopaedic Surgeon, The Hospital for Special Surgery, Clinical Associate Professor of Orthopaedic Surgery, Cornell University Medical College, Associate Attending Orthopaedic Surgeon, The New York Hospital, New York, New York

Franklin H. Sim, MD, Professor of Orthopaedic Surgery, Mayo Medical School, Consultant, Department of Orthopaedics, Mayo Clinic and Mayo Foundation, Rochester, Minnesota

Robert Stallbaumer, RN, Mid-America Center for Sports Medicine, Wichita, Kansas

Herbert H. Stark, MD, Clinical Professor of Orthopaedic Surgery, University of Southern California, School of Medicine, President and Chairman, Division of Orthopaedic Surgery, King/Drew Medical Center, Los Angeles, California

Marvin E. Steinberg, MD, Professor and Vice-Chairman, Department of Orthopaedic Surgery, University of Pennsylvania, Philadelphia, Pennsylvania

Steven W. Vequist, RPT, Mid-America Center for Sports Medicine, Wichita, Kansas

Arthur K. Walling, MD, Associate Professor, Department of Orthopaedic Surgery, College of Medicine, University of South Florida, Tampa, Florida

Terry L. Whipple, MD, Assistant Clinical Professor, The Medical College of Virginia, Richmond, Virginia

Kaye E. Wilkins, MD, Clinical Professor of Orthopedics, The University of Texas, Health Science Center at San Antonio, San Antonio, Texas

Kim M. Yearout, RPT, Mid-America Center for Sports Medicine, Wichita, Kansas

Norman P. Zemel, MD, Clinical Associate Professor, Department of Orthopaedics, University of Southern California, School of Medicine, Los Angeles, California

Robert E. Zickel, MD, Clinical Professor of Orthopedic Surgery, Columbia University, Deputy Director, Department of Orthopedics, St. Luke's-Roosevelt Hospital Center, New York, New York

Preface

The American Academy of Orthopaedic Surgeons *Instructional Course Lectures Volume XXXVII* contains topics selected from the lectures presented at the Academy's Annual Meeting held in San Francisco, California, in January 1987.

It is the second of the volumes to be published by the Academy, whose Board of Directors in 1985 decided that the Academy should assume publishing responsibilities for its own instructional courses. In making this decision, one important consideration was the timeliness of the volumes. The goal was to publish each volume in time to make it available for review and purchase at the following year's Annual Meeting.

To meet this goal, contributors to volume 37 were asked to submit their manuscripts shortly after the San Francisco meeting. Largely because of their responsiveness to this request, we have met the Academy's goal. We on the Instructional Course Committee hope this volume will serve as an important precedent to the timeliness of future volumes and that it will be a worthy contribution to the Academy's mission of providing its Fellows with educational and current orthopaedic literature.

Several important areas in orthopaedics are covered in volume 37, with the sections on avascular necrosis, nonunion of long bones, pelvic ring disruptions, and arthroscopic surgery providing thorough reviews of these topics.

Again, I would like to thank the contributors to this volume for their efforts in producing material that is both current and informative. I would also like to thank the members of the Committee on Instructional Courses. Without their contributions of time, energy, and expertise, the instructional course lectures program upon which this volume is based would not have been so successful and well organized. It is also appropriate, I think, to acknowledge the many instructional course lecturers whose efforts and knowledge are so vital to the continuing importance of the instructional courses.

Finally, I would like to thank several Academy staff members who so ably assisted me in producing this volume in such timely fashion. Marilyn L. Fox, PhD, managed the development, editorial, and production processes. Wendy O. Schmidt was the primary manuscript editor, planned the layout of illustrations, and indexed the book. Alice A. Michaels edited manuscripts, coordinated the word processing effort, and carried out the permissions process. Geraldine H. Dubberke and Catherine D. Smith contributed their word processing skills. Mark W. Wieting provided valuable guidance and oversight throughout the entire project.

Frank H. Bassett III, MD
Durham, North Carolina
Chairman
Committee on Instructional Courses

Lewis D. Anderson, MD
Mobile, Alabama

Joseph S. Barr, Jr., MD
Boston, Massachusetts

Walter B. Greene, MD
Chapel Hill, North Carolina

Paul P. Griffin, MD
Baltimore, Maryland

Contents

S E C T I O N   I

Neoplasms

1 A System of Staging Musculoskeletal Neoplasms   3   W.F. Enneking

S E C T I O N   II

Bone Banks and   2 Bone Banks and Allografts in Community Practice   13   A.A. Czitrom
Allografts   A.E. Gross
                                                                                   F. Langer
                                                                                   F.H. Sim

S E C T I O N   III

Avascular Necrosis   3 Blood Supply to Bone and Proximal Femur: A   27   C.L. Nelson
                        Synopsis
                     4 The Staging of Aseptic Necrosis   33   T.A. Lange
                     5 Management of Avascular Necrosis of the Femoral   41   M.E. Steinberg
                        Head—An Overview
                     6 Early Diagnosis of Avascular Necrosis of the   51   M.E. Steinberg
                        Femoral Head
                     7 Avascular Necrosis of the Femoral Head in   59   R.E. McCarthy
                        Children
                     8 Long-Term Follow-up of Total Hip Replacement   67   E.A. Salvati
                        in Patients With Avascular Necrosis   C.N. Cornell

S E C T I O N   IV

The Child's Foot   9 The Painful Foot in the Child   77   K.E. Wilkins
                     10 Surgical Correction of Clubfoot   87   D.W. McKay
                     11 Pathoanatomy and Surgical Treatment of the   93   N.C. Carroll
                        Resistant Clubfoot
                     12 Gait Analysis and Intoeing   107   F.M. Chang
                     13 The Flexible Flatfoot   109   F.M. Chang
                     14 Surgical Management of the Flatfoot   111   G.L. Glancy

S E C T I O N   V

Pelvic Ring   15 Assessment of Pelvic Stability   119   R.W. Bucholz
Disruptions   P. Peters
                     16 Initial Management of Pelvic Ring Disruptions   129   B.D. Browner
                                                                                   J.D. Cole
                     17 Pelvic Fractures: Diagnostic and Therapeutic   139   Y. Ben-Menachem
                        Angiography
                     18 Posterior Pelvic Disruptions Managed by the Use   143   D.C. Mears
                        of the Double Cobra Plate   C.P. Capito
                                                                                   H. Deleeuw

S E C T I O N   VI

Nonunion of   19 Historical Overview of Treatment of Nonunion   153   D. Paterson
Long Bones   20 The Use of Electricity in the Treatment of   155   D. Paterson
                        Nonunion
                     21 Nonunion of the Diaphysis of the Radius and Ulna   157   L.D. Anderson
                                                                                   F.N. Meyer

	22	Nonunion of the Humerus	161	C.H. Epps, Jr.
	23	Nonunion of the Tibia: Experience With Modified Phemister Bone Graft and With Compression Plates and Cancellous Bone Graft	167	P.G. Carnesale
	24	Nonunions of Fractures of the Proximal and Distal Thirds of the Shaft of the Femur	173	R.E. Zickel

S E C T I O N   VII

Arthroscopic Surgery	25	Arthroscopic Surgery of the Wrist	183	J.H. Roth G.G. Poehling T.L. Whipple
	26	Arthroscopy of the Elbow	195	W.G. Carson, Jr.
	27	Arthroscopic Meniscectomy	203	T.D. Rosenberg R.W. Metcalf W.D. Gurley
	28	Arthroscopic Meniscus Repair With a Posterior Incision	209	C.E. Henning J.R. Clark M.A. Lynch R. Stallbaumer K.M. Yearout S.W. Vequist
	29	Hip Arthroscopy Using the Lateral Approach	223	J.M. Glick

S E C T I O N   VIII

Injuries to Bone and Muscle	30	Problem Fractures and Dislocations of the Hand	235	N.P. Zemel H.H. Stark
	31	Classification of Ankle Fractures: Which System To Use?	251	A.K. Walling
	32	Management of Open Fractures in the Multiply Injured Patient	257	C.C. Edwards
	33	Injuries to the Muscle-Tendon Unit	275	W.E. Garrett, Jr.

S E C T I O N   IX

Professional Liability	34	Handling Malpractice Stress: Suggestions for Physicians and Their Families	285	M.C. Reineck
	35	Psychological Reactions to Medical Malpractice Suits and the Development of Support Groups as a Response	289	S.C. Charles

Index			293	

Neoplasms

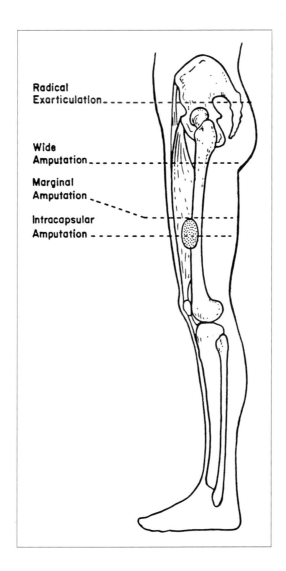

A System of Staging Musculoskeletal Neoplasms

William F. Enneking, MD

Introduction

The purposes of a staging system for musculoskeletal neoplasms are to (1) incorporate significant prognostic factors with progressive degrees of patient risk for local recurrence and distant metastases, (2) stratify the states to provide guidelines for surgical management, and (3) provide guidelines for adjunctive therapies. Over a number of years, staging systems for various classes of malignant tumors have been developed under the auspices of the American Joint Committee for Cancer Staging and End Results Reporting (AJC). The systems vary by cancer type depending on the natural course of the particular type of cancer. In 1980, a system for the surgical staging of musculoskeletal sarcoma was proposed, studied, and adopted by the Musculoskeletal Tumor Society[1] and subsequently adopted by the AJC.

The Staging System

The system adopted by the Musculoskeletal Tumor Society and the AJC is based on the interrelationship of three factors: grade (G), site (T), and metastases (M). Each of these factors is stratified by components that influence both prognosis and response to treatment. The changes in musculoskeletal neoplasms that form the basis of the staging system are classified as latent, active, aggressive, invasive, destructive, and metastatic. These changes together with their clinical, radiographic, and staging studies are summarized in Tables 1–1 and 1–2 and are discussed by grade, site, and metastasis.

Grade (G)

The grade is an assessment of the biologic aggressiveness of the lesion. It is not a purely histologic assessment (as in the 1, 2, 3, 4 grading of malignancies by Broders and associates[2]), nor a purely radiographic assessment (as in Lodwick's IA, IB, IC, II, and III radiographic classification of probabilities[3]) nor a purely clinical reflection of growth rate, doubling time, size, temperature, tissue pressure, or biochemical markers. This staging system is a blend of all of these assessments. The three stratifications of grade are G_0, G_1, and G_2. The identifying characteristics of grade are as follows:

G_0 **(benign)** Histologic characteristics are benign cy-

Table 1–1
Summary of the surgical staging system

Stage	Grade	Site	Metastasis
Benign tumors			
Stage 1, latent	G_0	T_0	M_0
Stage 2, active	G_0	T_0	M_0
Stage 3, aggressive	G_0	T_{1-2}	M_{0-1}
Malignant tumors			
Stage I, low-grade			
A: Intracompartmental	G_1	T_1	M_0
B: Extracompartmental	G_1	T_2	M_0
Stage II, high-grade			
A: Intracompartmental	G_2	T_1	M_0
B: Extracompartmental	G_2	T_2	M_0
Stage III, metastatic			
A: Intracompartmental, distant metastasis	G_{1-2}	T_1	M_1
B: Extracompartmental, distant metastasis	G_{1-2}	T_2	M_1

tologic findings, clearly differentiated cells, and low-to-moderate ratio of cell to matrix. The radiographic classification is Lodwick IA, IB, or IC, ranging from lesions with clear margins to those with capsular broaching and soft tissue extensions. Clinical findings include a distinct capsule, no satellites, no skips, rare metastases, variable growth rate, seen predominantly in adolescents and young adults.

G_1 **(low-grade malignant)** Histologic findings are Broder's grade 1 and some grade 2 with few mitoses, moderate differentiation, and distinct matrix. The radiographic classification is Lodwick II with indolent invasive features. Clinical findings are indolent growth, extracapsular satellites in the reactive zone, no skips, and only occasional distant metastases.

G_2 **(high-grade malignant)** Histologic findings are Broder's grades 2, 3, and 4 with frequent mitoses, poorly differentiated cells, and sparse and immature matrix. Anaplasia, pleomorphism, and hyperchromatism are high-grade cytologic features. The radiographic classification is Lodwick III, and the lesions are destructive and invasive. Clinical findings are rapid growth, symptomatic, both satellites and skips, occasional regional metastases, and frequent distant metastases.

The behavior of G_0 benign lesions may be latent, active, or aggressive. The histologic features of G_0 benign lesions are often poor indicators of their behavior, and thus the behavior of G_0 lesions is often better pre-

Table 1–2
Stages of musculoskeletal lesions

Stage	Grade, Site, Metastasis	Clinical Course	Isotope Scan
Benign			
1	$G_0 T_0 M_0$	Latent, static, self-healing	Background uptake
2	$G_0 T_0 M_0$	Active, progressing, expands bone or fascia	Increased uptake in lesion
3	$G_0 T_{1-2} M_{0-1}$	Aggressive, invasive, breaches bone or fascia	Increased uptake beyond lesion
Malignant			
I_A	$G_1 T_1 M_0$	Symptomatic; indolent growth	Increased uptake
I_B	$G_1 T_2 M_0$	Symptomatic mass; indolent growth	Increased uptake
II_A	$G_2 T_1 M_0$	Symptomatic; rapid growth	Increased uptake beyond radiographic limits
II_B	$G_2 T_2 M_0$	Symptomatic; rapid growth; fixed mass; pathologic fracture	Increased uptake beyond radiographic limits
III_A	$G_{1-2} T_1 M_1$	Systemic symptoms; palpable nodes; pulmonary symptoms	Pulmonary lesions; no increased uptake
III_B	$G_{1-2} T_2 M_1$	Systemic symptoms; palpable nodes; pulmonary symptoms	Pulmonary lesions; no increased uptake

*Lodwick radiographic classification.[3]

dicted by radiographic, staging, and clinical features (Table 1–2). The histologic characteristics of G_1 low-grade sarcomas are distinct from those of G_2 high-grade lesions, and their radiographic, staging, and clinical features support and confirm the histologic distinction. However, it may be difficult to distinguish G_0 lesions from G_1 lesions on purely histologic features, and, in many instances, the radiographic and particularly the staging studies may be of more value in differentiation than the histologic findings.

A promising new method of assessing grade is the determination of the nuclear DNA concentration (ploidy) by flow cytometry. Individual cell nuclei are stained with a specific fluorescent DNA dye, and the DNA concentration is assessed rapidly by fluorometric assay of the cells as they pass through a focused laser beam. Normal cells are euploid and so are most G_0 lesions. G_1 lesions have both abnormal numbers of cells in tetraploidy and may also show an abnormal cell line (aneuploid) quite distinctive from that of high-grade neoplasms. These correlations between ploidy and prognosis have been shown to be valid for other classes of neoplasia—particularly myelomas and lymphomas—and preliminary results suggest that this technique may be quite helpful in determining the prognosis of connective tissue lesions.[4]

In summary, surgical grading into G_0, G_1, or G_2 requires histologic, radiographic, and clinical correlation to achieve accuracy and reliability. Although certain histogenic types of sarcomas may be classified predominantly as G_1 or G_2 (Table 1–3), the characteristics of

each lesion must be assessed before a grade is assigned. For example, most parosteal osteosarcomas are G_1, but a few dedifferentiate into G_2 lesions and, as such, have a much more ominous prognosis. Conversely, although most classic osteosarcomas are G_2, occasionally one will be G_1 with a much more favorable prognosis.

Site (T)

The anatomic setting of the lesion has a direct relationship to the prognosis and the choice of surgical procedure. The three strata of anatomic settings are T_0, T_1, T_2. These classifications are determined primarily by clinical and radiographic techniques. Staging studies, such as isotope scanning, angiography, computed tomography (CT), magnetic resonance imaging (MRI), ultrasonography, and myelography, can make valuable contributions to the preoperative assessment of anatomic setting.

T_0 (intracapsular) The lesion remains confined within the capsule and does not extend beyond the compartment borders of its origin. While the boundaries of the capsule and/or the compartment of origin may be distorted or deformed, they both remain intact.

T_1 (extracapsular, intracompartmental) The lesion has extracapsular extensions into the reactive zone that are either continuous to the lesion or are isolated satellites. Both the lesion and the reactive zone about it are contained within an anatomic compartment bounded by the natural barriers to tumor extension: cortical bone, articular cartilage, joint capsule, or the dense fibrous

Radiographic Grade*	Angiogram	Computed Tomography
I_A	No neovascular reaction	Crisp, intact margin; well-defined capsule; homogeneous
I_B	Modest neovascular reaction	Intact margin, "expansile"; thin capsule; homogeneous
I_C	Moderate neovascular reaction	Indistinct, broached margin; extracapsular and/or extracompartmental extension; nonhomogeneous
II	Modest neovascular reaction; involvement of neurovascular bundle	Irregular or well-broached capsule but intracompartmental
II	Modest neovascular reaction; involvement of neurovascular bundle	Extracompartmental extension or location
III	Marked neovascular reaction; no involvement of neurovascular bundle	Broached pseudocapsule; intracompartmental
III	Marked neovascular reaction; involvement of neurovascular bundle	Broached pseudocapsule; extracompartmental
III	Hypervascular lymph nodes	Pulmonary lesions or enlarged nodes
III	Hypervascular lymph nodes	Pulmonary lesions or enlarged nodes

tissue of fascial septa, ligaments, or tendon sheath. To be classified as T_1, both the lesion and its pseudocapsule must be within the compartment. If the reactive zone extends outside of the compartment while the tumor remains within, the lesion is classified as extracompartmental (T_2). The anatomic compartments of both bone and soft tissue are shown in Table 1–4.

Three particular points about compartmentalization require elaboration. The skin and subcutaneous tissues are classified as a compartment even though there are no longitudinal boundaries. In the transverse dimension, however, the deep fascia forms an effective barrier between the subcutaneous and deeper tissues. The parosseous compartment is a potential compartment between cortical bone and overlying muscle. Lesions on the surface of bone that have not invaded either the underlying cortical bone or the overlying muscle, but have pushed them apart, are defined as intracompartmental. Lesions within muscular compartments that contain more than one muscle (for example, the volar compartment of the forearm) are considered intracompartmental despite the involvement of more than one muscle.

T_2 (extracapsular, extracompartmental) Lesions extending beyond compartmental barriers into the loosely bounded fascial planes and spaces with no longitudinal boundaries are extracompartmental, or T_2. Extracompartmental involvement may be either by extension of a previously intracompartmental lesion de novo into the extracompartmental tissues, or by inadvertent transmission of an intracompartmental lesion by trauma or surgical excision. Almost without exception, lesions (or their reactive zones) that abut or involve major neurovascular bundles are extracompartmental because of the extracompartmental location of these structures.

Metastasis (M)

In most staging systems for carcinomas, metastases are stratified as regional (N for nodes) or distant (M), since the prognosis and treatment is significantly different for these two sites of metastasis.

For sarcomas, metastatic involvement of either regional lymph nodes or distant organs has the same ominous prognosis and both are designated by M. There are only two strata of metastases for sarcomas: M_0 and M_1. M_0 indicates no evidence of either regional or distant metastases, while M_1 signifies either regional or distant metastases.

The three factors of grade, site, and metastasis are combined to form the criteria for the progressive stages of benign and malignant lesions (Table 1–1). Benign lesions are designated by the Arabic numerals 1, 2, or 3, corresponding to latent, active, or aggressive stages. The characteristics of stage 1, latent, stage 2, active, and stage 3, aggressive, lesions are shown in Table 1–2. Stages 1, 2, and 3 correspond closely to the Lodwick classification of radiographic features IA, IB, and IC.[3]

Stages of malignant lesions are designated by the Roman numerals I, II, or III, and these stages are synonymous with low-grade, high-grade, and metastatic. The three states of sarcomas are further stratified into

Table 1-3
Classification of histogenic sarcomas

Benign (G₀)	Malignant	
	Low-Grade (G₁)	High-Grade (G₂)
Osteoma	Parosteal osteosarcoma	Classic osteosarcoma
Osteoid osteoma	Endosteal osteosarcoma	Radiation sarcoma
Osteoblastoma		
Exostosis	Secondary chondrosarcoma	Primary chondrosarcoma
Enchondroma		Dedifferentiated chondrosarcoma
Chondroblastoma		Mesenchymal chondrosarcoma
Chondromyxofibroma		
Periosteal chondroma		
Fibroma	Fibrosarcoma, well-differentiated	Fibrosarcoma, undifferentiated
Fibromatosis	Malignant fibrous histiocytoma, well-differentiated	Malignant fibrous histiocytoma
Giant cell tumor, bone	Giant cell sarcoma, bone	Undifferentiated spindle cell sarcoma
Giant cell tumor, tendon sheath	Giant cell sarcoma, tendon	
	Epithelioid sarcoma	Synovial sarcoma
Neurofibroma		Neural sarcoma
Neurolemmoma		
Lipoma	Myxoid liposarcoma	Pleomorphic liposarcoma
Angiolipoma	Hemangiopericytoma	Angiosarcoma
Hemangioma	Hemangioendothelioma	
	Chordoma	Alveolar cell sarcoma
	Adamantinoma	
	Leiomyosarcoma	Rhabdomyosarcoma
		Ewing's sarcoma

A or B depending on whether the lesion is anatomically intracompartmental (A) or extracompartmental (B). The characteristics of these malignant lesions are shown in Table 1–2. The radiographic characteristics of stage I, low-grade lesions, correspond closely to stage II in the Lodwick classification, and stages II, high-grade, and III, metastatic, correspond to Lodwick's radiographic grade III.[3] Only after each lesion has been studied clinically and radiographically and has undergone biopsy for histogenic typing and cytologic grading can it be staged according to its characteristics. Some lesions tend to cluster in particular stages, for example, more than 90% of classic osteosarcomas are stage II$_B$. Others tend to be more evenly distributed: giant cell tumors of bone are approximately 10% stage 1, 65% stage 2, and 25% stage 3.

A particular lesion may undergo transition from one stage to another. Benign lesions that are stage 2, active, or even stage 3, aggressive, during adolescence frequently undergo involution into stage 1, latent, lesions after growth has ceased. On the other hand, certain benign lesions of any stage may undergo transformation into stage I, II, or III sarcomas. By definition, high-grade stage II and occasionally low-grade stage I lesions become stage III lesions after either regional or distant metastases develop. Certain factors have been implicated in the transition of benign or malignant lesions into higher-stage lesions. Radiation is thought to be responsible for transition of giant cell tumors, chondroblastomas, and other benign lesions into sarcomas. Repeated inadequate surgical interventions have been implicated in the evolution of low-grade fibrous lesions into high-grade fibrosarcomas and in the dedifferentiation of stage I parosteal osteosarcoma into stages II or III high-grade osteosarcoma.

Articulation With Surgical Treatment

Articulating the staging system with the surgical treatment of connective tissue tumors requires precise definitions of the stages and the treatment procedures. The traditional terms of incisional biopsy, excisional biopsy, resection, and amputation are difficult to define in biologic, anatomic, or physical terms. After a number of physical and surgical criteria were postulated, a method of defining treatment procedures was devised based on the surgical margin obtained and the remaining barriers to the lesion's extension.

The four oncologic surgical margins, the plane of dissection that achieves them, and the microscopic appearance of the tissue at the margin of the wound are

Table 1-4
Summary of anatomic sites

Intracapsular (T₀)	Extracapsular	
	Intracompartmental (T₁)	Extracompartmental (T₂)
Intraosseous	Intracortical	Extracortical extension
Intra-articular	Intra-articular	Extra-articular extension
Skin-subcutaneous	Skin-subcutaneous	Deep extension
Parosseous	Parosseous	Extension into bone or soft tissue
Intracapsular whether intracompartmental or extracompartmental	Intracompartmental soft tissue	Extracompartmental soft tissue; extracapsular by extension or origin
	Intracompartmental origin	Extracompartmental origin
	Ray, hand	Mid-hand, dorsal or palmar
	Ray, foot	Mid- or hind-foot
	Posterior calf	Popliteal fossae
	Anterolateral leg	Periarticular knee
	Anterior thigh	Femoral triangle
	Medial thigh	Obturator foramen, pelvis
	Posterior thigh	
	Buttocks	Sciatic notch, intrapelvic
	Volar forearm	Antecubital fossae
	Dorsal forearm	Periarticular elbow
	Anterior arm	Axilla
	Posterior arm	
	Deltoid	Periclavicular
	Periscapular	Paraspinal, head, neck

shown in Table 1–5. The four margins are described in surgical terms as intracapsular, marginal, wide, and radical, and they reflect the progressive barriers to tumor extension in their natural evolution: the pseudo-capsule, reactive zone, intracompartmental normal tissue, and compartmental boundaries. Although marginal, wide, and radical surgical margins may all be tumor-free, the residual reactive tissue at a marginal surgical margin often contains extensions or satellites. Also, the residual normal intracompartmental tissue beyond a wide margin occasionally contains skip lesions. For high-grade sarcomas, only a radical surgical margin with an intact barrier of normal tissue between the surgical margin and the reactive zone can be reliably called tumor-free.

The surgical margins of a tumor may be estimated by inspecting the cut surface of either bone or soft tissue. Tetracycline-labeling distinguishes reactive from normal bone and, thus, can visually identify the type of osseous margin. Often, specimens require histologic study to verify whether non-neoplastic tissue at a surgical margin is reactive or normal. The microscopic appearances of wide and radical surgical margins are histologically normal. In this case, the type of margin obtained is determined by whether or not the margin is beyond a compartmental barrier. The compartmental

Table 1-5
Musculoskeletal oncologic surgery

Clinical Data	Type of Surgical Margin			
	Intracapsular	Marginal	Wide	Radical
Plane of dissection	Within lesion	Within reactive zone, extracapsular	Beyond reactive zone; through normal tissue within compartment	Normal tissue, extracompartmental
Microscopic appearance	Tumor at margin	Reactive tissue with or without microsatellite tumors	Normal tissue with or without skip lesions	Normal tissue
Margin achieved by:				
Limb-salvage	Intracapsular piecemeal excision	Marginal en bloc excision	Wide en bloc excision	Radical en bloc resection
Amputation	Intracapsular amputation	Marginal amputation	Wide through-bone amputation	Radical exarticulation

barrier is recognized by gross inspection or radiographic examination of the specimen.

As shown in Table 1–5, each of the four surgical margins can be achieved by a local, limb-salvaging procedure or by an amputation, which makes eight possible oncologic procedures. The four types of limb-salvaging or local procedures are: (1) intracapsular excision: a debulking, or cytoreductive excision done piecemeal within the pseudocapsule; (2) marginal en bloc excision: an en bloc excisional biopsy, or shell-out done extracapsularly within the reactive zone; (3) wide en bloc excision: an en bloc excision done through normal tissue beyond the reactive zone but within the compartment of origin that leaves some portion of that compartment in situ, and (4) radical resection: an en bloc excision of the lesion and the entire compartment of origin that leaves no remnant of the compartment of origin. These surgical margins are diagrammed in Figure 1–1.

The terms excision and resection are coupled with

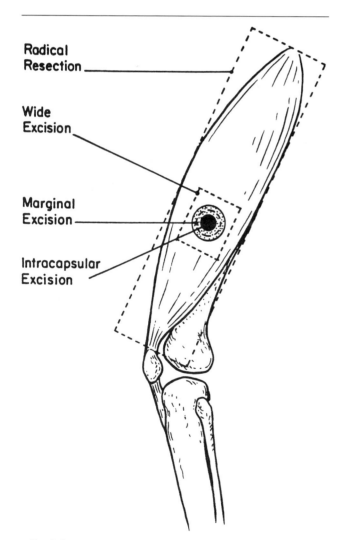

Fig. 1–1 Diagram of surgical margins in four limb-salvaging procedures (see Table 1–5).

wide and radical to emphasize the biologic differences between the two procedures. Wide excision and radical resection are correct terms but wide resection or radical excision are, by definition, incompatible terms. The correct use of these terms is important conceptually as well as semantically, because in Europe, "radical" margin is synonymous with tumor-free and thus can describe either marginal, wide, or radical surgical procedures. Therefore, in the European literature, excision and resection are used interchangeably, and "radical" refers to any local procedure with a tumor-free margin.

The other four types of oncologic procedures are amputations (see Table 1–5) that achieve various margins, and whose levels pass (1) within the pseudocapsule (intracapsular amputation); (2) through the reactive zone (marginal amputation); (3) through normal tissue proximal to the reactive zone but within the involved compartment, usually through bone (wide amputation); and (4) proximal to the involved compartment, usually a disarticulation (radical exarticulation, because it removes the entire compartment at risk). These surgical margins are shown in Figure 1–2.

Articulation of the stages in terms of the previously defined surgical margins and treatment procedures can be done with anatomic and biologic meaning rather than with less significant physical dimensions. The articulation for benign and malignant lesions is shown in Table 1–6.

Discussion

In preliminary trials by the Musculoskeletal Tumor Society, this staging system was shown to be practical, reproducible, and of significant prognostic value for sarcomas of both bone and soft-tissue origin.[5] Subsequent reports have shown its value in surgical planning and treatment evaluation.[5-9]

Some misconceptions arose from the original presentation of this system, in 1980, concerning the definitions of surgical margins and procedures. The common misconceptions concern the methods for describing the surgical margins and procedures for superficial lesions, extracompartmental lesions, and lesions that are inadvertently entered and subsequently excised. A superficial lesion in the skin or subcutaneous tissue that has not penetrated the deep fascia is intracompartmental. En bloc removal, with a plane of dissection beneath the deep fascia and through normal tissue surrounding the lesion, obtains an extracompartmental radical margin in depth (the surgical margin is outside a natural barrier, the deep fascia), but only a wide margin circumferentially (there are no natural barriers within skin and subcutaneous tissue, and so an extracompartmental radical margin is not possible in the defined sense). This ambiguity has been resolved by arbitrarily calling a surgical margin wide if it is less than

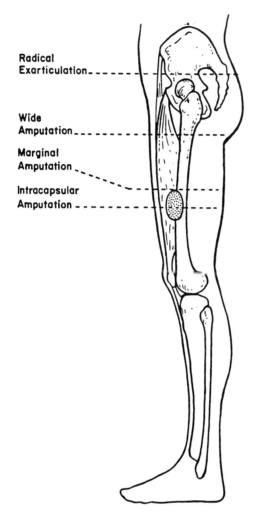

Radical
Exarticulation

Wide
Amputation

Marginal
Amputation

Intracapsular
Amputation

Fig. 1-2 Diagram of surgical margins in four amputation procedures (see Table 1-5).

5 cm about the reactive zone and radical if the margin is more than 5 cm. This dimension was chosen in light of previous experience with melanomas. Thus, a superficial I_A lesion excised en bloc to the deep fascia, with a surrounding margin of 2 cm, has been widely excised, while the same lesion with a 6-cm margin about it has been radically resected. Whether or not these physical dimensions are appropriate for the articulation of surgical margins and stages remains to be seen.

By definition, extracompartmental (B) lesions, whether by extension or origin, cannot be radically resected because the extracompartmental spaces and planes have no longitudinal barriers. For such lesions, a local procedure that removes the lesion en bloc with a surgical margin of normal tissue is a wide excision. Resection of an extracompartmental lesion that is radical in the transverse plane but not in the longitudinal plane is arbitrarily defined as a radical resection when the longitudinal margin is at the same level as the origin or insertion of the adjacent muscles. A lesion in the

subsartorial canal abutting the femoral neurovascular bundle that was removed en bloc, including the bundle, with a plane of dissection beyond the fascial boundaries of the canal (radical resection transversely), but with a proximal and distal surgical margin before the musculotendinous junctions of the sartorius, would have been widely excised, not radically resected. The same procedure with the proximal and distal margins at or beyond the musculotendinous junctions of sartorius would be a radical resection. If the lesion is removed en bloc by dissection within the canal, sacrificing the bundle, the excision is marginal. If the lesion is dissected away from the bundle, preserving the bundle, the procedure is designated either an intracapsular or marginal excision, depending on whether the dissection is within the pseudocapsule or the extracapsular reactive zone.

If a lesion involves two compartments, such as a lesion originating in bone and extending into the adjacent soft tissues, then both compartments must be removed totally en bloc to achieve a radical margin. For example, radical resection of a lesion of the distal femoral metaphysis that extends into the posterior thigh requires removal of the entire femur, hamstrings, and sciatic nerve en bloc. It is evident, then, that in certain instances the only practical way of achieving a radical margin is by amputation. This may be particularly true in certain anatomic sites, such as the popliteal fossae, femoral triangle, axillae, antecubital fossae, and flexor canal of the forearm, where a radical margin can be obtained by resection, but the functionless salvaged limb hinders rather than aids rehabilitation.

When lesions are entered surgically, the wound is contaminated and all the tissues exposed are at risk for recurrence of the lesion. If these exposed tissues are not removed, the margin is intracapsular. The procedure of removing exposed tissue is called a contaminated procedure if some of the exposed tissue remains in the wound. For example, if a lesion in the quadriceps is inadvertently entered, exposing the rectus femoris muscle, and the lesion is then widely excised with a cuff of normal tissue, the procedure is designated a contaminated wide excision, because some of the exposed more proximal rectus femoris remains in the wound. If, under the same circumstance, the entire quadriceps compartment is removed en bloc by extracompartmental dissection, then the procedure is an uncontaminated radical resection, so-called because after incisional biopsy, the entire tract at risk is appropriately excised en bloc to achieve wide or radical margins. Further, if the pseudocapsule is inadvertently entered during attempted excisional biopsy, a great deal more tissue must be removed to achieve an uncontaminated wide or radical margin. In certain instances, contamination may take place in such a way that the only method of achieving an uncontaminated wide or radical margin is by amputation; in other circumstances, for example with

Table 1-6
Articulation of stages with surgical margins

Tumor Stage	Grade, Site, Metastasis	Margin for Control
Benign		
1	$G_0 T_0 M_0$	Intracapsular
2	$G_0 T_0 M_0$	Marginal or intracapsular plus effective adjuvant
3	$G_0 T_{1-2} M_{0-1}$	Wide or marginal plus effective adjuvant
Malignant		
I_A	$G_1 T_1 M_0$	Wide, usually excision
I_B	$G_1 T_2 M_0$	Wide, consider amputation vs joint or neurovascular deficit
II_A	$G_2 T_1 M_0$	Radical, usually resection or wide excision plus effective adjuvant
II_B	$G_2 T_2 M_0$	Radical, consider exarticulation, wide excision, or amputation plus effective adjuvant
III_A	$G_{1-2} T_1 M_1$	Thoractomy, radical resection or palliative
III_B	$G_{1-2} T_2 M_1$	Thoractomy, radical exarticulation or palliative

pelvic involvement, obtaining an uncontaminated margin of any kind may be impossible.

Continuous refinement of these terms, definitions, and concepts is needed. For example, stratification of stage III should be seriously considered. It is becoming clearer that the prognosis of a patient who develops a solitary pulmonary metastasis from a G_0 or G_1 primary tumor years after local control of that tumor is significantly different from the patient who develops multiple metastases from a G_2 lesion at the onset or shortly after apparent local control of the primary lesion.[9] Meaningful stratifications would offer guidelines for the management of these lesions.

The final objective of this staging system—development of guidelines for adjunctive therapy—has yet to be realized. The effectiveness of adjuvant therapy continues to be judged by survival rates of various histogenic types of sarcomas without considering the influence on the survival rate of the sarcoma's stage, surgical margin, or adequacy of the surgical procedure performed. One decade after the widespread adoption of prophylactic chemotherapy, doubt continues as to whether the increase in survival rates during this period is the result of adjuvant chemotherapy or improvement in staging techniques that resulted in improved surgical control of the primary tumor. It is obvious that data concerning staging, surgical margins, and surgical procedures must be gathered to establish significant variables in assessing the various protocols for adjunctive management of musculoskeletal lesions.

References

1. Enneking WF: A system of staging musculoskeletal neoplasms. *Clin Orthop* 1984;204:9.
2. Broders AC, Hargrave R, Meyerding HW: Pathologic features of soft tissue fibrosarcoma. *Surg Gynecol Obstet* 1939;69:267.
3. Lodwick GC, Wilson AJ, Farrell C, et al: Determining growth rates of focal lesions of bone from radiographs. *Radiology* 1980;134:577.
4. Kreicbergs A, Boquist L, Borssén B, et al: Prognostic factors in chondrosarcoma. *Cancer* 1982;50:577–583.
5. Eriksson AI, Schiller A, Mankin HJ: The management of chondrosarcoma of bone. *Clin Orthop* 1980;153:44–66.
6. Boriani S, Bacchini P, Bertoni F, et al: Periosteal chondroma. *J Bone Joint Surg* 1983;65A:205–212.
7. Gherlinzoni F, Rock M, Picci P: Chondromyxofibroma. *J Bone Joint Surg* 1983;65A:198–204.
8. Gitelis S, Bertoni F, Picci P, et al: Chondrosarcoma of Bone. *J Bone Joint Surg* 1981;63A:1248–1257.
9. Sim FH: Diagnosis and treatment of bone tumors—A teaching approach, in Sim FH (ed): *Principles of Surgical Treatment*. Thorofare, NJ, Slack, 1983, pp 164–168.

Bone Banks and Allografts

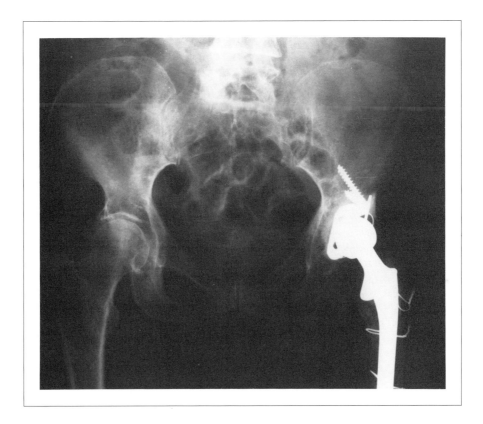

Bone Banks and Allografts in Community Practice

Andrei A. Czitrom, MD, FRCS(C), PhD

Allan E. Gross, MD, FRCS(C), PhD

Fred Langer, MD, FRCS(C), PhD

Franklin H. Sim, MD

Introduction

The use of preserved allograft bone in orthopaedic surgery has been documented by several groups specializing in the treatment of benign skeletal diseases or bone tumors.[1-6] The success of such programs depends on safe and effective bone banking.[7-10] Replacement of bone stock is increasingly required during revision and reconstructive surgery after failed total joint arthroplasty.[11,12] Since complex tissue banking is expensive, all large regional and institutional bone banks are limited to tertiary-care centers. These institutions cannot supply sufficient banked allograft bone on a national level. However, access to tertiary-care centers is limited and transfer of increasing numbers of patients to such centers is not practical. These considerations give a rationale for bone banking and the use of banked allograft bone at local community hospitals. This chapter describes methods of bone banking in community practice, delineates the use of banked allograft bone in general orthopaedics, reconstructive surgery, and tumor surgery, and discusses medicolegal considerations related to bone banking and the use of allografts in community practice.

Bone Banking

Although the logistics of bone banking in local community hospitals are different from those of complex banking procedures, the same general guidelines that ensure reliable preservation, safety, and availability apply as established previously for regional and institutional tissue banks.[13,14] Community bone banking requires safe, simple, and cost-effective methods of preservation. These criteria are best met by deep-freezing. The advantages of deep-frozen allografts (bank bone) over fresh autografts are unlimited quantity, no donor site morbidity, and maintained osteoconductive function. The disadvantages are the lack of osteogenic and osteoinductive function, slow healing rate, and potential sensitization of the recipient.

Donor Selection

There are no strict donor age limits for community bone banking. All disease-free bone can be used in some form or another. Bone from postmenopausal women should be used in morsellized form only. Bone is generally collected during surgery and frozen immediately after removal. In the case of cadaver or spare-part (traumatic amputation) harvesting, bone should be collected within 24 hours of death if the body or part is kept refrigerated (4 C) and within 12 hours if it is kept at room temperature (20 C).

The most important single step in selection is the exclusion of donors with the potential to transfer disease. General guidelines endorsed by the American Association of Tissue Banks[13] are to exclude all donors with the following conditions: infections (acute or chronic), malignancy, irradiation, systemic disease, venereal disease, hepatitis, slow virus disease, acquired immune deficiency syndrome (AIDS), history of drug abuse, intoxication or toxic substances in tissues, prolonged corticosteroid treatment, and unexplained death. When a case is questionable or any doubt exists, exclusion is the safest way to prevent transmission of disease.

Laboratory screening of donor blood is another important step to assure safety of bone transplantation. In community hospitals most donors will be patients undergoing surgical procedures. Therefore, blood testing can be carried out preoperatively. The following tests are required: (1) VDRL test (for syphilis); (2) hepatitis B antigen and antibody (for hepatitis B); (3) HIV antibody (for AIDS); and (4) blood group. In addition, in the case of cadaver harvesting, blood samples for culture (aerobic and anaerobic) must be obtained from three different sites. Harvested bone should be stored temporarily and must not be used until the results of the blood tests are known. Bone from donors with positive serologic test results must be discarded. The blood group result is important for the purpose of matching certain patients at risk (Rh-negative women of childbearing age) to avoid possible Rh-sensitization.[15]

Informed consent should be obtained from both donor and recipient. For live donors the consent should include the laboratory screening tests. Denial of consent for the screening tests outlined above disqualifies the donor (this may become a problem because of the fear of AIDS testing).

Procurement

The major source of bone in community banking is the operating room because many orthopaedic procedures require excision of bone. The most common source is femoral heads excised during hip arthroplasty. However, significant quantities of bone can be obtained from femoral condyles and tibial plateaus during knee arthroplasty, wedges removed at osteotomy, excisions of bone (patella, radial head), and ribs resected during thoracotomy. In addition, large amounts of bone become available in cases of traumatic amputation in which replantation is not feasible. Cadaver harvesting permits the procurement of large quantities of bone but is generally not within the capabilities of community hospitals. Methods of cadaver harvesting have been described in detail previously.[14]

Donor bone must be screened meticulously before transplantation. This involves microbiologic and histopathologic testing. After harvest and before storage, aerobic and anaerobic cultures are taken from the surface and marrow sections. A routine section of a representative area obtained by core biopsy is processed for histopathologic testing. The results of these studies should be evaluated in the same manner as the serologic tests before release of the bone for use. If pathologic abnormalities are detected, the bone must be discarded.

Storage and Retrieval

Harvested bone is packaged under sterile conditions in the operating room. The triple-wrapping technique is recommended. It is acceptable to use glass, polyethylene, or plastic containers combined with towels. Labeling should be simple and informative. The label should include donor information, date of procurement, and identification number. It is useful to add the surgeon's name, size of bone (small, medium, large femoral head), sex of donor (for simple quality estimate), and the blood group.

Temporary storage of bones should be at −70 C in a special area of the freezer or in a separate freezer if one is available. Upright freezers are recommended because they make sorting and retrieval more convenient. Bones in temporary storage are not used until screening (serologic and bone) is complete. If screening test results are positive or if a living donor develops an infection after procurement, all bones from that donor must be discarded.

Final storage is also at −70 C. Household freezers (−20 C) are not recommended because of the possibility of slow autolysis at this temperature. The final storage area should contain only bone that meets the criteria for use (i.e., is screening-negative).

When bones are taken from storage for use, the coverings should be removed under sterile conditions in the operating room. Repeat cultures (aerobic and anaerobic) are done before thawing. The bones are placed in warm (50 C) antibiotic solution (saline with 50,000 units of bacitracin or Betadine solution) before use.

Storing bones for two to three years at −70 C is acceptable, but it is better to store them for less than one year to minimize the possibility of infection. Infection in the freezer should be monitored every six months by taking samples from the inside freezer walls with swabs, and assessing random samples of stored bones (by submitting 5% of stored specimens in toto for microbiologic and histopathologic screening).

Sterilization is not obligatory for community bone banks provided that all guidelines for exclusion, screening, and sterile procurement are met. However, sterilization is required for cadaver harvests done outside of operating rooms and can be an additional safety measure against infection in all cases. The authors have had extensive experience with gamma irradiation (25 Gy from a ^{60}Co source) and recommend this method for hospitals where facilities exist. To date the authors' clinical and experimental work has shown no detrimental effects of this method on the biologic and mechanical properties of bank bone. Sterilization is optional and by no means a substitute for proper screening and sterile procurement.

Simple manual record-keeping is adequate for community banking. A local bone bank committee that includes a pathologist, a microbiologist, and an infection control nurse is helpful. Using radiographs and microcomputers for increased efficiency is optional, not essential.

Cost and Safety

The guidelines given above are realistic in terms of the feasible range for most community hospitals. Evidence for the cost-effectiveness and safety of these procedures is provided in Table 2–1, which compares published data related to capital expenditures and complications from allografts in large, institutional banks and a small community bank.[16-18] It is clear from these data that community banking requires minimal expenditures and is as safe as institutional banking.

Table 2–1

Comparison of cost and safety of community bone banking with institutional bone banking*

Clinical Data	Institutional Bank	Community Bank
Cost		
Capital	$165,000	$5,000
Processing	$2,500 per graft	3 hr of wages/wk
Years	1983–1984	1982–1984
Femoral heads		
Total allografts	78	180
Discarded grafts	2	29
Implanted grafts	58	101
Procedures	47	77
Infections	1	0
Complications from grafts	0	0

*Adapted from Friedlaender,[16] Tomford, Ploetz, and Mankin,[17] and Hart, Campbell, and Kartub.[18]

The Use of Allograft Bone

Indications for the use of allograft bone are guided by biologic and biomechanical principles. Deep-frozen bank bone does not provide live cells for osteogenesis and is poor in its ability to induce new bone formation by host cells. However, it is effective as a scaffold for bony ingrowth (osteoconductive function) when placed against live, bleeding host bone surfaces that are fertile in terms of bone formation potential. In these situations, allograft bank bone provides mechanical support in areas of bone deficiency. The graft may function (1) as a filler (filling cavities), (2) as a buttress (preventing collapse), (3) as a strut (maintaining continuity), or (4) as augmentation (spreading autograft bone). These are general principles that apply to many common clinical situations in which bank bone can be used successfully.

General Orthopaedics

Guidelines for the use of allograft bone have emerged from a clinical study of 183 patients. A successful result was defined simply as the bone fulfilling the function for which it was intended. We realize that there are many other factors that determine success in each case. Bank bone was used in the following situations:

To Fill a Bone Cavity A successful result was achieved in 30 of 32 cases. These included unicameral bone cysts, benign bone tumors managed by curettage and grafting, and large degenerative cysts adjacent to arthritic joints. When the bone is used to fill a cavity, it is imperative that the lining of the cavity be curetted to bleeding bone.

As a Buttress Allograft bone was successful in 95 of 101 cases. The uses included buttressing the articular surface in acute tibial plateau and os calcis fractures (15 of 17 cases successful), buttressing the tibial tuberosity anteriorly during a Macquet osteotomy (50 of 51 cases successful), and Cloward grafting for anterior cervical fusions (30 of 33 cases successful).

Nonunion Bank bone was used seven times with only four successful outcomes.

To Enhance Primary Union or Arthrodesis Bank bone was used ten times with only six cases achieving union in difficult fractures and arthrodeses.

To Augment the Quantity of Autograft Bone In repeat spinal fusions for scoliosis in adults in which the bone graft was to be spread over a large area and only a small amount of host iliac crest bone was available, the autograft bone was mixed with bank bone. Bank bone served as a vehicle to spread the autograft bone with bone-inductive properties. Successful spinal fusion was achieved in 31 of 33 cases by radiologic criteria.

On the basis of their clinical experience, the authors have defined guidelines for the use of bank bone in general orthopaedics. Bank bone can be used to fill a bone cavity, as a buttress, and to augment the quantity of autograft bone. It should not be used in nonunions or to enhance primary unions and arthrodeses.

Reconstructive Surgery

In the past ten years it has become apparent that failed total joint arthroplasties may be associated with loss of bone stock. It is now accepted that revision arthroplasty should be carried out with supplemental bone grafting when indicated. The quantity and shape of the bone required to restore bone stock make it difficult or impossible to use iliac crest bone. Thus, banked allograft bone must be available.[11,12] Three common clinical indications for the use of banked allograft bone in implant revision arthroplasty of the hip are protrusio, acetabular dysplasia, and proximal femoral deficiency (Table 2–2).

Protrusio A central or superomedial protrusio may be associated with a loose acetabular prosthesis (Fig. 2–1). This deficit must not be treated with an increased volume of cement. The bone stock must be restored by either morsellized cancellous allograft bone or, on occasion, a solid bone fragment. Some of these defects are so large that two or three femoral heads may be needed to obtain enough bone for morsellization. Solid bone pieces are usually fixed with large cancellous screws. There are several choices of acetabular implant that can be used, both uncemented or cemented.

Dysplasia In some acetabular revisions it is difficult to obtain good coverage of the new cup because of superolateral bone loss from loosening or failure to obtain good coverage during the primary procedure because of lack of bone grafting (Fig. 2–2). In this situation intact femoral head segments can provide

Table 2–2

Indications and techniques for acetabular and femoral reconstructions with allograft bone

Deficit	Graft	Implant
Protrusio	Morsellized allograft, intact femoral head	Uncemented cup, screw-in, press-fit, or bicentric; cemented cup and protrusio ring
Dysplasia	Intact femoral head segment	Uncemented cup, screw-in, press-fit, or bicentric; cemented cup and protrusio ring
Proximal femur	Proximal femur or proximal tibia	Long-stem femoral component: uncemented; cemented to allograft and host (in elderly patient); cemented to allograft alone

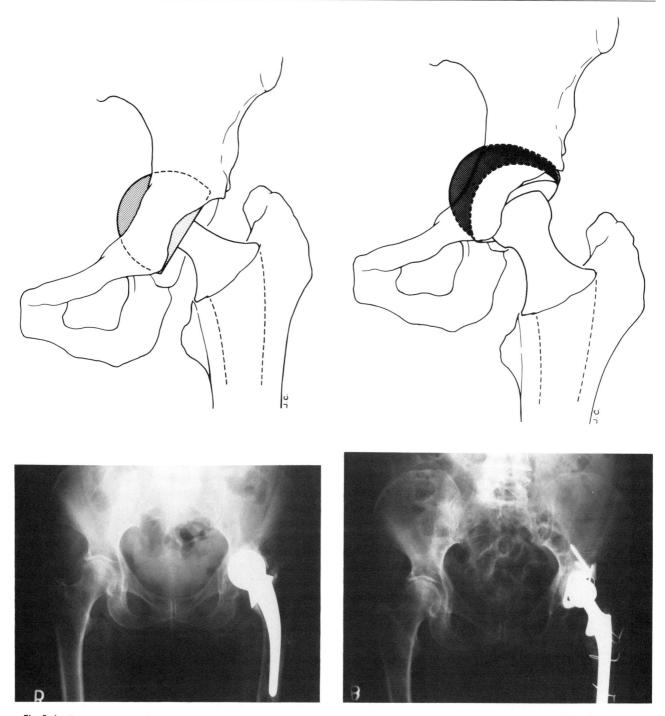

Fig. 2-1 Reconstruction of protrusio. **Top left:** Diagram of protrusio with acetabular implant protruding beyond the ilio-ischial line. **Top right:** Diagram of reconstruction with morsellized allograft bone or intact femoral head segment. **Bottom left:** Roentgenogram of a 74-year-old woman shows superomedial protrusio five years after a cemented hemiarthroplasty performed for a fractured neck of femur. **Bottom right:** Appearance three years after reconstruction using morsellized allograft bone and a Muller protrusio ring.

good coverage of the acetabular implant. These shelf grafts are fixed with cancellous screws. The junction of the shelf allograft and the pelvic wall is autografted with cancellous bone. Cemented or uncemented acetabular implants can be used in combination with the shelf graft.

Proximal Femoral Deficiency Loss of proximal femoral bone stock in an implant that has undergone previous revision leads to loss of abductor strength, marked lurch, and leg-length discrepancy (Figs. 2–3 and 2–4). This deficiency can be remedied with frozen banked allograft bone if suitable bone segments are available. The

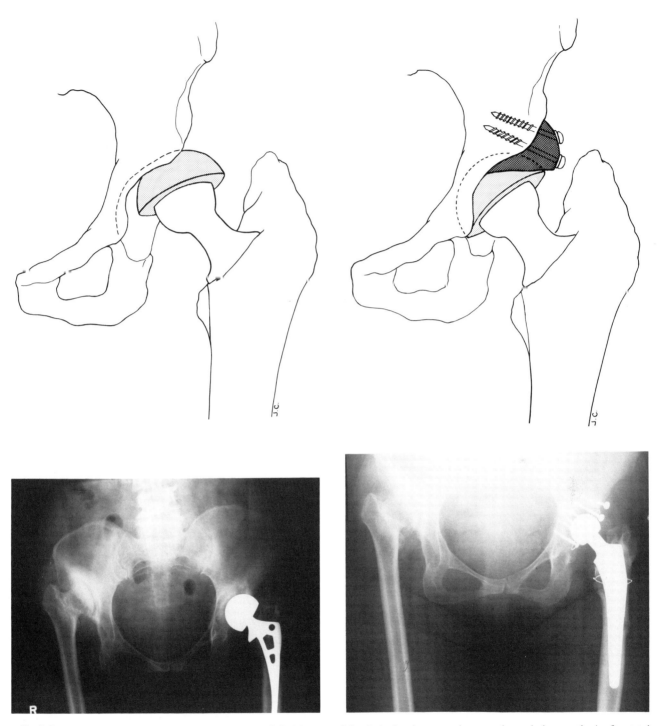

Fig. 2-2 Reconstruction of acetabular dysplasia. **Top left:** Diagram of dysplasia showing a poorly covered acetabular prosthesis after total hip replacement. **Top right:** Diagram of reconstruction with a femoral head segment used to provide coverage of the new cup. **Bottom left:** Roentgenogram of a 60-year-old woman shows a poorly covered bicentric prosthesis. **Bottom right:** Appearance two years after revision with uncemented femoral and acetabular components and a femoral head segment used as a shelf graft to provide coverage. The graft is held by two lag screws while the Natural-Loc cup is held by four special screws made for the acetabular component.

graft may be long enough to require only the calcar (2 cm) or a significant amount of proximal femur. Anything less than 2 cm should not be grafted. The best bone for this situation is strong cortical bone from a proximal femoral allograft or a proximal tibial allograft that can be shaped easily into a proximal femoral form. A long-stem femoral component should be used with most of these grafts. In older patients, cement can be

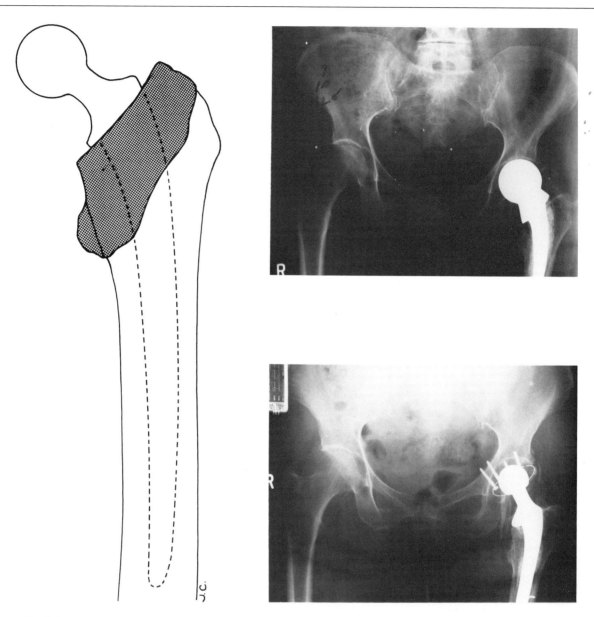

Fig. 2-3   Reconstruction of proximal femoral deficiency. **Left:** Diagram of reconstruction with a small proximal femoral allograft and a long-stem femoral component. **Top right:** Roentgenogram of a 58-year-old woman three years after a cemented hemiarthroplasty showing loss of the calcar secondary to stress shielding. **Bottom right:** Appearance three years after revision with a proximal femoral allograft and a long-stem femoral component.

used in both the allograft and the host. In younger patients, cement should not be used in the host femur. Cement may be used in the allograft since the bone is dead. The junction of host and allograft bone should always be autografted. If there is rotational instability at the junction of host and allograft, stabilization may be achieved by cement in the older patient and by a plate or a step-cut in the younger patient.

The use of allografts for the reconstruction of bone stock in revision hip surgery demands attention to the following basic principles: (1) host bone is never sacrificed or devascularized; (2) in younger patients cement is used in the allograft but never in host bone; (3) the

allograft-host junctions are always supplemented with autograft bone; and (4) bone from postmenopausal women is used in morsellized form only.

Tumor Surgery

The diagnosis of bone tumors is hampered by their diversity and by the number of non-neoplastic lesions that simulate tumors (Table 2–3). Surgical treatment, whether resection or amputation, is defined by the margins achieved as described by the Musculoskeletal Tumor Society (Table 2–4). The staging system is useful in individualizing the extent of the surgical procedure to the biologic aggressiveness of the tumor. Most be-

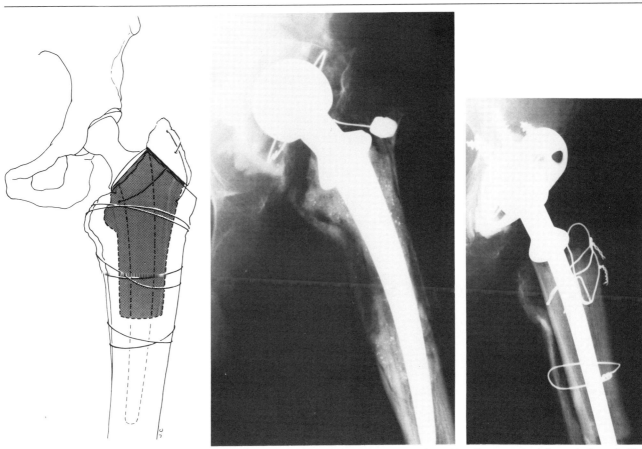

Fig. 2–4 Reconstruction of a proximal femoral deficiency. **Left:** Diagram of reconstruction with a large proximal femoral allograft. The patient's residual proximal femur is wired around the allograft. **Center:** Roentgenogram of a 50-year-old man with hemophilia shows loss of the proximal femur after multiple hip reconstructions. **Right:** Appearance three years after revision with a large proximal femoral allograft.

nign and low-grade malignant lesions can be managed by relatively conservative procedures, whereas high-grade lesions require more aggressive treatment.

Allografts have been useful in the reconstruction of the skeleton after excision of tumors. Major uses include (1) filling defects in bone after curettage or simple excision, (2) major intercalary and articular allograft reconstruction after limb-sparing tumor resection, and (3) reconstruction of bony defects in metastatic disease. In a community setting the allograft bank bone is utilized primarily to fill defects after curettage of nonaggressive benign lesions. Major segmental and articular reconstructions after excision of tumors or in metastatic disease require major institutional bone banks and thus are not usually within the scope of community practice.

Curettage and Grafting of Benign Lesions For benign bone tumors, the disease can be controlled and function preserved in the bone and neighboring joint by curettage or simple excision (Fig. 2–5). The tumor must be completely removed and the osseous structure restored by filling the cavity with bone grafts. The single most important factor in effective curettage is adequate exposure. This requires a large cortical window and com-

plete excision of the tumor by removing 50% or more of the circumference of the bone. Curettage through a small hole in the cortex routinely leads to recurrence. After tumor removal, the margins must be thoroughly scraped with a sharp curette, followed by the use of a dental burr to extend the margins beyond the reactive zone of the tumor. Local adjuvant treatment with phenol may be used to further extend the margin. If this is done, the soft tissues are packed with petrolatum gauze and moist sponges and the tumor cavity is filled with phenol for 30 to 45 seconds. The phenol, which coagulates protein, is effective in reaching the crevices in the cortical bone to which the tumor has permeated. The phenol is removed and the cavity rinsed with 95% acid alcohol and then lavaged vigorously with large amounts of isotonic saline. A variation of this procedure is excision curettage, in which a margin is created around most of the tumor while curettage is carried out in the subchondral region in an attempt to preserve the joint. After curettage or excision many cavities are large and require tight packing with bone grafts morsellized in a bone mill.

Bone allografts represent a satisfactory alternative or addition to bone autografts in filling these defects.

Table 2-3
Classification of 6,221 Primary Tumors of Bone at the Mayo Clinic*

Benign Tumors	No. of Cases	Malignant Tumors	No. of Cases
Hematopoietic (No. = 2,572; 41.4%)			
—	—	Myeloma	2,245
—	—	Reticulum cell sarcoma	327
Chondrogenic (No. = 1,300; 20.9%)			
Osteochondroma	579	Primary chondrosarcoma	367
Chondroma	162	Secondary chondrosarcoma	52
Chondroblastoma	44	Dedifferentiated chondrosarcoma	51
Chondromyxoid fibroma	30	Mesenchymal chondrosarcoma	15
Osteogenic (No. = 1,199; 19.3%)			
Osteoid osteoma	158	Osteosarcoma	962
Benign osteoblastoma	43	Parosteal osteogenic sarcoma	36
Unknown Origin (No. = 607; 9.8%)			
Giant cell tumor	264	Ewing's sarcoma	299
(Fibrous) histiocytoma	7	Malignant giant cell tumor	20
—	—	Adamantinoma	17
—	—	(Fibrous) histiocytoma	35[†]
Fibrogenic (No. = 234; 3.8%)			
Fibroma	72	Fibrosarcoma	158
Desmoplastic fibroma	4	—	—
Notochordal (No. = 195; 3.1%)			
—	—	Chordoma	195
Vascular (No. = 99; 1.6%)			
Hemangioma	69	Hemangioendothelioma	25
—	—	Hemangiopericytoma	5
Lipogenic (No. = 5)			
Lipoma	5	—	—
Neurogenic (No. = 10)			
Neurilemmoma	10	—	—
Total benign tumors	1,447	Total malignant tumors	4,774

*Classification based on that advocated by Lichtenstein.[23] Adapted with permission from Dahlin DC: *Bone Tumors: General Aspects and Data on 6,221 Cases,* ed 3. Springfield, Charles C Thomas, 1978, p 7.
†Not included in data totals.

Table 2-4
Grading system for surgical procedures in the treatment of bone tumors*

Grade	Margin	Local Treatment	Amputation
1	Intralesional	Curettage or debulking	Debulking or amputation
2	Marginal	Marginal excision	Marginal amputation
3	Wide	Wide local excision	Wide through-bone amputation
4	Radical	Radical local resection	Radical disarticulation

*Reprinted with permission from Enneking WF, Spanier SS, Goodman MA: A system for the surgical staging of musculoskeletal sarcoma. *Clin Orthop* 1980;153:106–120.

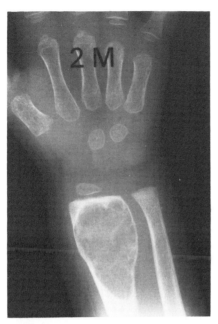
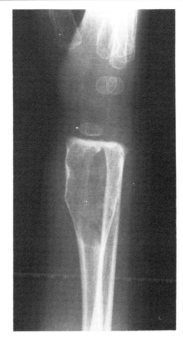
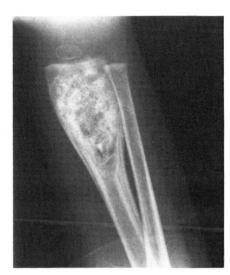
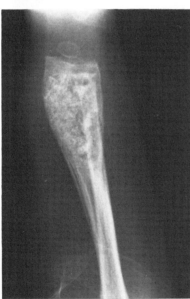

Fig. 2-5 Example of curettage and grafting of a benign lesion. **Left and Center:** Antero-posterior and lateral roentgenograms of the distal radius in a 2-year-old boy show a lytic, destructive lesion with thinning and expansion of the cortex. Open biopsy yielded a diagnosis of aneurysmal bone cyst. **Right and Bottom:** Appearance after excision by curettage and reconstruction with morsellized allograft bone.

Healing and blending of the allograft with host bone is often rapid. This incorporation can be enhanced by the addition of host autogenous bone at a 3:1 ratio of allograft to autograft. Recurrence rates are similar regardless of the type of bone graft used. The grafts have no effect on recurrence but indicate a more radical and adequate excision. Factors other than the type of graft influence the postoperative result: among these are the aggressiveness of the lesion, the patient's age and sex, the location of the tumor, the thoroughness of the curettage, and the completeness of packing with bone graft.

Major Segmental and Articular Reconstruction Recent devel-

opments in musculoskeletal oncology have been attributed to the ability to perform limb-sparing resections for malignant neoplasms.[19] The goal of the resection is to achieve local control of the tumor with an appropriate surgical margin. This frequently results in a large osseous and soft-tissue defect. The aim of the reconstruction is to restore maximum function. Salvage of a mobile joint may be achieved with either an osteochondral allograft or a custom-made prosthetic replacement. Segmental or arthrodesis reconstruction at the knee, hip, or shoulder can be performed with an autogenous bone graft (vascularized or nonvascular) or an intercalary allograft. Prosthetic reconstruction has the advantage of maintenance of motion and immediate functional restoration. It is indicated in older patients, those with high-grade malignancies, and those with limited life expectancies. Although the early results have been satisfactory, long-term prosthetic survival is of legitimate concern. Therefore, increased emphasis has been placed on biologic reconstructive alternatives. Osteochondral allograft replacement has significant complication rates,[3,4] but with improved patient selection, allograft banking, and surgical techniques, this method is becoming increasingly useful. Osteoarticular allograft reconstruction should be considered in patients who are young, are not overweight, have benign or low-grade malignant lesions, and who are unwilling to accept an arthrodesis. Chemotherapy and radiation therapy retard allograft incorporation but do not contraindicate its use. Allograft reconstruction is better indicated for benign and low-grade malignant tumors. This method of reconstruction requires a major bone bank and facilities that are usually only available in tertiary-care institutions.

Reconstruction of Bony Defects in Metastatic Disease Metastatic bone disease is the most common type of malignant bone tumor. It often appears as a destructive process with a pathologic fracture. Conventional reconstruction with implants and bone cement often fail if the area of bone loss is extensive. Many patients survive for relatively long periods and their functional requirements demand an effective reconstructive technique. This can usually be achieved by using bone allografts to replace segments of bone loss (Fig. 2–6). The use of banked bone in metastatic disease is indicated when bone loss is extensive. The allograft is used as a segmental graft for diaphyseal, metaphyseal, or articular disease. The metaphyseal allograft is supplemented by a joint implant. The medullary cavity of the allograft is filled with bone cement to help with screw and implant-stem fixation. The form of fixation is determined by the most effective means of restoring biomechanical strength according to the same principles used for fracture fixation.

During the last three years the authors used bone allografts for metastatic disease in 28 patients ranging in age from 35 to 85 years (mean, 55 years). There were ten femoral or hip reconstructions, six shoulder reconstructions, six humeral reconstructions, five pelvic reconstructions, and one elbow reconstruction. Five patients survived for less than four weeks, six for less than six months, 15 for six to 18 months, and two for more than two years. Complications consisted of one infection in a heavily irradiated extremity. In no case did the graft break or resorb and in no case did the tumor recur within the graft.

The advantages of bone allografts in the surgical treatment of metastatic disease can be summarized as follows: (1) they allow a wide excision of the tumor area; (2) they can easily be made to custom-fit the defect; (3) they are strong and retain their configuration; and (4)

tumor recurrence within an allograft is unlikely. It is evident that this type of allograft reconstruction requires a large bone bank supplying a variety of bone segments and thus may not be feasible in many community hospitals.

Medicolegal Considerations

In the establishment of a community bone bank, there are important safety considerations related to liability risks. These are particularly important in the case of cadaver harvesting but also apply when bone from live donors is used. They demand exacting donor health criteria, extensive disease screening of donors, and quality control of the harvested bone. The Uniform Anatomical Gift Act (UAGA)[20–22] was a response to these concerns and has established a basic legal framework for transplantation. The provisions of this act in relation to major regional and institutional bone banking have been reviewed previously.[7,9,14] The UAGA has almost eliminated legal problems in regard to postmortem donation of body parts. However, since some states have made variations in the provisions of the UAGA when adopting their own acts, the physician must refer to specific state provisions before proceeding.

In the case of living donors, the major source of femoral head allografts for a "limited" bone bank, the UAGA does not apply. The donation of a femoral head at the time of hip arthroplasty is legally determined by the donor. The usual standards of good medical practice, including obtaining the informed consent of the recipient, apply. Moreover, most states require informed donor consent before an AIDS blood test is conducted.

Beyond the regulatory requirements is the issue of legal liability. Transplantation can raise questions concerning negligence. Although the UAGA provides immunity from civil or criminal liability for anyone acting in good faith under the act, civil litigation can still be begun for (1) negligent treatment before the death of the donor; (2) donation involving negligence and taking effect while the donor is alive rather than at death; (3) negligent treatment of the live donor; (4) not obtaining informed consent; (5) improper storage or banking methods; and (6) improper preoperative or postoperative surgical care. If an AIDS screening test is not done, there is a great potential for liability.

Another possible problem area is the theory of strict product liability or implied warranty for the allograft. This problem has been minimized by the increasing number of state statutes defining organ transplantation as a "service" and thus avoiding strict liability or implied warranty based on the "sale" of a product. Individuals involved in the transplantation process in states where the law does not define transplantation as a "service" must refer to the law of the jurisdiction in which the procedures are performed.

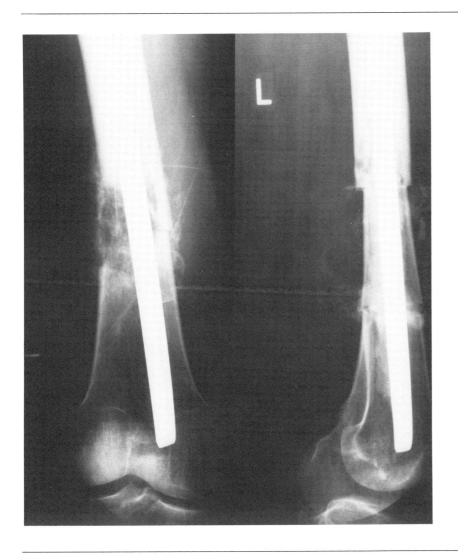

Fig. 2-6 Allograft reconstruction in metastatic disease. **Left:** Roentgenogram shows a metastatic lesion from renal cell carcinoma in the femur of a 50-year-old man treated with an intramedullary nail. Revision was required because of persistent pain and instability. **Right:** Roentgenogram shows reconstruction with segmental allograft and rigid intramedullary fixation with new nail and cement.

Summary

The increasing volume of orthopaedic reconstructive procedures requiring replacement of bone stock justifies the initiation of programs of bone banking in community hospitals. Provided that strict criteria are followed to assure rigorous screening of donor bone and the reliable preservation of bone graft material, community banking is safe and cost-effective. Banked allograft bone can be used successfully in a wide variety of orthopaedic procedures performed in community hospitals. In general, the best uses are filling bone cavities, buttressing, and augmenting the quantity of autograft bone. In revision reconstructive surgery of the hip, bank bone is used to replace bone stock in protrusio, acetabular dysplasia, and proximal femoral deficiency. The best and most common indication for the use of bank bone in tumor surgery is after curettage or excision of benign lesions. Allografts may be used to reconstruct bony defects after excision of malignant tumors and in the surgical treatment of metastatic disease. These instances require larger bone bank facilities than those commonly available in a community hospital setting. Medicolegal considerations related to bone banking and the use of allografts in community practice include the regulatory requirements outlined in the UAGA, questions concerning negligence liability, and theories of strict product liability. Overall, good medical practice and obtaining informed consents will minimize legal risks related to bone banking and transplantation in a community setting.

References

1. Spence KF, Sell KW, Brown RH: Solitary bone cyst: Treatment with freeze-dried cancellous bone allograft: A study of one hundred and seventy-seven cases. *J Bone Joint Surg* 1969;51A:87–96.
2. Volkov MV, Imamaliyev AS: Use of allogenous articular bone implants as substitutes for autotransplants in adult patients. *Clin Orthop* 1976;114:192–202.

3. Mankin HJ: Allograft transplantation in the management of bone tumors, in Uhtoff H (ed): *Current Concepts of Diagnosis and Treatment of Bone and Soft Tissue Tumors.* New York, Springer, 1984, pp 142–162.

4. Gross A, McKee N, Farine I, et al: Reconstruction of skeletal defects following en-bloc excision of bone tumors, in Uhtoff H (ed): *Current Concepts of Diagnosis and Treatment of Bone and Soft Tissue Tumors.* New York, Springer, 1984, pp 163–174.

5. Ottolenghi CE: Massive osteo and osteo-articular bone grafts: Technique and results of 62 cases. *Clin Orthop* 1972;87:156–164.

6. Parrish FF: Allograft replacement of all or part of the end of a long bone following excision of a tumor. *J Bone Joint Surg* 1973;55A:1–22.

7. Friedlaender GE: Bone-banking. *J Bone Joint Surg* 1982;64A:307–311.

8. Doppelt SH, Tomford WW, Lucas AD, et al: Operational and financial aspects of a hospital bone bank. *J Bone Joint Surg* 1981;63A:1472–1481.

9. Tomford WW, Doppelt SH, Mankin HJ, et al: 1983 Bone bank procedures. *Clin Orthop* 1983;174:15–21.

10. Malinin TI, Martinez OV, Brown MD: Banking of massive osteoarticular and intercalary bone allografts—12 years' experience. *Clin Orthop* 1985;197:44–57.

11. Harris WH: Allografting in total hip arthroplasty: In adults with severe acetabular deficiency including a surgical technique for bolting the graft to the ilium. *Clin Orthop* 1982;162:150–164.

12. Gross AE, Lavoie MV, McDermott P, et al: The use of allograft bone in revision of total hip arthroplasty. *Clin Orthop* 1985;197:115–122.

13. American Association of Tissue Banks: Guidelines for the banking of musculoskeletal tissues: *Am Assoc Tissue Banks Newslett* 1979;3:2–32.

14. Friedlaender GE, Mankin HJ: Bone banking: Current methods and suggested guidelines, in Murray DG (ed): *AAOS Instructional Course Lectures, XXX.* St. Louis, CV Mosby Co, 1981, pp 36–55.

15. Johnson CA, Brown BA, Lasky LC: Rh immunization caused by osseous allograft. *N Engl J Med* 1985;312:121–122.

16. Friedlaender GE: Personnel and equipment required for a "complete" tissue bank. *Transplant Proc* 1976;8:235–240.

17. Tomford WW, Ploetz JE, Mankin HJ: Bone allografts of femoral heads: Procurement and storage. *J Bone Joint Surg* 1986;68A:534–537.

18. Hart MM, Campbell ED, Kartub MG: Bone banking: A cost effective method for establishing a community hospital bone bank. *Clin Orthop* 1986;206:295–300.

19. Sim FH, Bowman WE, Wilkins RM, et al: Limb salvage in primary malignant bone tumors. *Orthopedics* 1985;8:574–581.

20. Sadler AM, Sadler BL, Stason EB: The Uniform Anatomical Gift Act: A model for reform. *JAMA* 1968;206:2501–2506.

21. Curran WJ: The Uniform Anatomical Gift Act. *N Engl J Med* 1969;280:36–37.

22. Sadler AM Jr, Sadler BL, Stason EB, et al: Transplantation—a case for consent. *N Engl J Med* 1969;280:862–867.

23. Lichtenstein L: Classification of primary tumors of bone. *Cancer* 1951;4:335.

Avascular Necrosis

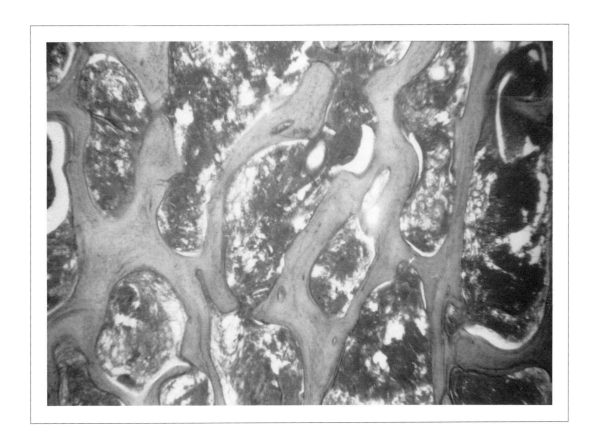

Blood Supply to Bone and Proximal Femur: A Synopsis

Carl L. Nelson, MD

Blood Supply to Bone

The arterial blood supply is abundant, high in oxygen content, and multiple. It is usually classified according to anatomic location: diaphyseal (nutrient), periosteal, metaphyseal, epiphyseal (Fig. 3–1).

Diaphyseal (Nutrient) Arteries

The nutrient, or diaphyseal, artery (dual in the human femur) enters the nutrient foramen nearest the most rapidly growing epiphysis and is directed toward the slowest growing epiphysis. The nutrient artery then divides into ascending and descending branches that spiral around the central venous sinus. The ascending and descending branches further divide to produce multiple parallel branches; these vessels terminate by anastomosis with the terminal metaphyseal branches. There are also separate branches of the nutrient artery that supply the bone marrow independently.

Throughout their course, the longitudinal parallel branches of the nutrient artery give off transverse branches that form an endosteal network. The transverse branches from the parallel branches of the nutrient artery are of three types: (1) short branches that penetrate the middle one third of the cortex, (2) recurrent branches that penetrate the inner one fourth of the cortex and loop back into the medullary canal, and (3) transfixing branches that pass through the cortex to anastomose with the periosteal branches[1] (Fig. 3–2).

The nutrient arteries, through their transverse branches, supply the diaphyseal marrow cavity as well as the inner one third of the cortex.

Intracortical Circulation of the Diaphysis

According to Trias and Fery,[2] the intracortical circulation consists of two networks that anastomose with

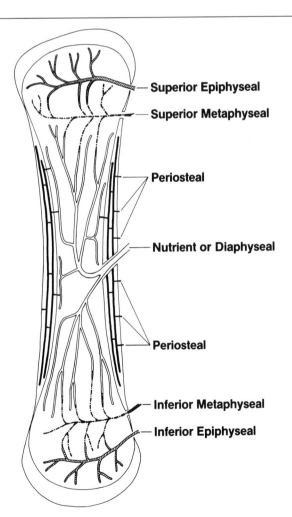

Fig. 3-1 Anatomic classification of the blood supply to bone.

Superior Epiphyseal
Superior Metaphyseal
Periosteal
Nutrient or Diaphyseal
Periosteal
Inferior Metaphyseal
Inferior Epiphyseal

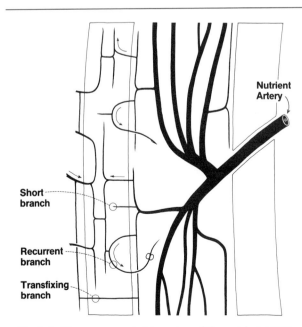

Fig. 3-2 Transverse cortical branches of the nutrient artery.

Nutrient Artery
Short branch
Recurrent branch
Transfixing branch

one another (Fig. 3–3). The longitudinal system extends through the cortex and is a network of uniform capillaries that are continuous with the periosteal and endosteal networks. These interconnecting networks have several functions. They serve as reservoirs of blood, in regulation of blood pressure, and in distribution of nutrients. These vessels form an anatomic unit within a bone.

The second vascular system in the cortex is transverse. After a straight course through the inner third of the cortex, the transverse vessels anastomose in the middle third of the cortex with the longitudinal system. Both the longitudinal and the transverse anatomic system anastomose freely with each other and with the periosteal vessels and endosteal networks.

The transverse system predominates in the middle third of the cortex. In the adult, the transverse system is represented by the haversian bone in growing diaphysis. Where haversian bone is rare, the transverse system is practically absent. In the adult, the transverse system continues into the haversian canals and anastomoses with the perpendicular system, which permeates the whole cortex.

The arterial flow in the cortex is centrifugal, although Trueta and Harrison[3] originally described it as centripetal. Rhinelander[4] and Trias and Fery[2] stated that the blood may flow in either direction, depending on physiologic conditions. It appears that in the mature animal the direction of arterial flow is predominately centrifugal, while in the immature animal, the contribution of the periosteum is much greater. Because the two cortical systems are profusely anastomosed to each other and to the periosteal and endosteal networks, the blood can flow in either direction, depending on physiologic conditions.

Understanding this concept enables one to understand the differences between the child and the adult in their reactions to such conditions as osteomyelitis, trauma, and avascular changes.

In summary, the network of longitudinal vessels is the principal blood supply system to cortical bone, while the transverse system functions primarily to mediate the blood flow in and out of the longitudinal system.

Periosteal Arterioles

The periosteal arterioles enter at fascial attachments to supply the cortex locally. Loosely attached periosteum does not convey afferent blood vessels to mature bone. Consequently, loosely attached periosteum can be elevated with relative impunity, while fascial attachments should be preserved.

Venous and Capillary Systems

Veins are more numerous than arteries and have a volumetric capacity six to eight times greater than the arteries. After maturity, the metaphysis is drained by the metaphyseal veins. The diaphysis is drained to the periosteum by the cortical venous channels and periosteal capillary venae comitantes at fascial attachments.

Indirect venous drainage occurs through the large, tortuous central venous sinus (Fig. 3–4).

Metaphyseal and Epiphyseal Arteries

The metaphyseal arteries enter all sides of the metaphysis through multiple foramina at ligamentous at-

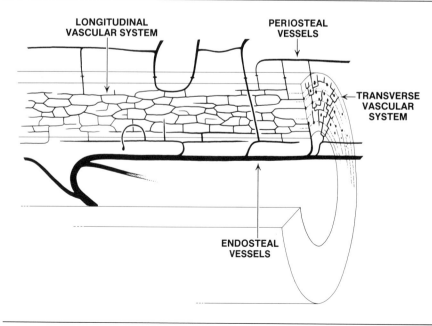

Fig. 3–3 Intracortical circulation.

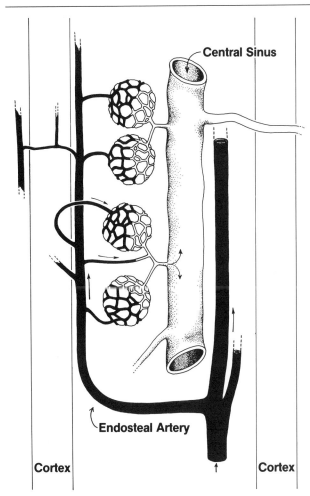

Fig. 3–4 Indirect venous drainage.

The normal blood supply of long bones has three primary constituents: (1) the afferent vascular system, (2) the efferent vascular system, and (3) the intermediate vascular system of compact bone.

The Afferent Vascular System

The epiphysis and metaphysis have separate circulations that are divided by the epiphyseal growth plate until they unite at maturity.

The periosteum of the diaphysis contains a highly vascular osteogenic layer that provides appositional growth. At maturity, the periosteal osteogenic layer becomes atrophic and has no blood vessels, but this layer may be reactivated by injury.

At maturity, the diaphysis is supplied on all sides by the metaphyseal arteries that enter at ligamentous attachments. All portions of the cancellous structure of the metaphysis are well vascularized and no vascular problems follow fracture or osteotomy.

The diaphysis has three sources of blood supply: (1) the nutrient artery (dual in human femur), (2) metaphyseal arteries (proximal, distal) which anastomose at each end of the medulla, to form (3) the medullary arterial supply—the major supply to all of the diaphyseal cortex.

The periosteal arterioles enter at fascial attachments, to supply only the external third of the cortex locally.

The Efferent Vascular System

The metaphysis is drained by the metaphyseal veins while the diaphysis is drained to the periosteum by the cortical venous channels from the deep cortex to periosteal venules, periosteal capillaries in continuity with capillaries of the superficial cortex, and venae comitantes of the periosteal arterioles.

The efferent vascular system blood flow is centrifugal through the cortex from the medulla to the periosteum.

The medullary contents with hematopoietic elements are drained by the large emissary veins. When there is a large nutrient canal, the emissary veins completely traverse the cortex and the venae comitantes of the nutrient artery.

Intermediate Vascular System of Compact Bone

There is no true capillary network between the afferent and efferent vascular systems like that present in the soft tissues. The ultimate vascular channels in cortex are blood vessels of capillary size that run one or two to a canal through rigid bony canals. The cortical canaliculi convey nutriments to the osteocytes in a fluid

tachments. The epiphyseal arteries, unlike the metaphyseal arteries, arise from the circumferential arterial network next to the epiphysis and enter the epiphysis near the margin of the articular cartilage. In children, the growth plate is the functional boundary between the epiphyseal and metaphyseal blood supply, while in the adult, there is anastomosis between the two. Although these blood supplies do anastomose in the adult, there appears to be a functional distinction between the epiphysis and metaphysis. This functional difference presupposes a permanent difference in neurovascular control, which is supported by the existence of persistent pressure differences between the epiphysis and the metaphysis.

Microcirculation of Bone
Afferent and Efferent System of Rhinelander[4]

The blood supply to bone supplies the epiphysis and metaphysis, which are composed chiefly of trabecular (cancellous or spongy) bone, and the diaphysis, which is composed primarily of cortical (compact) bone.

compartment that is separate from the surrounding blood vessels.

Blood Supply of Healing Mature Bone

When injury occurs, the normal supply increases and remains dominant. A new and transitory extraosseous blood supply is derived from the surrounding soft tissues for early nourishment of periosteal callus and detached bony fragments.

Since fascial attachments convey the blood supply to bone (via periosteal arterioles), they should not be disturbed surgically. The loosely attached periosteum does not convey afferent blood vessels to bone and can be surgically elevated.

Blood Supply of the Femoral Head

The medial and lateral circumflex arteries give rise to arterial branches that form a ring at the base of the femoral neck. The metaphyseal and epiphyseal arteries arise from this ring of arterial branches. The posterior portion of the arterial ring is usually formed by the medial circumflex artery and the anterior portion is formed by the lateral circumflex artery. Branches from the ring ascend (ascending cervical or retinacular), penetrate the capsule at its attachment to the femur (intertrochanteric line anteriorly and the neck posteriorly), and vessels from these branches form the metaphyseal and epiphyseal arteries of the proximal femur.

Trueta and Harrison[3] stated in their classic article that although the metaphyseal and epiphyseal arteries anastomose when the epiphyseal plate disappears, each area retains some circulatory autonomy.

Trueta and Harrison[3] chose to name the arteries of the proximal femur by their site of entry into bone: (1) epiphyseal arteries—medial and lateral, and (2) metaphyseal arteries—superior and inferior.

The lateral epiphyseal artery and both groups of metaphyseal arteries (superior and inferior) usually arise from the medial femoral circumflex artery. The medial epiphyseal artery is a continuation of an artery within the ligamentum teres, arising either from the obturator artery or the medial femoral circumflex artery.

The lateral epiphyseal arteries vary in number from two to six and enter the head posterosuperiorly to lie within a ligamentous fibrous sheath, supplying two thirds to four fifths of the epiphysis. These superior retinacular arteries provide the major blood supply to the head of the femur. The medial epiphyseal artery runs laterally from the ligamentum teres, enters the femur through the foramen capitalis, and anastomoses with the lateral epiphyseal vessels.

The epiphyseal vessels are arranged in a series of arterial arcades directed toward the articular surface circumferentially. The arcades of epiphyseal vessels arch to meet mirror image vessels and form the anastomosing arches. These arches appear "as if a series of fountains were arranged in such a fashion that the spray from any one fell into the rising columns of its neighbors on all sides."[3]

There are usually two to three superior metaphyseal arteries arising from vessels that also give origin to the lateral epiphyseal vessels. The superior metaphyseal arteries enter the bone some distance from the articular cartilage, follow the epiphyseal plate, and then anastomose with the inferior metaphyseal arteries that enter the bone near the articular cartilage.

Before the metaphyseal vessels enter the femoral head, they have frequent interconnecting anastomoses in the subsynovial tissues to the circulus articularis vasculosus of Hunter. On the neck of the femur, the circle tends to be deficient anteriorly and the vascular border is most evident superiorly and inferiorly.

Trueta and Harrison[3] also noted that in the adult there is often a visible demarcation of the epiphysis and metaphysis because of the two different types of marrow—red and yellow. The epiphysis is often occupied by yellow marrow that appears as inactive fat with vessels of small capillary size. Yellow marrow does not have the sinusoids that are characteristic of red marrow.

Articular Cartilage

Although the articular cartilage is avascular, it comes in contact with capillary vessels on deep attached surfaces and at its peripheral margin.

Precapillary loops, arising in the marrow, pass through canals in the subchondral bone and form a single broad loop. Capillary loops at the deep surface of the calcified cartilage and postcapillary venules return to the precapillary loops through the canals to the marrow. This system is different from any other in the marrow circulation and appears to be specific to the chondroosseous junction.

Intramedullary Pressure

Intravenous circulation has been difficult to study because of its complexity and the limited method of investigation. Currently, most studies are done by introducing a trochar into bone and recording intramedullary pressure. Most agree that the data produced are from a small hematoma at the tip of the trochar. The cancellous bone pressures recorded (intramedullary pressures) are interstitial pressures probably equivalent to pressures in the capillary.

The recorded intramedullary pressure shows a pulse pressure synchronous with cardiac contraction and an

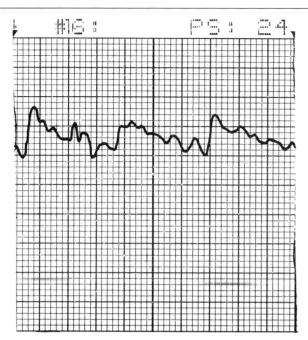

Fig. 3-5 Intramedullary pressure recording showing normal undulations.

undulation related to breathing (Fig. 3–5). The pressure varies with the animal and the region of bone studied. The intramedullary pressure is not the same in the diaphysis, metaphysis, or epiphysis of the same bone, which implies a functional autonomy by region.

The intramedullary pressure is related to blood pressure, although an individual with hypertension will not have an abnormal intramedullary pressure. The intramedullary pressure is increased by muscular contraction, ligation of the femoral artery, and femoral vein occlusion. Vagus nerve stimulation and adrenaline decrease intramedullary pressure. The femoral head intramedullary pressure is higher than the pressure at the trochanteric level, and pressures higher than 30 mm Hg are considered abnormal.

Blood Flow to Bone

A bone blood flow of 10 ml/min/100 g is considered normal and is regulated by vasomotor nerves to the intravenous vessels, by hormones, and by blood constituents, such as hydrogen ions, carbon dioxide, and oxygen. Cardiac output and muscle contraction also influence blood flow to bone.

There is a direct relationship between bone blood flow and intramedullary pressure in the arterial vessels. A decrease in arterial flow results in decreased intramedullary pressure. On the venous side, however, occlusion of the femoral vein produces intravenous hypertension and accelerated blood flow. Thus, venous blood flow is indirectly related to intramedullary pressure.

"In physiological circumstance, there is a real parallel between flow and pressure, but this parallel may disappear in pathological conditions."[1]

References

1. Ficat RP, Arlet J: Anatomy of bone circulation, in Hungerford DS (ed): *Ischemia and Necrosis of Bone*. Baltimore, Williams & Wilkins, 1980.
2. Trias A, Fery A: Cortical circulation of long bones. *J Bone Joint Surg* 1979;61A:1052–1059.
3. Trueta J, Harrison MH: The normal vascular anatomy of the femoral head in adult man. *J Bone Joint Surg* 1953;35B:442–461.
4. Rhinelander FW: The normal microcirculation of diaphyseal cortex and its response to fracture. *J Bone Joint Surg* 1968;50A:784–800.

The Staging of Aseptic Necrosis

Thomas A. Lange, MD

The staging of the clinical and pathologic changes that occur in aseptic necrosis has not changed appreciably since its initial description by Marcus and associates[1] in 1973. Before then, there was no generally accepted ordering of events in the evolution of femoral head changes. In 1966, Malka[2] cited three "periods" of the disease described by the French authors Serre and Simon. The first period was "onset," during which pain starts. The physical findings were described as relatively normal, as were the radiographic findings. The second period was "roentgenologic change" when, after two to six months of pain, the femoral head radiograph takes on the classic appearance of flattening and increased density. The third and final period in the evolution of aseptic necrosis was "complications," described as formation of "radiolucent geodes" or "sequestrum" formation and articular incongruity. These "periods" in aseptic necrosis, however, did not address the subtle asymptomatic beginnings subsequently described by Marcus and associates[1] and Springfield and Enneking[3] as the "silent hip."

The Enneking staging system of aseptic necrosis of the femoral head developed out of the recognition that radiographic and pathologic changes occur in the contralateral hip of patients with symptoms caused by a collapsed femoral head. This early asymptomatic or "silent" period was divided arbitrarily into stages I and II on the basis of radiographic and pathologic changes.[1,3] The onset of pain heralds a pathologic fracture in the subchondral bone, and ushers in stage III. Stage III is distinguished radiographically from stage IV by a relatively round femoral head. In stage IV, subchondral collapse is evident. The final stages, stages V and VI, show the development of degrees of secondary degenerative arthritis. This brief overview of the six stages makes it apparent that this system is neither purely clinical nor purely radiologic, but attempts to weave into some order all events including pathologic changes.

Stage I is clinically asymptomatic; the head is still spherical and appears grossly normal. It differs radiographically from a normal hip by virtue of areas of thickened trabeculae scattered throughout the head (Fig. 4–1). Pathologic core biopsy specimens reveal viable bone annealed to necrotic trabeculae, explaining the radiographic changes. The marrow spaces may be populated with histiocytes and mononuclear inflammatory cells.[1]

Stage II remains clinically asymptomatic and requires that the head be spherical and the articular cartilage

normal. The radiographic appearance has a characteristic "rind" of reactive bone that defines the infarct area, which may appear wedge-shaped or cystic (Fig. 4–2, *top left* and *top right*). Histologically, the trabeculae within the "defined" infarct are acellular, lacking any osteocytes. The adjacent marrow is equally acellular. Even the previously noted inflammatory cells are gone (Fig. 4–2, *bottom left*).

Stage III begins with the onset of groin pain, most often during weightbearing. An anteroposterior radiograph may appear to be normal although a frog-leg lateral view may reveal a fracture between the subchondral bone of the head and the supporting trabeculae. This transversely oriented fracture appears as a crescent-shaped radiolucency, giving rise to the term "crescent" sign (Fig. 4–3, *top left*).

This stage probably corresponds with the "period of onset" described by Serre and Simon and cited by Malka.[2]

The zone of the infarct develops increased density because of mineral deposition in some of the marrow spaces between thickened trabeculae from previous cycles of repair.

Histologically the infarct zone has thickened acellular bony trabeculae and eosinophilic-staining amorphous debris in the marrow spaces. In a cut coronal section, separation of the subchondral bone from underlying trabeculae is seen at either margin of the primary compression trabeculae (Fig. 4–3, *top right* and *bottom left*). The articular cartilage, however, remains intact and viable because of diffusion of synovial nutrients.

Table 4–1
Staging system of Ficat and Arlet*

Stage	Joint line	Head Contour	Trabeculae
I	Normal	Spherical	Normal or osteoporotic
II	Normal	Spherical	Diffuse porosis/ sclerosis or wedge sclerosis
III	Normal or increased	Early collapse or "out of round"	Sequestrum appearance
IV	Decreased	Marked collapse	Extensive destruction

*Reproduced with permission from Hungerford DS: Bone marrow pressure, venography and core decompression in ischemic necrosis of the femoral head, in *The Hip: Proceedings of the Seventh Open Scientific Meeting of the Hip Society*. St. Louis, CV Mosby Co, 1979, pp 218–237.

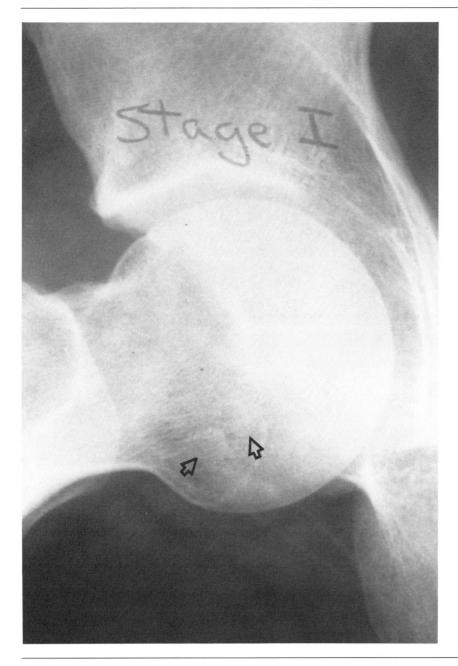

Fig. 4-1 Lateral radiographic view of an asymptomatic hip in a patient with alcohol-induced aseptic necrosis on the symptomatic side. The small patchy densities (arrows) seen in the trabecular bone suggest that this is stage I.

In stage IV of the Enneking staging system, the radiograph reveals lateral collapse of the subchondral bone so that flattening of the head is apparent (Fig. 4–4, *top*). The zone of the infarct becomes more radiodense with the deposition of mineral in the necrotic marrow spaces that began in stage III. Grossly, a permanent wrinkle develops in the articular cartilage, which remains otherwise healthy to this point (Fig. 4–4, *bottom*).

Histologically, the infarct zone contains more of the thickened acellular bony trabeculae and acellular eosinophilic-staining amorphous debris, some of which is calcified, in the marrow spaces (Fig. 4–5, *top*). Outside of the infarct there is a zone of dense fibrous repair tissue that seems to limit vascular ingrowth. The tra-becular bone adjacent but peripheral to the fibrous zone has several layers of repair with only the outermost containing osteocytes. The marrow spaces are filled with hypervascular granulation (Fig. 4–5, *bottom*).

Clinically, during this stage the pain increases in amount and duration and the gait is definitely antalgic.

Stage V insidiously evolves from stage IV without any distinct clinical or radiographic features to mark its onset. Most patients in this stage have continuous pain and choose to use external support for ambulation. Radiographically, in addition to progressive head flattening (Fig. 4–6), there is evidence of acetabular cartilage wear. Histologically the articular cartilage is worn, shredded, and repaired by fibrocartilage in various areas.

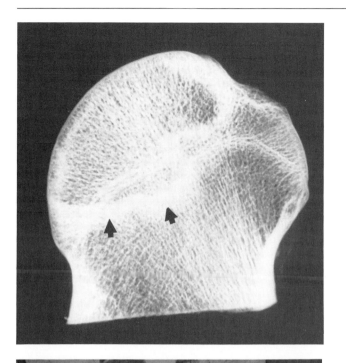

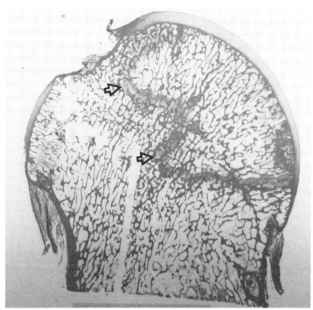

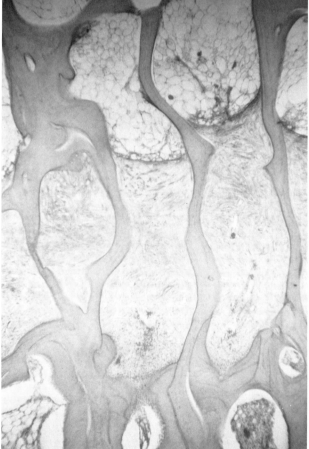

Fig. 4-2 Stage II femoral head. **Top left:** Micrograph of a slab section demonstrating the thickened trabeculae that form a "rind" of bone that defines the infarct zone (arrows). **Top right:** In this macrosection the articular cartilage and subchondral bone appear to be intact. There is an irregular outline of the infarct zone defined by thickened trabeculae and densely staining fibrous tissue (arrows). **Bottom left:** Low-power micrograph of the fibrous zone that defines the infarct. Acellular bone and marrow are at the top. The densely packed fibrous connective tissue in the intratrabecular spaces is in the middle. At the bottom the bony trabeculae are widened by several layers of repair bone annealed to the original necrotic trabeculae. The marrow spaces have elements of viable marrow at the outer perimeter of the zone of demarcation in stage II (hematoxylin and eosin, × 40). (Reproduced with permission from the W. Thaxton Springfield Center for Orthopaedic Study and Research, University of Florida, Gainesville.)

Stage VI (Fig. 4–7) is uncommon because the severe pain normally prompts the patient to undergo arthroplasty long before radiographically apparent joint de- struction. Osteophytes and degenerative cysts predom- inate in the radiographic and gross pathologic appearance. Except for the severe head flattening, and

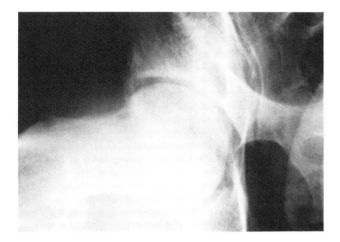

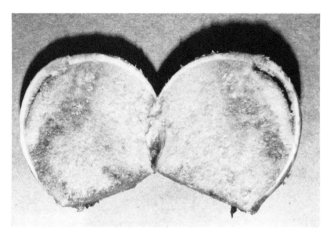

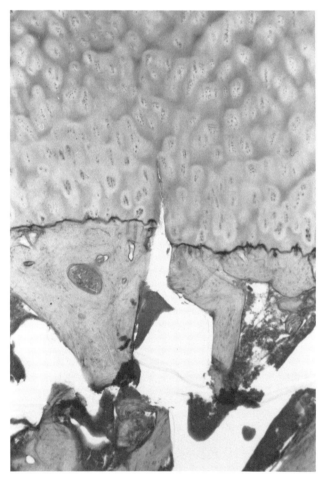

Fig. 4-3 Stage III, painful femoral head. **Top left:** Lateral view shows a faint radiolucent zone immediately beneath the subchondral bone opposite the acetabular fovea. This radiolucency is known as the "crescent" sign. **Top right:** This bivalved femoral head demonstrates the separation of subchondral bone from underlying infarcted trabeculae. The dark cleft corresponds with the radiographic crescent sign. **Bottom left:** At the extreme margin of the crescent sign, the cleft in the subchondral bone supports viable articular cartilage. Note that there is very slight displacement of the tidemark and early propagation of the fracture into the articular cartilage. (Bottom left figure reproduced with permission from the W. Thaxton Springfield Center for Orthopaedic Study and Research, University of Florida, Gainesville.)

in some cases the virtual absence of a definable head, the radiographic changes are primarily those of advanced degenerative arthritis.

The clinical and radiologic changes are diagrammatically summarized in Figure 4–8.

Since the publication of the Enneking staging system in 1973, others have proposed and published staging systems based primarily on radiographic changes. Among these is the Sugioka classification, which is based on radiographic changes only. Sugioka and associates[4] used the following grading system: grade I, necrosis just visible, femoral head still round; grade II, flattening of the head; grade III, markedly collapsed head without narrowing of the joint space; and grade IV, advanced changes of the head with narrowing of the joint space. All four grades were assigned after the clinical onset of

Table 4-2
Radiologic classification of ischemic necrosis of the femoral head*

Clinical Data	Simple Necrosis		Necrosis Complicated by Collapse	
	Stage I	Stage II	Stage III	Stage IV
Joint line	Normal	Normal	Normal	Narrowed
Femoral head contour	Normal	Normal	Flattened subchondral infraction collapse	Collapsed
Trabeculae	Normal or very slight osteoporosis	Osteoporosis; mixed sclerosis/porosis	Sequestrum formation	Destruction of superior pole
Diagnosis				
By radiograph	Impossible	Probable	Certain	Very difficult to distinguish among arthrosis, flammatory arthritis, and necrosis
By functional exploration of bone	Hemodynamic, probable; histopathologic, certain	Hemodynamic, probable; histopathologic, certain	Confirmation	Hemodynamic insufficient; combined biopsy necessary

*Adapted from Ficat and Arlet.[6]

Table 4-3
Mechanistic staging of osteonecrosis*

Stage	Description	Radiographic Findings
0	Fat embolism 1. Intraosseous vascular occlusion 2. Inflammatory 3. Focal intravascular coagulation	Normal
I	Osteonecrosis	Normal to patchy, small areas of increased density
II	Revascularization	Round head; "sclerotic" area adjacent to articular surface
III	Collapse and deformity	Crescent sign and collapse
IV	Degenerative change	Joint incongruity

*Derived from the data of Jones.[9,10]

pain since the rotational osteotomy described was performed for relief of pain. Sugioka and associates did not address any asymptomatic stages but based their grades on pain relief and progression of deformity.

A more commonly used staging system is that of Ficat and Arlet, which was made popular by Hungerford.[5] The early version shown in Table 4–1 was purely radiologic. Again, all stages were based on the presumption of a painful hip. This staging system was later expanded.[6,7] The revised system included probabilities of diagnosis on the basis of radiographs and supplemental intraosseous pressure readings and core biopsy material (Table 4–2). This was a valid attempt to correlate pathophysiologic and hemodynamic changes with the radiographic stages but it failed to correlate clinical symptoms with the above stages. A physician using the Ficat and Arlet system must remember that the stages are primarily radiographic and are in symptomatic hips.

The most recent modification of this system[8] includes stage 0 to represent the preclinical and preradiologic-

change stage of the disease. This was the first acknowledgment of a preclinical stage, an important concept.

Two additional staging systems warrant inclusion in this discussion. That of Jones,[9,10] which might be considered mechanistic in style, has five stages from 0 to IV (Table 4–3).

Stage 0 (fat embolism) has three phases. Phase I is "mechanical" and initiated by intraosseous vascular occlusion. Phase II is "chemical" and results from a toxic inflammatory response in the marrow caused by free fatty acids. Phase III is "thrombotic" and is caused by focal intravascular coagulation.

Stage I (osteonecrosis) is the time of the infarct in the head. This may be asymptomatic and roentgenograms are normal but bone scan or tomographic findings may be abnormal. In stage II (revascularization) the lengthy process of repair begins. Small lesions are repaired while others progress to stage III (collapse), which coincides with the onset of symptoms. Stage IV (degeneration) follows if treatment fails to arrest the collapse.

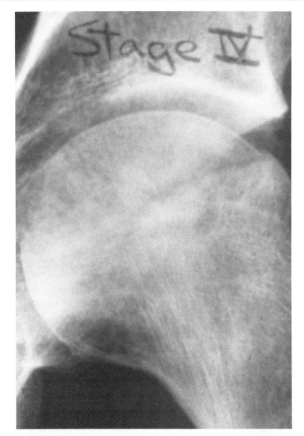

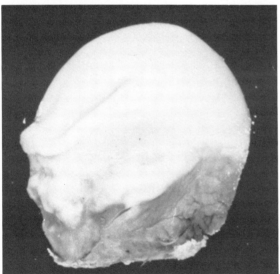

Fig. 4–4   Symptomatic stage IV femoral head. **Top:** This is the painful hip illustrated in Figure 4–1 that led to the discovery of the "silent hip" seen in stage I. Note the lateral step-off immediately under the corner of the acetabulum. **Bottom:** Gross appearance reveals the permanent wrinkle in the articular cartilage caused by the collapse of the underlying subchondral bone. (Bottom figure reproduced with permission from the W. Thaxton Springfield Center for Orthopaedic Study and Research, University of Florida, Gainesville.)

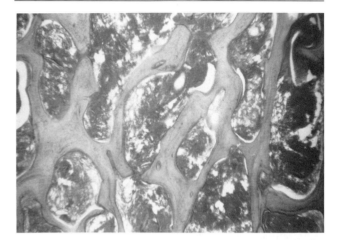

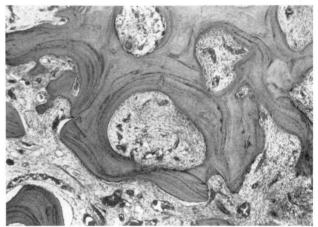

Fig. 4–5   Stage IV femoral head. **Top:** Low-power view reveals the densely packed amorphous eosinophilic material between the thickened necrotic trabeculae (hematoxylin-eosin, × 40). **Bottom:** Section from area immediately outside of the infarct zone demonstrates the hypervascularity that develops in the attempt to revascularize the femoral head. The concentric cement lines suggest that several periods of repair have occurred. (Reproduced with permission from the W. Thaxton Springfield Center for Orthopaedic Study and Research, University of Florida, Gainesville.)

The final staging system to consider is that of Steinberg and associates.[11] It expands the six Enneking stages into seven by including a stage 0 in which both the radiograph and the bone scan are normal but in which magnetic resonance imaging or other diagnostic modalities may establish a diagnosis before clinical and radiographic changes are apparent. In stage I the radiograph is normal but the bone scan is abnormal. Stages II through V are divided into mild, moderate, and severe phases to denote the degree of radiographic involvement of the femoral head (Table 4–4).

From this discussion it should be apparent that it is not universally accepted that the onset of pain in the hip implies a pathologic subchondral bone fracture. Some authors, including Ficat and Arlet in France and Hungerford in the United States, believe that the pain may be related to intraosseous pressure or perhaps in-

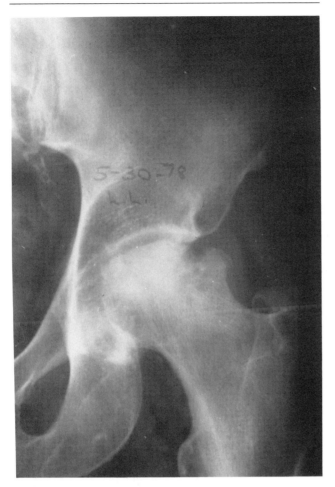

Fig. 4-6 Anteroposterior radiograph of a patient with symptomatic avascular necrosis in which significant collapse and marked increased density in the femoral head have occurred. These changes are consistent with stage V aseptic necrosis.

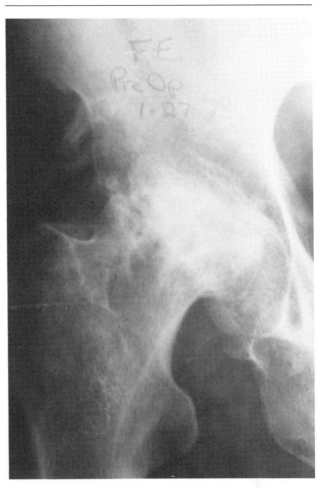

Fig. 4-7 Anteroposterior radiograph of a patient with severe continuous pain depicts stage VI avascular necrosis in which extreme femoral head collapse and loss of joint space are prominent features.

traosseous inflammation rather than to a subchondral fracture. This seemingly minor intellectual disagreement is the basis for quite different treatment recommendations. If one accepts that subchondral collapse causes the pain, then efforts to save the head in its original configuration by core decompression or bone grafting are probably in vain. Conversely, if radiography fails to demonstrate a fracture, then core decompression[7] may be expected to relieve the pain of intraosseous hypertension.

Perhaps one reason for the failure of core decompression in some painful spherical heads is that the subchondral fracture is too subtle to be detected. On the other hand, the successes of core decompression in some painful heads may imply that not all Enneking stage I and II femoral heads are asymptomatic before collapse.

The selective use of magnetic resonance imaging[12,13] and bone scanning[14,15] may enhance our ability to diagnose aseptic necrosis early in the asymptomatic hip at risk so that core decompression or other prophylactic

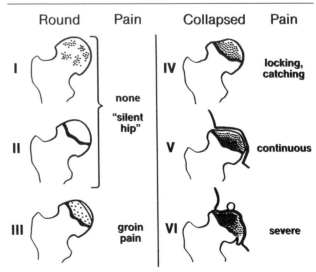

Fig. 4-8 The six stages in the Enneking staging system. At left, the first three stages in which the radiographic appearance of the femoral head is round. At right, the three stages in which collapse is evident on the anteroposterior radiograph. Corresponding to the radiographic appearance are the symptoms associated with the progression of the stages. Stages I and II are asymptomatic and are indicated as the "silent hip."

Table 4-4

Radiographic evaluation and staging of the hip in avascular necrosis of the femoral head*

Stage	Characteristics
0	Normal radiograph; normal bone scan
I	Normal radiograph; abnormal bone scan
II	Sclerosis and/or cyst formation in femoral head A. Mild (<20%) B. Moderate (20% to 40%) C. Severe (>40%)
III	Subchondral collapse (crescent sign) without flattening A. Mild (<15%) B. Moderate (15% to 30%) C. Severe (>30%)
IV	Flattening of head without joint narrowing or acetabular involvement A. Mild (<15% of surface and <2 mm of depression) B. Moderate (15% to 30% of surface or 2 to 4 mm of depression) C. Severe (>30% of surface or >4 mm of depression)
V	Flattening of head with joint narrowing and/or acetabular involvement A. Mild B. Moderate } determined as above plus estimate of C. Severe } acetabular involvement
VI	Advanced degenerative changes

*Reproduced with permission from Steinberg ME: Early results in the treatment of avascular necrosis of the femoral head with electrical stimulation. *Orthop Clin North Am* 1984;15:163–175.

therapies can be initiated. Determining the efficacy of diagnostic studies in the early detection of aseptic necrosis and comparing the results of treatment at various stages of the disease using different modalities will require a commonly accepted staging system. The various theories all have their proponents. I hope this summary of published staging systems for aseptic necrosis will allow prospective studies to report results on the basis of either a specific radiographic staging system that includes the clinical symptoms or a system that incorporates pain so that valid comparisons of treatment will become possible. In the future, as our understanding of this intriguing condition improves, we can look forward to a unifying staging system.

Acknowledgment

Supported in part by the John L. McClellan Memorial Veterans Administration Medical Center, Little Rock, Arkansas.

References

1. Marcus ND, Enneking WF, Massam RA: The silent hip in idiopathic necrosis. *J Bone Joint Surg* 1973;55A:1351–1366.
2. Malka S: Idiopathic aseptic necrosis of the head of the femur in adults. *Surg Gynecol Obstet* 1966;23:1057–1065.
3. Springfield DS, Enneking WF: Idiopathic aseptic necrosis, in *Bones and Joints*. Baltimore, Williams & Wilkins, 1976, chap 5, pp 61–87.
4. Sugioka Y, Katsuki I, Hotokebuchi T: Transtrochanteric rotational osteotomy of the femoral head for the treatment of osteonecrosis. *Clin Orthop* 1982;169:115–126.
5. Hungerford DS: Bone marrow pressure, venography and core decompression in ischemic necrosis of the femoral head, in *The Hip: Proceedings of the Seventh Open Scientific Meeting of the Hip Society*. St. Louis, CV Mosby Co, 1979, pp 218–237.
6. Ficat RP, Arlet J: Necrosis of the femoral head, in Hungerford DS (ed): *Ischemia and Necrosis of Bone*. Baltimore, Williams & Wilkins, 1980, chap 4.
7. Hungerford DS: Treatment of ischemic necrosis of the femoral head, in Evarts CM (ed): *Surgery of the Musculoskeletal System*. New York, Churchill Livingstone, 1983, vol 3, chap 1.
8. Ficat R: Treatment of avascular necrosis of the femoral head, in *The Hip: Proceedings of the 11th Open Scientific Meeting of the Hip Society*. St. Louis, CV Mosby Co, 1983, pp 279–295.
9. Jones JP Jr: Fat embolism and osteonecrosis. *Orthop Clin North Am* 1985;16:595–633.
10. Jones JP Jr: Osteonecrosis, in McCarty DJ (ed): *Arthritis and Allied Conditions*, ed 10. Philadelphia, Lea and Febiger, 1985, 1356–1373.
11. Steinberg ME, Brighton CT, Hayken GD, et al: Early results in the treatment of avascular necrosis of the femoral head with electrical stimulation. *Orthop Clin North Am* 1984;15:163–175.
12. Mitchell MD, Kundel HL, Steinberg ME, et al: Avascular necrosis of the hip: Comparison of MR, CT, and scintigraphy. *AJR* 1986;147:67–71.
13. Bassett LW, Gold RH, Reicher M, et al: Magnetic resonance imaging in the early diagnosis of ischemic necrosis of the femoral head: Preliminary results. *Clin Orthop* 1984;214:237–248.
14. Dumler F, Vulpetti AT, Guise ER Jr, et al: Scintigraphy in the early diagnosis of osteonecrosis of the femoral head in chronic hemodialysis and transplantation. *Clin Nephrol* 1977;8:349–353.
15. Turner JH: Post-traumatic avascular necrosis of the femoral head predicted by preoperative technetium–99m antimony-colloid scan. *J Bone Joint Surg* 1983;65A:786–796.

Management of Avascular Necrosis of the Femoral Head—An Overview

Marvin E. Steinberg, MD

Introduction

At the present time, no method of treating avascular necrosis (AVN) of the femoral head is completely satisfactory. A number of different approaches have been advocated, and the choice of which to use depends in part on the stage at which the condition is diagnosed and in part on the personal preference of the investigator. In many, if not most of these cases, definitive data concerning the results of treatment are not yet available.

The most common cause of AVN is trauma. Displaced subcapital and high transcervical fractures are associated with a high incidence of AVN as well as nonunion. There are significant differences between posttraumatic and nontraumatic AVN. The traumatic variety is usually associated with a healing fracture; some type of metallic fixation device is generally present; and the condition is unilateral. It occurs in a much older patient population and may be associated with either nonunion at the fracture site or degenerative changes in the hip joint. There is usually involvement of most of the femoral head, and weightbearing has been limited for a prolonged period. In part because of these factors, early diagnosis is usually difficult and AVN is often diagnosed only after gross collapse of the femoral head. In such cases, attempts to preserve the femoral head are generally unsuccessful and are not indicated. If pain and disability are not too great, symptomatic treatment may be all that is required. If pain and disability are significant, the patient generally requires an arthroplasty. In an elderly individual with a relatively normal acetabulum, a femoral endoprosthesis, either unipolar or bipolar, can be used. When definite acetabular abnormality is present, either on preoperative radiographs or at the time of surgery, total hip replacement is the treatment of choice. Since total hip replacement usually produces better and more predictable results than femoral endoprostheses do, endoprostheses are now rarely used in late reconstruction.

Posttraumatic AVN also occurs in younger individuals who have sustained fractures, dislocations, or fracture-dislocations of the hip, but this is much less common.

Nontraumatic AVN primarily affects young adults and is bilateral in more than 50% to 60% of cases. The goal is to preserve, not to replace, the femoral head. Although we have no completely satisfactory treatment for this condition, results are best with early treatment.

A primary goal, therefore, must be early diagnosis, as discussed elsewhere in this volume.[1]

Evaluating Results

Why is there so much difference of opinion as to the effectiveness of various techniques for treating AVN? In large part this results from the methods used to evaluate postoperative results and the differing durations of follow-up. In my experience, it is not possible to determine definitive results at one year, as many have attempted to do. I believe that a case must be followed up for a minimum of two years. Many hips that seem to be doing well at one year experience later collapse and degeneration. If a hip remains stable for approximately two or three years, a sudden change in its status is unlikely.

An objective and comprehensive system for evaluating results must also be used. Older systems, which place the hip in one of four or five categories and which do not actually measure the extent of involvement, may be quite misleading. When such a system is used, changes may indeed take place that are not identified. The staging and evaluation system shown in Table 5–1 grades the hip by both type and extent of involvement. With this system, even subtle degrees of progression can be detected.[2]

Nonsurgical Treatment

A number of orthopaedic surgeons continue to treat AVN nonsurgically, hoping that spontaneous healing of the lesion will occur. Some advocate symptomatic care, limiting the activity level and the degree of weightbearing by the amount of pain. Others limit the patient to either partial weightbearing or nonweightbearing at the time the diagnosis is made. How effective is this approach? Surprisingly, little has been published on this subject. In children, a significant degree of spontaneous healing does occur after Legg-Calvé-Perthes' disease, and it is therefore tempting to assume that the same will take place in the adult. In a retrospective study, my associates and I reviewed the sequence of events in 48 hips with nontraumatic AVN that were treated nonsurgically.[3] Follow-up ranged from six months to ten years. Careful radiologic assessment showed that the condition progressed in ten of 12 hips

Table 5–1
Staging of avascular necrosis of the femoral head

Stages	Characteristics
0	Normal radiograph; normal bone scan
I	Normal radiograph; abnormal bone scan
II	Sclerosis and/or cyst formation in the femoral head (mild, < 20%; moderate, 20% to 40%; severe, > 40%)
III	Subchondral collapse (crescent sign) without flattening (mild, < 15%; moderate, 15% to 30%; severe, > 30%)
IV	Flattening of femoral head without joint narrowing or acetabular involvement (mild, < 15% of surface and < 2 mm of depression; moderate, 15% to 30% of surface or 2 to 4 mm of depression; severe, > 30% of surface or > 4 mm of depression)
V	Flattening of the femoral head with joint narrowing and/or acetabular involvement (mild, < 15% of surface and < 2 mm of depression plus estimate of acetabular involvement; moderate, 15% to 30% of surface or 2 to 4 mm of depression plus estimate of acetabular involvement; severe, > 30% of surface or > 4 mm of depression plus estimate of acetabular involvement)
VI	Advanced degenerative changes

Table 5–2
Progression by stage of involvement

Stage	No. of Hips	Hips With Progression	
		No.	%
0 to II	16	13	81
III	11	9	82
IV	10	10	100
V and VI	18	17	94
Total	55	49	89

allowed to bear weight as tolerated, and in 35 of 36 hips treated with either limited weightbearing or non-weightbearing. Overall, progression occurred in 92% of cases. Limiting the amount of weight placed on the involved hip did not appear to affect the result.

We subsequently evaluated 55 hips, including the original 48, and classified them by stage of involvement at the time that the diagnosis was first made (Table 5–2). Of the hips diagnosed before radiographic evidence of collapse, 81% showed progression. Of those with subchondral collapse, indicated by a crescent sign but without flattening of the articular surface, 82% progressed. All hips with some degree of femoral head flattening initially progressed. Of those seen after the appearance of more advanced degenerative changes, such as joint line narrowing or acetabular involvement, 95% showed radiographic progression. The overall progression rate was 89%.[3]

These studies lead to the conclusion that once the diagnosis is clinically apparent, most cases progress.

This does not appear to be influenced by the degree of weightbearing permitted. The results were, however, somewhat better in patients seen in the very earliest stages. There are, of course, a certain number of patients in whom small areas of avascularity of the femoral head remain asymptomatic and heal satisfactorily, as in cases of subclinical pulmonary emboli. Many, if not most, of these cases are never diagnosed.

Prophylactic Surgery

Once the clinical diagnosis has been made, consideration should be given to the prophylactic measures available. At the present time these include drilling or "core decompression," grafting, osteotomy, and electrical stimulation.

Drilling or Decompression

Simple drilling or "forage" has been used for some time, but the results in general have not been entirely satisfactory. Ficat and Arlet[4] in France and Hungerford[5] in the United States have popularized the technique of "core decompression." The rationale and technical details of this procedure will not be described in detail here. Initially, these authors reported good to excellent results in 80% to 90% of early cases. Thus, this approach was greeted with some degree of enthusiasm. Not all investigators, however, have had such gratifying results. Camp and Colwell[6] reported a much lower success rate and a high number of complications with this procedure. My own experience with approximately 175 of these procedures has been somewhere between these two extremes. Since I combine grafting with decompression, my technique and results are discussed below. At the present time, this is my preferred method for managing early cases of AVN of the femoral head.

Bone Grafting

The many types of grafting procedures include the use of cancellous bone, cortical bone, muscle-pedicle bone grafts, bone grafts with a microvascular anastomosis, and osteochondral allografts.

Almost 40 years ago Phemister[7] described the use of a cortical graft inserted from a lateral approach into the femoral head and neck. This technique was expanded by Bonfiglio and associates.[8-10] In addition to opening up channels for vascular ingrowth, the cortical strut graft provided mechanical support to the articular surface of the femoral head during the healing process and thus retarded collapse. This approach, as well as almost every other grafting procedure, also decompresses the femoral head. Satisfactory long-term results were reported in 78% of cases by Bonfiglio and associates, but others have generally not been able to duplicate this high degree of success.[11]

Many techniques are available for the insertion of a

cancellous graft into the area of the lesion. Anterior, posterior, and lateral approaches have been employed. My surgical approach is similar to that described by Ficat and Arlet[4] and Hungerford,[5] except that instead of leaving the large central channel empty, I place a very loose fitting cylinder of cancellous bone in it to act as a scaffolding for bone repair. The graft is taken from the relatively normal bone of the intertrochanteric region and thus does not require a separate surgical site (Figs. 5–1 and 5–2). Because this graft fits very loosely and is placed in only one of three channels, its presence does not eliminate the effect of decompression. This technique has yielded satisfactory results in approximately 50% of cases treated before the onset of femoral head collapse. In some cases no progression occurred, whereas in others there was some progression before the condition appeared to stabilize. In many instances femoral head replacement was avoided or at least postponed. In others, however, the condition did progress and patients required arthroplasty between one and two years after the procedure. Compared to the natural course of this condition without any surgical intervention, these results must be viewed as at least partly successful.

Meyers and associates[12,13] employed a bone graft with an intact muscle-pedicle in an attempt to revascularize the necrotic area. Although they were satisfied with the results, others have not been able to duplicate them.

Gilbert and associates[14] in France and Urbaniak and associates[15] in the United States have used a microvascular grafting technique.

Through a lateral approach, the necrotic bone in the femoral head is removed and packed loosely with cancellous graft. A section of fibula is then placed through the lateral femoral cortex into the femoral head and

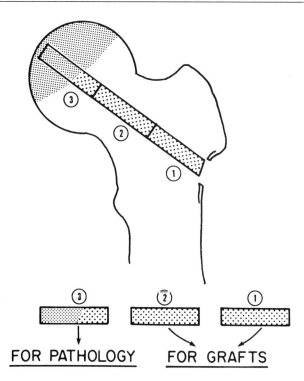

Fig. 5–2 Schema of technique for decompression and grafting showing retrieval of grafts and histologic specimen.

neck. Blood supply to the region is ensured by a microvascular anastomosis between the nutrient artery and vein of the fibula and local vessels. Preliminary results of this technically difficult procedure have been encouraging and it should be kept in mind as a promising option in the treatment of this disease.

There has been interest in removing the necrotic segment along with its overlying articular cartilage and replacing them by means of an osteochondral allograft.[13,16,17] The operation is technically demanding and many problems are yet to be solved. Only a small number of such procedures have been done and I consider this technique to be experimental at the present time. This approach may present a reasonable option for the patient who already has some degree of surface collapse if the technical details can be worked out satisfactorily.

Osteotomy

Other procedures that fit into the general category of prophylactic surgery include the various osteotomies of the proximal femur. Merle d'Aubigné and associates[18] initially reported good results with flexion/extension osteotomies performed before 1963. In a later report, however, this group conceded that after longer follow-up 40% of their cases had to be considered failures and that all eventually showed progressive changes.[19] Recently there has been renewed interest in the role of osteotomy. New techniques have included varus, valgus, flexion, and extension osteotomies. Although many

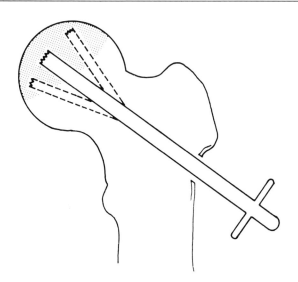

Fig. 5–1 Schema of technique for decompression and grafting showing placement of trephines.

of the investigators believe that these procedures provide better results than a nonsurgical approach, the reported data are limited and the follow-up is relatively short-term.[20-23] Although many theories have been used to explain why these osteotomies should work, the exact mechanisms are uncertain. One common denominator is that a certain degree of intraosseous decompression is effected simply by transecting the bone. Another is that a new and perhaps healthier segment of articular cartilage is brought into the region of major weightbearing. The amount of angulation that can be produced by this type of osteotomy is relatively small and it is generally impossible to shift weightbearing from a diseased to a healthy area of the femoral head.

Sugioka and associates[24-26] described a new type of osteotomy involving rotation of the femoral head along the axis of the neck. They have performed more than 300 procedures and follow-up has been longer than ten years. They have had gratifying results in a high percentage of cases, including many with gross collapse of the femoral head. Using this technique, the femoral head can be rotated up to 90 degrees, thus allowing a much more effective repositioning of normal bone and cartilage into the weightbearing region of the femoral head (Figs. 5–3 and 5–4).

This procedure is technically demanding. Their indications, technical details, and follow-up care must be duplicated carefully if their results are to be achieved. It is essential that the circulation to the femoral head and neck be preserved and that the osteotomy be performed in the intertrochanteric region, not at the base of the neck. Such a deviation from the original technique perhaps explains the high percentage of failure reported by others. This technique should be reevaluated in the hope that other investigators can indeed duplicate the results of Sugioka and associates. If this can be done, this technique may be a valuable addition to our treatment of AVN. It may be applicable not only to the early stages of AVN but also to later stages in which a certain degree of femoral head collapse has already taken place.

Electrical Stimulation

Because of the osteogenic effects of selected types of electrical stimulation and their value in healing established nonunions, there has been interest in applying this technique to the treatment of AVN. Bassett and associates[27] and Eftekhar and associates[28] reported promising results with pulsed electromagnetic fields applied externally without previous surgery.

My associates and I have used a direct-current cathode wrapped around a bone graft and inserted directly into the femoral head as a supplement to decompression and grafting (Fig. 5–5). Although the final evaluation of this study has not been completed, early results show no evidence that the addition of electrical current enhances the results obtained by decompression and bone grafting alone.[29] At the present time we are evaluating another type of electrical signal, capacitive coupling, as an adjunct to decompression and grafting. Although we remain optimistic, no results are yet available.

At the present time electricity in the treatment of AVN, either alone or as an adjunct to surgery, should not be considered a proven technique for general use.

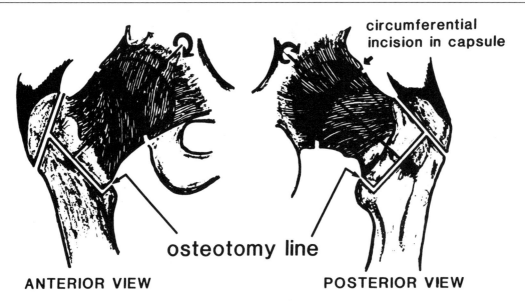

circumferential incision in capsule

osteotomy line

ANTERIOR VIEW   **POSTERIOR VIEW**

Fig. 5–3   Schema of the transtrochanteric rotational osteotomy of Sugioka. (Reproduced with permission from Sugioka Y: Transtrochanteric anterior rotational osteotomy of the femoral head in the treatment of osteonecrosis affecting the hip. *Clin Orthop* 1978;130:191–201.)

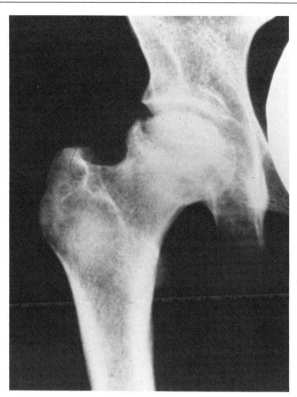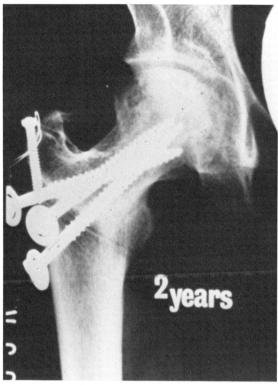

Fig. 5–4   Radiographs of hip before (at left) and two years after (at right) transtrochanteric osteotomy. (Reproduced with permission from Sugioka Y: Transtrochanteric anterior rotational osteotomy of the femoral head in the treatment of osteonecrosis affecting the hip. *Clin Orthop* 1978;130:191–201.)

Arthroplasty

The approaches described so far are considered "prophylactic surgery" and have as their goal the preservation of the spherical and structurally intact femoral head. These procedures work best in the early stages of the disease. Once collapse has occurred, the chance of salvaging the femoral head is extremely small. When radiographs demonstrate anything beyond a minimal degree of collapse, or when the patient has developed even moderate discomfort, limp, or decreased motion, such preventative measures are generally no longer indicated. At this point the patient is usually given symptomatic care until pain and disability warrant reconstructive surgery. The most common approach then is to consider some type of arthroplasty, such as cup arthroplasty, surface replacement arthroplasty, femoral endoprosthetic replacement, or total hip replacement.

Cup Arthroplasty

Before the development of total hip replacement, cup arthroplasty was the primary technique for reconstruction of the badly involved hip. For many reasons, this procedure was almost completely abandoned once total hip replacement became established. Patients with AVN, in particular, did badly because the necrotic seg-

ment of the femoral head often collapsed beneath the cup. Recently, however, there has been renewed interest in this procedure in a somewhat modified form.

In France, Kerboul and associates[19] and L. Sedel (oral communication) have used the "adjusted" cup arthroplasty as a temporizing procedure in this condition. Instead of moving freely on both the femoral and acetabular sides of the joint, the cup is fitted tightly over the femoral head so that there is little motion at that point. Most of the motion, then, occurs between the cup and the acetabulum. Satisfactory short-term results have been reported.

Carl Nelson has used a modification of this technique in a small number of patients with AVN (oral communication). The cup is cemented onto the femoral head, which is then replaced into the relatively normal acetabulum. This approach gives the patient a reasonably well-functioning joint and has postponed the need for total hip replacement arthroplasty. Both of these approaches merit consideration.

Surface Replacement Arthroplasty

At one time it was thought that surface replacement arthroplasty might prove to be a useful alternative to total hip replacement, especially in the young adult. A number of patients with AVN underwent surface re-

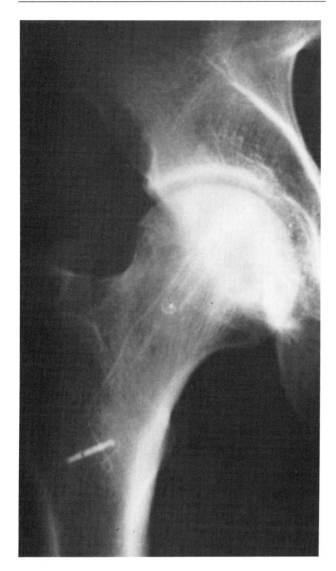

Fig. 5–5   Radiograph of a right hip four years after decompression and grafting with supplemental electrical stimulation. The lesion has not progressed and the patient is doing well clinically.

placement but, unfortunately, the five-year failure rate was unacceptable and this approach has been abandoned in the treatment of AVN at most centers.[30,31] There are certain theoretical advantages to this approach, however, and experimentation continues to refine and improve the technique.[32]

Femoral Endoprosthetic Replacement

Before the advent of total hip replacement, the classic approach to advanced AVN was replacement of the femoral head by an endoprosthesis. The results with uncemented prostheses were not entirely satisfactory. The high percentage of failures was attributed to motion within the femoral canal, protrusio acetabuli, or both. After the development of total hip replacement, the number of endoprostheses inserted for AVN di-

minished significantly. In the past several years, however, there has been increasing concern about the high failure rate of total hip replacement in young, heavy, active adults. Accordingly, interest has focused on other options, especially on the role of the femoral endoprosthesis. It was postulated that using a cemented or a biologic ingrowth component would eliminate most problems related to motion of the femoral stem within the shaft. Furthermore, it was presumed that using a bipolar component would significantly decrease problems on the acetabular side. In an attempt to evaluate the efficacy of femoral endoprosthetic replacement in patients with AVN, my colleagues and I reviewed 36 prostheses in 31 patients less than 50 years of age whose acetabuli appeared normal on radiographs. Twenty-nine of these hips had AVN. The patients' mean age was 38.3 years and the mean follow-up was 7.1 years.

The overall incidence of revision in this group was 47%, with an average time to revision of 5.4 years. Thirty-eight percent of these prostheses required revision at five years and 56% at ten years. Of the prostheses that had not been replaced at the time of evaluation, 11% were considered excellent, 47% good, 21% fair, and 21% poor. The mean Harris score was 74%. The causes of failure were loosening within the medullary canal of the femur, protrusio acetabuli, or both (Fig. 5–6).

It must be noted that this was a retrospective study. Most of the femoral prostheses were not cemented into place, the importance of the precise fit of the ball into the acetabulum was not emphasized to the extent that it is today, and the majority of these devices were unipolar rather than bipolar. The few bipolar components in this group, however, did not seem to fare better than the solid prostheses and protrusio acetabuli was not eliminated (Fig. 5–7). These findings were confirmed by Desman and associates,[33] Heiner and associates,[34] and D.S. Hungerford (oral communication). Although the use of cemented or biologic ingrowth components and precise fitting of the prosthesis to the acetabulum will certainly improve the results, the inherent problems will not be solved. Even normal acetabular cartilage does not tolerate a metallic prosthesis well, and most patients who require femoral head replacement no longer have normal cartilage.

Total Hip Replacement

It is my general impression that even in these particularly high-risk patients, results with total hip replacement are better that those with femoral endoprostheses. In an attempt to evaluate this more objectively, my colleagues and I reviewed and combined the data from five recent studies of total hip replacement in younger adults.[35-39] The mean age and duration of follow-up in this group of patients were similar to those in the endoprosthesis study. At approximately five years, the revision rate for the total hip replace-

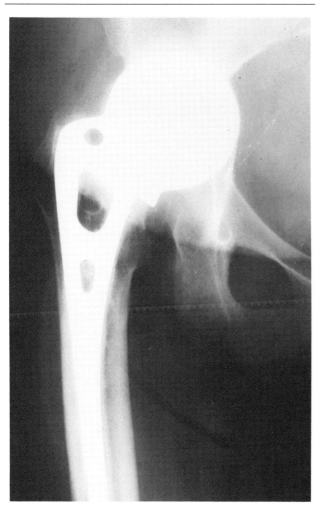

Fig. 5-6 Radiograph of failed Austin Moore prosthesis inserted for AVN. Note protrusio acetabuli and loosening of femoral component.

ments was 13% compared with 47% for the femoral endoprostheses. Results were rated good to excellent in 81% of the total hip replacements and in 58% of the femoral endoprostheses. Although it might be argued that with modern devices and technology, the results with femoral endoprostheses could be improved, the same argument applies to total hip replacements. Ac-

cordingly, it is our feeling that we should not be too hasty about substituting the femoral endoprosthesis for total hip replacement in this group of patients.

Miscellaneous Procedures

Two other procedures that might be considered under special circumstances are hip fusion and the Girdlestone pseudarthrosis.

Fusion

Hip fusion may be a reasonable option in a young, active, heavy man with unilateral disease. It is, of course, important to examine the patient carefully to be sure that the opposite hip is not involved at the time of the proposed surgery and that it is not likely to become involved in the future. Thus, the patient with posttraumatic AVN involving only one hip might be a suitable candidate. Although fusion of an avascular head is more difficult than fusion of a viable head, with modern techniques it should present no major difficulties. The advantages and disadvantages of this procedure should, of course, be explained to the patient before it is undertaken.

Girdlestone Pseudarthrosis

In a small number of patients in whom neither fusion nor replacement arthroplasty is indicated, the Girdlestone pseudarthrosis may be more suitable. This procedure might be considered, for example, in a patient with sepsis complicating AVN, or in a patient who requires pain relief but who is nonambulatory for other reasons and who cannot tolerate a hip fusion.

Determination of Procedure by Stage of Involvement

Which procedure to use depends largely on the stage of hip involvement. Of the various staging systems for AVN, I have found the one shown in Table 5–1 to be the most valuable.

Before the collapse of the femoral head (stages 0, I, and II, Table 5–3), treatment options include non-

Table 5-3
Treatment of AVN of the femoral head

Stage	Description	Treatment
0, I, and II	Prior to collapse	Nonsurgical; decompression; grafting; osteotomy; possibly electrical stimulation
III and IV-A	Early collapse	Same as for earlier stages, but results are less satisfactory
IV-B and IV-C	Later collapse without acetabular involvement	Nonsurgical; rotational osteotomy (Sugioka); femoral endoprosthesis; cup arthroplasty; total hip replacement
V and VI	Collapse with acetabular involvement	Nonsurgical; total hip replacement; fusion (in selected cases); Girdlestone pseudarthrosis (in selected cases)

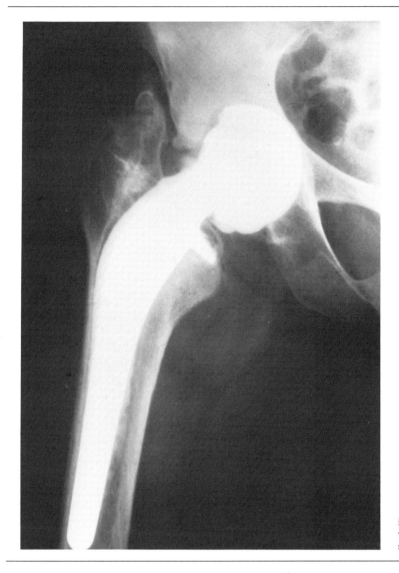

Fig. 5–7 Radiograph of painful bipolar prosthesis inserted approximately two years earlier in young woman with femoral collapse secondary to AVN. Note protrusio acetabuli as well as loosening of femoral component.

surgical management, decompression, bone grafting, osteotomy, and perhaps electrical stimulation. I favor decompression combined with bone grafting, using a loosely fitted cancellous graft.

For patients with early collapse of the femoral head (stages III and IV-A), the same procedures should be considered. The results, however, are likely to be less satisfactory and nonsurgical management is more common. There may also be a greater rationale for the use of the transtrochanteric rotational osteotomy at this stage.

When definite flattening of the femoral head is present, but before the appearance of acetabular involvement (stages IV-B and IV-C), most preventative measures are of little value. (One of the few surgical techniques that might be considered is rotational osteotomy, which has proven itself capable of femoral head preservation in many instances, even in cases of limited collapse.) If pain and disability are not too great,

most patients at this stage can be treated nonsurgically. Increasing pain and disability eventually make hip arthroplasty necessary. Although there are a few surgeons who advocate cup arthroplasty, femoral endoprosthetic replacement and total hip replacement are the treatments of choice.

Once definite involvement of the acetabulum has occurred (stages V and VI), supportive measures should be continued until such time as arthroplasty is required. I cannot advocate inserting a femoral prosthesis into an abnormal acetabulum, and total hip replacement is, therefore, the procedure of choice at this stage.

Summary

The most common cause of AVN of the femoral head is a displaced subcapital or transcervical fracture. Circumstances here differ significantly from those encountered in the patient with nontraumatic AVN, especially because the traumatic variety is seen most often in the elderly population. Attempts to preserve the femoral head are generally not indicated and the treatment of choice for the hip with sufficient pain and disability is either endoprosthetic replacement or total hip replacement.

In contradistinction, nontraumatic AVN occurs primarily in younger adults and is often bilateral. In these patients the goal is to preserve, not to replace, the femoral head. "Conservative" or nonsurgical management has generally been unsuccessful. Results with established surgical procedures have been inconsistent and frequently disappointing, often because they have been instituted too late. Although no approach is completely effective, in general the earlier treatment begins, the better the results will be. Early diagnosis, therefore, is essential. This depends on a heightened clinical awareness of this condition. The importance of various imaging techniques, including high-quality plain radiographs, technetium scans, and magnetic resonance imaging must be stressed. Newer procedures for the treatment of early AVN are being developed and evaluated. These currently include the use of vascularized grafts, osteochondral allografts, transtrochanteric rotational osteotomy, and electrical stimulation. I hope that one or more of these approaches will prove useful in preserving the femoral head. Until such time, I shall continue to use bone grafting with decompression to treat hips with limited involvement.

When definite collapse of the femoral head has occurred and when pain and disability are sufficient to require surgical intervention, the treatment of choice is arthroplasty. Although many still favor the use of a bipolar femoral endoprosthesis, I believe that total hip replacement provides more consistent, more durable, and better results.

Whichever arthroplasty is chosen, I anticipate continually improving results with advances in technique and component design.

References

1. Steinberg ME: Early diagnosis of avascular necrosis of the femoral head, in Bassett FH (ed): American Academy of Orthopaedic Surgeons *Instructional Course Lectures, XXXVII*. Park Ridge, IL, American Academy of Orthopaedic Surgeons, 1988, pp 51–57.

2. Steinberg ME, Hayken GD, Steinberg DR: A new method of evaluation and staging of avascular necrosis of the femoral head, in Arlet J, Ficat RP, Hungerford DS (eds): *Bone Circulation*. Baltimore, Williams & Wilkins, 1984, pp 398–403.

3. Steinberg ME, Hayken GD, Steinberg DR: The "conservative" management of avascular necrosis of the femoral head, in Arlet J, Ficat RP, Hungerford DS (eds): *Bone Circulation*. Baltimore, Williams & Wilkins, 1984, pp 334–337.

4. Hungerford DS (ed): *Ischemia and Necrosis of Bone*. Baltimore, Williams & Wilkins, 1980.

5. Hungerford DS: Bone marrow pressure, venography, and core decompression in ischemic necrosis of the femoral head, in *The Hip: Proceedings of the Seventh Open Scientific Meeting of the Hip Society*. St. Louis, CV Mosby Co, 1979, pp 218–237.

6. Camp JF, Colwell CW Jr: Core decompression of the femoral head for osteonecrosis. *J Bone Joint Surg* 1986;68A:1313–1319.

7. Phemister DB: Treatment of the necrotic head of the femur in adults. *J Bone Joint Surg* 1949;31A:55.

8. Bonfiglio M: Aseptic necrosis of the femoral head in dogs: Effect of drilling and bone grafting. *Surg Gynecol Obstet* 1954;98:591–599.

9. Boettcher WG, Bonfiglio M, Smith K: Non-traumatic necrosis of the femoral head: II. Experiences in treatment. *J Bone Joint Surg* 1970;52A:322.

10. Bonfiglio M, Voke EM: Aseptic necrosis of the femoral head and non-union of the femoral neck. *J Bone Joint Surg* 1968;50A:48.

11. Marcus ND, Enneking WF, Massam RA: The silent hip in idiopathic aseptic necrosis: Treatment by bone-grafting. *J Bone Joint Surg* 1973;55A:1351–1366.

12. Meyers MH, Harvey JP Jr, Moore TM: Treatment of displaced subcapital and transcervical fractures of the femoral neck by muscle-pedicle-bone graft and internal fixation: A preliminary report on one hundred and fifty cases *J Bone Joint Surg* 1973;55A:257–274.

13. Meyers MH: The treatment of osteonecrosis of the hip with fresh osteochondral allografts and with the muscle pedicle graft technique. *Clin Orthop* 1978;130:202–209.

14. Gilbert A, Judet H, Judet J, et al: Microvascular transfer of the fibula for necrosis of the femoral head. *Orthopedics* 1986;9:885.

15. Urbaniak J, Nunley JA, Goldner RD, et al: Treatment of aseptic necrosis of the femoral head by vascularized fibular graft. Presented at the Eighth Combined Meeting of the Orthopaedic Associations of the English-Speaking World, Washington, D.C., May 3–8, 1987.

16. Meyers MH, Jones RE, Bucholz RW, et al: Fresh autogenous grafts and osteochondral allografts for the treatment of segmental collapse in osteonecrosis of the hip. *Clin Orthop* 1983;174:107–112.

17. Meyers MH: Resurfacing of the femoral head with fresh osteochondral allografts: Long-term results. *Clin Orthop* 1985;197:111–114.

18. Merle d'Aubigné R, Postel M, Mazabraud A, et al: Idiopathic necrosis of the femoral head in adults. *J Bone Joint Surg* 1965;47B:612.

19. Kerboul M, Thomine J, Postel M, et al: The conservative surgical treatment of idiopathic aseptic necrosis of the femoral head. *J Bone Joint Surg* 1974;56B:291–296.

20. Wagner H, Bauer W: Five-year follow-up of intertrochanteric osteotomy for ischemic necrosis of the femoral head. Presented at the Symposium on Osteotomy of the Hip and Knee, Boston, Massachusetts, May 14–16, 1986.

21. Millis MM: Biplane intertrochanteric osteotomy for osteonecrosis. Presented at the Symposium on Osteotomy of the Hip and Knee, Boston, Massachusetts, May 14–16, 1986.

22. Maistrelli GL, Fusco U, Avai A, et al: Osteonecrosis of the hip treated by intertrochanteric osteotomy: A four- to 15-year follow-up. Presented at the 54th Annual Meeting of the American Academy of Orthopaedic Surgeons, San Francisco, California, Jan 26, 1987.

23. Jacobs MA, Hungerford DS, Krackow KA, et al: Results of intertrochanteric hip osteotomies for avascular necrosis. Presented at the 54th Annual Meeting of the American Academy of Orthopaedic Surgeons, San Francisco, California, Jan 26, 1987.

24. Sugioka Y: Transtrochanteric anterior rotational osteotomy of the femoral head in the treatment of osteonecrosis affecting the hip: A new osteotomy operation. *Clin Orthop* 1978;130:191–201.

25. Sugioka Y, Katsuki I, Hotokebuchi T: Transtrochanteric rotational osteotomy of the femoral head for the treatment of os-

teonecrosis: Follow-up statistics. *Clin Orthop* 1982;169:115–126.

26. Sugioka Y: Transtrochanteric rotational osteotomy in the treatment of idiopathic and steroid-induced femoral head necrosis, Perthes' disease, slipped capital femoral epiphysis, and osteoarthritis of the hip: Indications and results. *Clin Orthop* 1984;184:12–23.

27. Bassett CAL, Schink-Ascani NM, Lewes SN: Treatment of femoral head osteonecrosis with pulsed electromagnetic fields (PEMFS), in Arlet J, Ficat RP, Hungerford DS (eds): *Bone Circulation*. Baltimore, Williams & Wilkins, 1984, pp 343–354.

28. Eftekhar NS, Schink-Ascani MM, Mitchell SN, et al: Osteonecrosis of the femoral head treated by pulsed electromagnetic fields (PEMFs): A preliminary report, in Hungerford DS (ed): *The Hip: Proceedings of the Eleventh Open Scientific Meeting of the Hip Society*. St. Louis, CV Mosby Co, 1983, pp 306–330.

29. Steinberg ME, Brighton CT, Hayken GD, et al: Early results in the treatment of avascular necrosis of the femoral head with electrical stimulation. *Orthop Clin North Am* 1984;15:163–175.

30. Amstutz HC: The THARIES hip resurfacing technique. *Orthop Clin North Am* 1982;13:813–832.

31. Steinberg ME: Symposium on Surface Replacement Arthroplasty of the Hip: Summary and conclusions. *Orthop Clin North Am* 1982;13:895–902.

32. Amstutz HC, Kabo M, Hermans K, et al: Porous surface replacement of the hip with Chamfer cylinder design. *Orthop Trans* 1987;11:59.

33. Desman SM, Lachiewicz PF: Results of the bipolar endoprostheses in avascular necrosis of the femoral head. Presented at the 54th Annual Meeting of the American Academy of Orthopaedic Surgeons, San Francisco, California, Jan 26, 1987.

34. Heiner JP, Evarts CM: Total hip arthroplasty: Biological fixation: A preliminary report. Presented at the 54th Annual Meeting of the American Academy of Orthopaedic Surgeons, San Francisco, California, Jan 26, 1987.

35. Chandler HP, Reineck FT, Wixson RL, et al: Total hip replacement in patients younger than thirty years old: A five-year follow-up study. *J Bone Joint Surg* 1981;63A:1426–1434.

36. Collis DK: Cemented total hip replacement in patients who are less than fifty years old. *J Bone Joint Surg* 1984;66A:353–359.

37. Dorr LD, Takei GK, Conaty JP: Total hip arthroplasties in patients less than forty-five years old. *J Bone Joint Surg* 1983;65A:474–479.

38. Ranawat CS, Atkinson RE, Salvati EA, et al: Conventional total hip arthroplasty for degenerative joint disease in patients between the ages of forty and sixty years. *J Bone Joint Surg* 1984;66A:745–752.

39. Welch RB, Wynne G: Total hip replacement in the younger patient. *Orthop Trans* 1984;8:374.

Early Diagnosis of Avascular Necrosis of the Femoral Head

Marvin E. Steinberg, MD

There is no precise way to define an "early" diagnosis of avascular necrosis (AVN). From a radiologic standpoint, an early diagnosis must be made before flattening of the femoral head or subchondral collapse has occurred and, ideally, before any radiographic changes whatsoever are apparent. From a functional standpoint, early AVN should be considered that stage at which preservation of an intact femoral head is still possible.

The importance of early diagnosis must be stressed. Because AVN occurs primarily in younger adults and is frequently bilateral, the goal is to preserve rather than to replace the femoral head. Early diagnosis permits early treatment, which in turn should provide a better chance to save the femoral head. Although current treatment methods are not nearly as effective as we would like them to be, new and better methods will make earlier diagnosis increasingly important.

History

In assessing the patient with suspected AVN, the first step is taking a careful history. In general, symptoms are nonspecific and in many patients this condition is entirely asymptomatic in its earlier stages. When symptoms do develop, they usually consist of pain, a limp, and possibly a decrease in range of motion. Pain sometimes develops before there is radiographic evidence of collapse and occasionally before any radiographic abnormalities are apparent. This may result from increased intraosseous pressure or microfractures.[1,2] Often, however, symptoms first appear during the later stages of the disease. They may be associated with subchondral collapse or gross flattening of the articular surface.

In most instances, predisposing factors can be elicited during the course of history-taking. In some cases, a direct cause-and-effect relationship exists. In others, the causative factors are less clear-cut and it is perhaps best to think in terms of association rather than cause and effect.

The most common cause of AVN of the femoral head is trauma, especially when trauma results in a displaced high cervical fracture. A few cases are related to traumatic dislocation. Rarely, AVN follows hip trauma without fracture or dislocation. In these instances, the pathogenesis is unclear.

A second group of cases are those without any antecedent trauma. These occur less often than the traumatic variety, but have engendered considerably more interest because their pathogenesis is complicated and frequently uncertain, to make an early diagnosis is difficult, and their management is frustrating. Although a number of causative factors have been implicated, the most common are systemic corticosteroids, excessive use of alcohol, and sickle cell disease. In addition, it should be noted that in most series 20% to 25% of cases have no clearly defined causative factors and are considered to be idiopathic.[3-5]

During history-taking the physician must inquire about other areas of bony involvement and must bear in mind that if this disorder has been diagnosed in one femoral head, the chance of the other being involved is more than 50%. Less commonly, shoulder, knee, and tarsal or carpal involvement occurs. It is also essential that the history rule out other possible causes of hip symptoms or abnormalities that might be confused with AVN.

Physical Examination

Findings on physical examination are nonspecific. During the early stages, examination of the hip is entirely within normal limits. As the condition progresses, some pain on motion may be present. Later, the range of motion may decrease and the patient may demonstrate a limp. Shortening of the limb occurs after gross collapse of the femoral head. During the physical examination, other possible causes of hip abnormalities or symptoms (for example, radiation of pain to the hip and thigh originating in the lumbosacral region) must be ruled out. Signs of a generalized arthritic phenomenon or other systemic disorder must also be sought.

Laboratory Tests

In most cases laboratory findings are within normal limits. Although one common theory of the pathogenesis of AVN involves an alteration in circulating lipids, this is rarely detected by serologic testing. In some instances, however, other associated or predisposing conditions, such as sickle cell disease, may be diagnosed. Laboratory tests play a major role, which must not be overlooked, in ruling out other causes of hip abnormality.

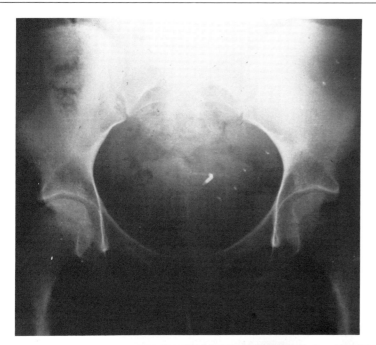

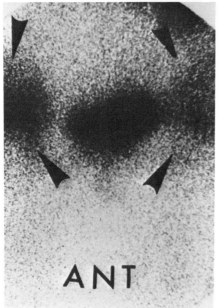

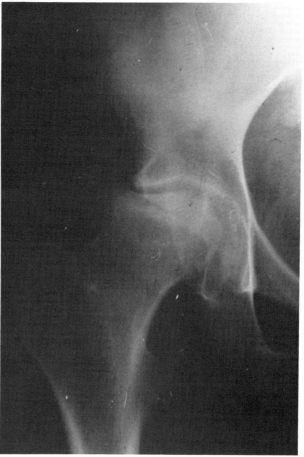

Fig. 6–1 A young renal transplant patient with minimal pain in the right hip. **Top left:** Anteroposterior radiograph appears normal. **Bottom left:** Technetium bone scan done at this time shows increased isotope uptake about the right hip. **Bottom right:** Three months later, a routine radiograph shows gross collapse of the femoral head.

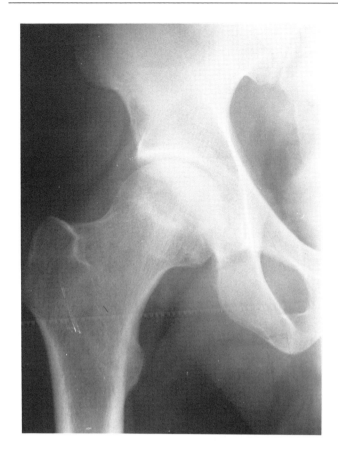

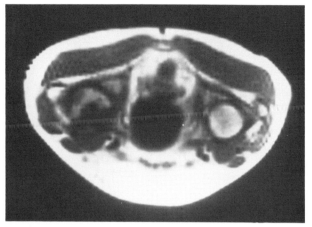

Fig. 6–2 In a case of typical AVN, a radiograph (**left**) shows stage II involvement of the femoral head with areas of radiolucency and sclerosis and MRI (**right**) shows decreased signal intensity in involved areas.

Imaging

Perhaps the most interesting and most useful among the methods of diagnosing early AVN are the various imaging techniques currently available. These include routine radiographs, tomograms or laminograms, computed tomographic (CT) scans, technetium bone scans, single-photon emission computed tomography (SPECT), and magnetic resonance imaging (MRI).

Radiographs

Routine radiographs are, of course, the first line of diagnosis. These must be of extremely high quality and must be taken in both the anteroposterior and lateral projections. Early in the course of the disease, these are within normal limits. Later they may show some osteopenia or possibly mottling, which is also referred to as the appearance of "cysts and sclerosis." Later, when subchondral collapse occurs, a radiolucent crescent may be seen just beneath the subchondral bone and parallel to the articular surface. Some of these changes are essentially pathognomonic of AVN if other conditions have been ruled out clinically. Later still, there is flattening of the femoral head. In the final stages, degenerative changes of the articular cartilage lead to joint narrowing and involvement of the acetab-

ulum. It must be remembered that the early changes are within the bone of the femoral head. This enables one to distinguish AVN from the various forms of arthritis that affect the femoral head and acetabulum simultaneously and with which AVN is sometimes confused.

Technetium Bone Scans

Technetium bone scans have been used for several years and are quite helpful. These may be within normal limits, especially during the early phases of the disease. When abnormal, the picture usually shows increased uptake of isotope, that is, a "hot" scan. Occasionally there is an area of decreased uptake or a "cold" region over the center of the femoral head. Sometimes both of these findings appear in the same hip with decreased uptake over the center of the lesion and increased uptake surrounding it. Decreased uptake of isotope is caused by diminished circulation or decreased metabolic activity of bone. Increased uptake is caused by increased bone formation or circulation, usually in association with a reparative process at the margin of the lesion. There are, of course, many conditions that produce increased uptake of isotope and this is a nonspecific finding. If the plain radiograph is normal, however, there are few conditions that produce a "cold"

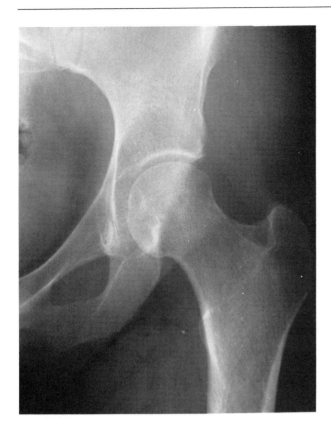

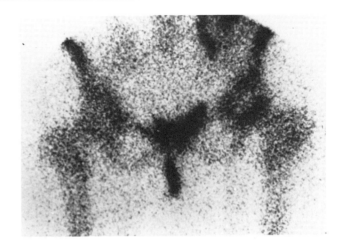

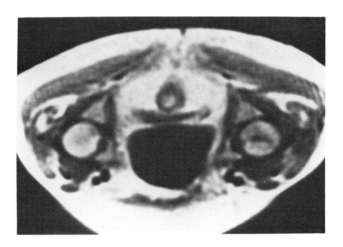

Fig. 6–3 A young women with end-stage renal disease who had multiple arthralgias. **Top left:** Radiograph of the right hip shows only osteoporosis. **Top right:** Bone scan is consistent with AVN and shows decreased uptake over the femoral head and increased uptake in surrounding areas. **Bottom right:** Results of MRI are typical of AVN although the changes are more subtle than those shown in Figure 6–2, *right.*

femoral head, and AVN is much more likely. As with any other test, both false-negatives and false-positives occur.[6,7]

MRI

MRI is being used with increasing frequency in the diagnosis of AVN. It is sensitive to the very earliest changes in this condition and can detect abnormalities in fat and bone marrow that occur before changes in bone. MRI abnormalities are not entirely specific and a number of other conditions may give a similar picture. The specificity of this test is currently being evaluated. At the present time, however, it is perhaps the best single means for the early diagnosis of AVN of the femoral head.[8-11]

Other Imaging Techniques

Tomograms or laminograms have been used for some time to supplement plain radiographs. They occasionally show early changes in the femoral head more clearly. Although they may still be of some value when CT scans and MRI are not readily available, we rarely use tomograms at this time. CT scanning allows AVN to be diagnosed before routine radiographs or laminograms in certain cases. Because CT abnormalities depend on changes in bone density, they cannot be relied on in the very earliest stages of AVN. Like laminograms, we now use them infrequently. If the diagnosis cannot be made on the basis of high-quality anteroposterior and lateral plain radiographs of the hip, a technetium bone scan and MRI should be done. In almost all cases in

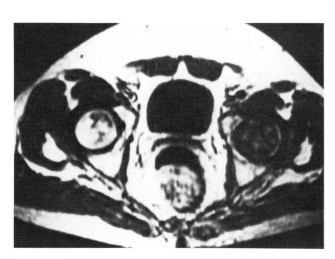

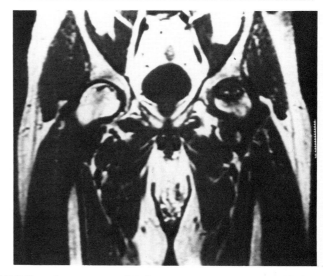

Fig. 6–4   MRI in a patient with bilateral AVN. Newer, more powerful (1.5 T) equipment was used. **Left:** Transverse or axial section. **Right:** Coronal section.

which the disease is indeed present, one or both of these studies will be abnormal.[10,11]

Recently, there has been some interest in the role of SPECT in the early diagnosis of AVN. This technique combines some of the better features of the CT scan and the technetium bone scan. Theoretically, it should prove valuable. At the present time, experience with this technique is quite limited and we are uncertain as to what its role will be.

Examples and Comparison of Imaging Techniques

The first case demonstrates the usefulness of the technetium bone scan in establishing an early diagnosis before the appearance of radiographic abnormalities. Patient 1 was a young woman who had undergone a renal transplantation and was being treated with corticosteroids and azathioprine. At the time of the initial studies, her right hip was minimally symptomatic and the physical findings were normal. The plain radiographs (Fig. 6–1, *top left*) were interpreted as being within normal limits. The technetium bone scan performed at the same time (Fig. 6–1, *bottom left*) showed a markedly increased uptake of isotope about the right hip. On this basis, a tentative diagnosis of AVN was made. MRI was not available at this time. Three months later, gross collapse of the hip was apparent on routine films (Fig. 6–1, *bottom right*), confirming the diagnosis.

The second case shows the typical MRI picture of AVN of the femoral head. Patient 2 was a previously healthy young man who developed AVN of the right hip associated with excessive alcohol intake. Plain radiographs showed stage II involvement with areas of radiolucency and increased density (Fig. 6–2, *left*). The MRI pattern was clearly abnormal and showed the de-

crease in signal intensity (dark areas) typical of this condition (Fig. 6–2, *right*).

The third case illustrates the role of MRI in confirming the diagnosis of AVN early in the course of the disease. Patient 3 was a young woman with end-stage renal disease who developed multiple transitory arthralgias. The pain eventually settled in her right hip. Plain radiographs of this hip showed only osteoporosis (Fig. 6–3, *top left*), similar to that seen in other joints. A bone scan (Fig. 6–3, *top right*) was interpreted as consistent with AVN as it showed decreased uptake over the femoral head and increased uptake in adjacent areas. The MRI pattern (Fig. 6–3, *bottom right*) was typical of AVN, although changes were more subtle than those seen in Figure 6–2, *right*. Tissue obtained at the time of decompression and bone grafting confirmed the diagnosis.

MRI is a relatively new and expensive technique. These studies are not yet routinely available in all areas. It is also a rapidly changing field, and within the last few years "new generations" of equipment have replaced older ones. These have tremendously improved the detail, resolution, and capabilities of this technique, enabling us to detect even more subtle changes in bone and soft tissue. The fourth case demonstrates the quality of images made with the latest generation of MRI equipment in a patient with bilateral AVN (the left hip was more involved than the right hip). Figure 6–4, *left*, shows a transverse section through both femoral heads. This is the same plane routinely examined by earlier, less powerful units, as shown in the previous illustrations. Note, however, the increased detail. Figure 6–4, *right*, shows a coronal section that demonstrates with even greater clarity the changes in the femoral heads.

These coronal sections could not be easily obtained with earlier equipment. At the present time, they are proving so useful that they have virtually eliminated the need for transverse or axial sections in diagnosing AVN of the femoral head.

Table 6–1 compares the sensitivity, specificity, and accuracy of MRI and technetium scans in 66 hips of patients with AVN. The percentages of true results and false-positive and false-negative results with each technique are shown. This study indicates that MRI in this group of patients was both more sensitive and more accurate than the technetium scan, although somewhat less specific.

Figure 6–5, *left*, shows the accuracy of each of the various imaging techniques used to evaluate patients with AVN. These data are based on the interpretations of MRI, technetium scans, CT scans, tomography, and plain films of 55 hips with biopsy-proven AVN. Although MRI appeared to be the most accurate (96%), other techniques also gave a high percentage of accurate diagnoses. It should be noted, however, that many of these hips had well-established disease and that

the physician interpreting the studies knew that AVN was suspected or had been diagnosed.

Figure 6–5, *right*, compares the accuracy of MRI, CT, and bone scans in 14 hips with early AVN, evaluated before any abnormalities were noted on plain radiographs. In these cases MRI appeared to be significantly more accurate than either bone scans or CT. This is an important observation as these patients with normal radiographic findings are those for whom it is most difficult and yet most important to develop methods of early diagnosis. Note that two percentages, 86% and 100%, are listed for MRI. In one patient, whose technetium scan was abnormal bilaterally, the first MRI study was interpreted as being within normal limits, whereas the second study, performed two months later, was consistent with bilateral AVN. Plain radiographs at both times were normal. This indicates that, although MRI would appear to be the single best technique for the early diagnosis of AVN, false-negatives occasionally occur and that in some instances a technetium scan may detect abnormalities before MRI.

Other Diagnostic Techniques

Ficat and Arlet[1] and Hungerford[2] have written extensively on the use of intraosseous pressure measurements and intraosseous venography. I have not relied on these techniques and cannot cite personal experience. They are invasive or semi-invasive and often require a general or spinal anesthetic. In view of the excellent results being obtained with modern imaging techniques, their value is questionable at this time.

Another technique described by a small number of investigators is selective or "superselective" angiography of the femoral head. Experience with this tech-

Table 6-1
Sensitivity, specificity, and accuracy of MRI and technetium bone scans in 66 hips with AVN

Results	MRI	Technetium Scan
Findings (%)		
True-positive	76	68
True-negative	15	17
False-positive	6	4
False-negative	3	11
Sensitivity	96	86
Specificity	71	79
Accuracy	91	85

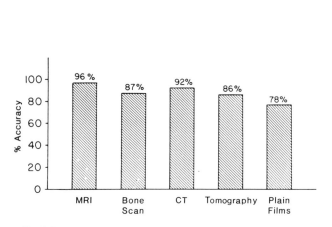

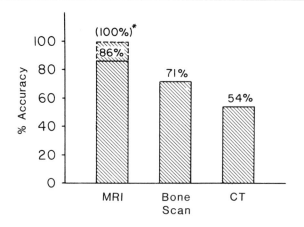

*(Repeated MRI read as positive in 2 cases, 2 months after initial negative reading)

Fig. 6-5 Diagnostic accuracy of various imaging techniques in 55 hips with biopsy-proven AVN (**left**) and in 14 hips with early AVN (**right**).

nique is limited, but the few who have mastered it believe that it may indeed assist in making an early diagnosis.[12] Although I have no experience with this technique, I believe that it, too, is a semi-invasive study with, at best, a limited application in unusual cases.

The ultimate diagnostic test, of course, is a careful histologic examination of tissue removed from the femoral head. On occasion, when the diagnosis is in doubt, an isolated biopsy might be considered. If this is done with a small-bore instrument, only a limited sample of tissue will be available for evaluation and it may not be possible to make the diagnosis. In most instances, a diagnosis can be made with a high degree of accuracy, using the non-invasive methods described earlier. If one then elects to treat the patient with a surgical approach that involves removal of tissue from the femoral head, histologic examination will serve to confirm (or dispute) a diagnosis already made and acted on clinically.

Summary and Conclusions

Early diagnosis is important because it leads to early treatment and a better chance of saving the femoral head. The first, and perhaps the most important step, in making an early diagnosis is a heightened clinical awareness of this condition. The physician must be familiar with the nonspecific symptoms, physical findings, and laboratory tests, as well as with the various predisposing factors associated with avascular necrosis. Other causes of hip abnormality or symptoms must be ruled out, as AVN is in part a diagnosis of exclusion. Imaging techniques, which are extremely useful in the early diagnosis of this condition, include good-quality plain radiographs, technetium bone scans, and especially MRI. Technetium bone scans and MRI are quite sensitive, although not entirely specific, and must be used in conjunction with a comprehensive clinical evaluation of the patient.

References

1. Hungerford DS (ed): *Ischemia and Necrosis of Bone*. Baltimore, Williams and Wilkins, 1980.
2. Hungerford DS: Bone marrow pressure, venography, and core decompression in ischemic necrosis of the femoral head, in *The Hip: Proceedings of the Seventh Open Scientific Meeting of the Hip Society*. St. Louis, CV Mosby Co, 1979, pp 218–237.
3. Steinberg ME: Avascular necrosis of the femoral head, in Tronzo RG (ed): *Surgery of the Hip Joint*. New York, Springer-Verlag, 1987, vol 2, pp 1–29.
4. Jacobs B: Epidemiology of traumatic and nontraumatic osteonecrosis. *Clin Orthop* 1978;130:51–67.
5. Cruess RL: Osteonecrosis of bone: Current concepts as to etiology and pathogenesis, *Clin Orthop* 1986,208.30–39.
6. Alavi A, McCloskey JR, Steinberg ME: Early detection of avascular necrosis of the femoral head by 99m technetium diphosphonate bone scan: A preliminary report. *Clin Orthop* 1977;127:137–141.
7. D'Ambrosia RD, Shoji H, Riggins RS, et al: Scintigraphy in the diagnosis of osteonecrosis. *Clin Orthop* 1978;130:139–143.
8. Thickman D, Axel L, Kressel HY, et al: Magnetic resonance imaging of avascular necrosis of the femoral head. *Skeletal Radiol* 1986;15:133–140.
9. Bassett LW, Gold RH, Reicher M, et al: Magnetic resonance imaging in the early diagnosis of ischemic necrosis of the femoral head: Preliminary results. *Clin Orthop* 1987;214:237–248.
10. Mitchell DG, Rao VM, Dalinka MK, et al: Avascular necrosis of the femoral head: Correlation of MR imaging, radiographic staging, radionuclide imaging, and clinical findings. *Radiology* 1987;162:709–715.
11. Mitchell MD, Kundel JL, Steinberg ME, et al: Avascular necrosis of the hip: Comparison of MR, CT, and scintigraphy. *Am J Radiogr* 1986;147:67–71.
12. Théron J: Superselective angiography of the hip: Technique, normal features, and early results in idiopathic necrosis of the femoral head. *Radiology* 1977;124:649–657.

Avascular Necrosis of the Femoral Head in Children

Richard E. McCarthy, MD

Avascular necrosis (AVN) in children is similar in many ways to that seen in adults. The most common disease associated with the avascular appearance is Legg-Calvé-Perthes' disease. AVN can be regarded as a common denominator with many causes and Legg-Calvé-Perthes' disease as the most common idiopathic form. Its prolonged course with intermittent, repeated vascular insults is analogous to the AVN found in alcohol- or steroid-ingesting adults. In both adults and children, isolated vascular insults are the common feature in AVN caused by trauma such as fractures or dislocations, but certain anatomic features make the pediatric hip more susceptible to the development of AVN of either type.

Blood Supply

The posterolateral portion of the femoral head is supplied by the intertrochanteric vessels and the inferomedial portion through the artery of the ligamentum teres. The superomedial portion has the worst supply and is the most susceptible to avascular states. At birth, the cartilaginous proximal femur is supplied by both medial and lateral circumflex arteries with a small contribution from the ligamentum teres.[1] A few small vessels cross the physis from the metaphysis to the epiphysis peripherally, but these tend to close down by 18 months of age, leaving two separate zones. The developing ossification center receives its blood supply from the posterosuperior branches of the medial circumflex artery.

Before the age of 3 years, both the medial and lateral circumflex vessels contribute blood supply to the epiphysis. After this age the lateral circumflex artery supplies only the metaphysis and the trochanteric apophysis. The artery of the ligamentum teres has not reached the depth of the epiphysis and will not until 9 to 10 years of age.[2] Trueta[2] felt that the artery of the ligamentum teres makes a greater contribution to the cartilaginous epiphysis between the ages of 3 to 8 in blacks than it does in whites, possibly helping to explain the lower incidence of Legg-Calvé-Perthes' disease among blacks. The primary and almost the only supply to the growing epiphysis comes through the posterosuperior and posteroinferior arterial branches of the solitary medial circumflex artery. Because of this limited supply, the proximal femur from 3 to 8 years of age is susceptible to vascular injury or insult.[3,4]

Types of Avascular Necrosis

The femoral head can appear to be avascular in a number of pediatric conditions. Legg-Calvé-Perthes' disease is the most common form of idiopathic AVN in children. Systemic illnesses such as hypothyroidism, sickle cell disease, and Gaucher's disease frequently have a similar avascular radiologic appearance. Deformities of the epiphysis associated with multiple epiphyseal dysplasia or Morquio's syndrome may also appear to be avascular and, along with the previously named illnesses, can develop bilaterally. Bilateral Legg-Calvé-Perthes' disease is rare (10% to 12% of cases[5]) and, unlike bilateral AVN from other causes, the hips are in different stages of healing.

Direct insults to the blood supply, such as occur with fractures through the proximal femur,[6–9] prolonged traumatic dislocations,[10,11] bone cysts of the femoral neck,[12] abnormal casting positions of the femur,[13] or intracapsular tamponade (from infection or hematoma),[14,15] may produce avascular changes. This category of AVN may be considered "traumatic" to differentiate it from the more common "idiopathic" type. The avascular-appearing changes in the femoral head associated with the treatment of congenital hip dislocation also fall into this category because of the direct insult to vascular flow.

Recently, AVN has been noted in a few pediatric patients undergoing chemotherapy for neuroblastoma[16] and also in a small number of children receiving steroids for systemic illnesses.[17,18] The relationship between these illnesses and AVN is unknown.

Etiology

The exact etiology of AVN in most cases remains unclear; however, the pathomechanics leading to osseous collapse must be preceded by loss of structural integrity in the area of maximum stress concentration.[18] Usually this is brought about by loss of vascular supply (through laceration, occlusion, embolus, or compartment syndrome), followed by osteoblast cell death and subsequent osteoid resorption through osteoclastic activity. In Legg-Calvé-Perthes' disease, this mechanism repeats itself many times. Dead woven bone can be observed on dead lamellar bone. The woven bone, in turn, is resorbed by a new influx of osteoclasts with osteogenic cells following (Fig. 7–1). This pattern sup-

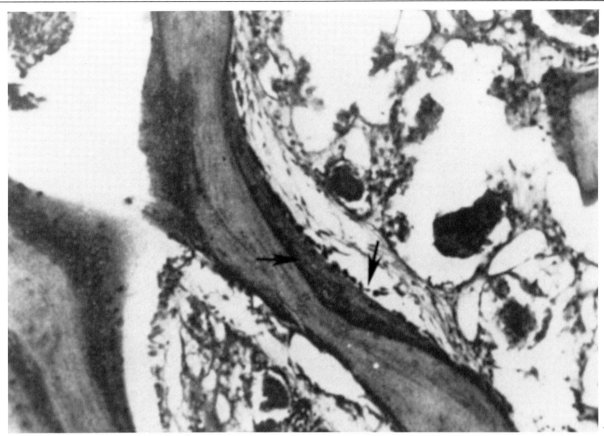

Fig. 7–1 Dead lamellar bone has been partially resorbed and added to by woven bone that has lost its blood supply and died (arrow at left). The osteogenic cells along the edge (arrow at right) are beginning another phase of addition to the trabecula. This picture supports the theory of multiple infarctions as the cause of idiopathic avascular necrosis. (Reproduced with permission from Jensen OM, Lauritzen J: Legg-Calvé-Perthes' disease: Morphological studies in two cases examined at necropsy. *J Bone Joint Surg* 1976;58B:332–338.)

ports the theory of multiple vascular insults as the cause of Legg-Calvé-Perthes' disease. The postulated contributory factors leading to Legg-Calvé-Perthes' disease are beyond the scope of this discussion,[19-22] but a systemic disease, possibly hormonal in nature, seems to predispose to vascular compromise of the femoral head.

Since the vascular anatomy leaves the developing femoral head precariously supplied during most of youth and since a variety of factors can bring about an insult to the blood supply, it is easy to understand how a traumatic event, even one as slight as normal weight-bearing, can collapse the weakened osteoid and produce AVN (precarious blood supply + vascular insult ± predisposing factors + trauma = AVN).

Pathologic Stages and Classification

The pathologic stages of AVN in children vary according to the etiology of the vascular insult. The stages of disease progression in Legg-Calvé-Perthes' disease have been well studied.[5,22-24] Avascular necrosis from other, nontraumatic causes progresses similarly. Such

AVN characteristically progresses slowly from the early radiologic signs of joint widening to the end stages of regeneration. Enchondral ossification ceases with the initial disruption of blood supply, regarded by some as an infarction.[5,22,25] Woven bone is then laid down on the dead trabeculae by the repair cells (osteoblasts). These, in turn, are robbed of their blood supply through a subsequent infarction, producing the characteristic pattern of dead woven bone on dead trabeculae with copious amorphous necrotic granulation tissue between the trabeculae. The next ingrowth of repair tissue is slowed by this debris, prolonging the healing process. Resorption of dead bone through osteoclastic action is part of the repair process and causes the subchondral bone to weaken. This leads to a crescent-sign fracture when the trabeculae collapse on one another with weightbearing forces. The resorption process (osteolysis) continues through the fragmentation phase and radiologically appears as lytic areas in the epiphysis. Metaphyseal lytic areas (cysts) may also develop beneath the area of the devascularized epiphysis.

Regeneration begins with a remodeling of the epiphysis into a shape determined by pressure influences from the acetabulum. In younger children (less than 8 years old), the acetabulum itself has the capability of remodeling and enlarging over the deformed head. The femoral neck also remodels by broadening to support the enlarged head.

In the final phases of healing, there may be further changes in the head and acetabulum from mutual malpositioned pressure influences. These, coupled with physeal growth arrest, can produce a flattened head, short neck, and relative trochanteric overgrowth (Fig. 7–2).

"Traumatic" vascular insults causing AVN do not usually progress through these pathologic stages. The end result after regeneration may appear to be the same (Fig. 7–2), but the stages are much more like those seen in the adult with an initial increased radiologic density progressing to regeneration without a fragmentation phase. In most children with femoral neck fractures who develop AVN, radiologic evidence of AVN appears within one year of the fracture.[8,14] It is heralded by loss of definition in the epiphyseal plate, indicating premature closure, and progresses in a pattern similar to that in the adult. Ratliff[26] identified three radiologic patterns of necrosis for traumatic AVN in femoral neck fractures (Fig. 7–3). Type I involvement has diffuse AVN of the proximal fragment (epiphysis and metaphysis). Diffuse, segmental, or no collapse occurred as a result of revascularization. Type II AVN involves only the epiphysis, either partially or completely; the metaphysis was spared. Type III has the appearance of AVN involving only the femoral neck without avascular changes in the epiphysis. Patients with type I AVN have the worst prognosis and those with type III the best.

Both Catterall[27] and Salter[28] classified Legg-Calvé-Perthes' disease on the basis of radiologic criteria. Both systems depend on the degree to which the femoral head is involved in the avascularity. Catterall types I and II (Salter type A) involve less than 50% of the epiphysis with retention of the medial and lateral columns that support the femoral head through the reparative process. In Catterall types III and IV (Salter type B) the avascularity extends to include a larger portion of the head; metaphyseal reaction and the loss of the lateral support lead to early collapse. At-risk signs, which can help but not absolutely predict the outcome of the disease, include lateral subluxation, or extrusion of the epiphysis, along with Gage's sign, a horizontal physis, or loss of motion. These are important indications of a bad prognosis.

Diagnostic Methods

Newer techniques such as bone scanning and magnetic resonance imaging offer certain advantages in establishing the diagnosis and may some day help to predict outcome. Nuclear counters can produce an image profile that allows a more accurate comparison of the

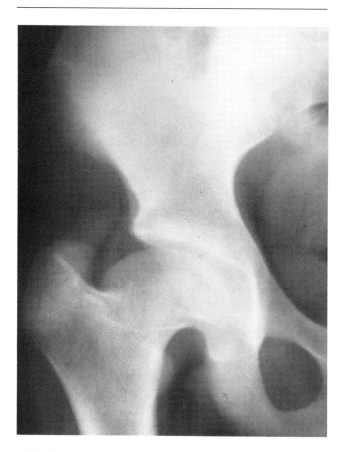

Fig. 7-2 The regenerative phase may result in the appearance of a short femoral neck, flattened head, and trochanteric overgrowth whether the AVN was of idiopathic or traumatic origin.

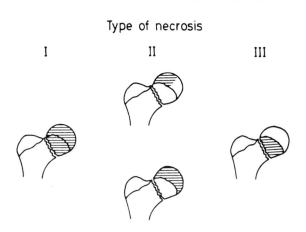

Fig. 7-3 The three types of avascular necrosis associated with femoral neck fractures in children. Type I is diffuse through the metaphysis and epiphysis and has the worst prognosis. Type II involves only the epiphysis, partially or completely. Type III AVN involves only the femoral neck. (Reproduced with permission from Lloyd-Roberts GC, Ratliff AHC: *Hip Disorders in Children*. London, Butterworths, 1978, p 174.

blood flow to the femoral head in the early phases of the scan (Fig. 7–4). An avascular pattern on the scan may permit an earlier diagnosis than is possible with plain films. Some feel that nuclear scanning makes possible the staging of disease and the determination of prognosis.[29,30]

Magnetic resonance imaging produces coronal and axial views (Fig. 7–4) so that the positive image of the lipid content in the normal epiphysis can be compared with the darker, negative image seen in the avascular epiphysis[31-33] (and P. Scoles, personal communication, January 1987). This is a sensitive early indicator of avascularity but does not help in determining the extent of involvement or the rate of revascularization. Some of the advantages of magnetic resonance imaging in children are the lack of ionizing radiation to the growing skeleton, the elimination of contrast injections, two-plane imaging, and the early diagnosis obtained. The disadvantages include problems related to malpositioning that can lead to misinterpretation. For instance, with slight pelvic obliquity the normal dark growth plate may appear on the same axial cut as the opposite light epiphysis and be interpreted as abnormal.[34] Sedation is necessary because of the long period required for image acquisition and, at present, the expense is exorbitant compared to other methods.

Magnetic resonance imaging can help to determine congruency and containment of the femoral head but, at present, no new accepted classification system has been developed.

Treatment

The goal of any treatment should be the prevention of deformity that might lead to degenerative hip disease.[35] What prognosticators can we use to predict hip deformity in youngsters? When the avascular process is caused by Legg-Calvé-Perthes' disease, we know there is a poor prognosis for older patients with the onset of symptoms after 9 years of age, especially those with the Salter B (Catterall types III or IV) classification.[27,36,37] The at-risk signs are helpful early indicators of a poor result, that is, a loss of sphericity or congruency by the completion of healing. When the avascularity has a traumatic cause, the prognosis depends on the degree of head involvement and the age of the child at the time of the incident. In younger children there will be more deformity should the avascularity arrest growth. We know that patients with femoral neck fractures and total collapse of the femoral head (resulting in a Ratliff type I involvement) have a poor prognosis; other types fare better.

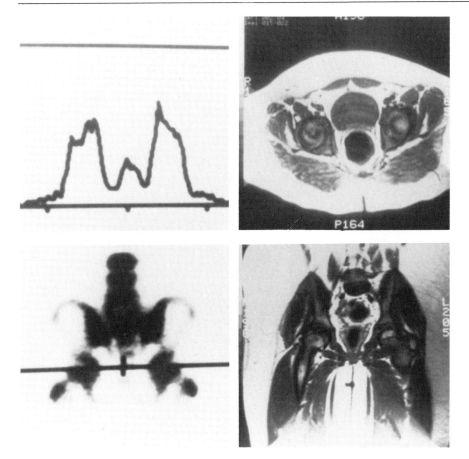

Fig. 7–4 Computer-enhanced nuclear counters can provide an image profile that gives a more accurate count and picks up subtle decreases in the activity of the femoral head such as occur in AVN (**left**). Magnetic resonance imaging produces a darker image in the avascular hip that can be visualized coronally (**top right**) and axially (**bottom right**). The patient's right hip has an avascular appearance in this example.

Treatment must be individualized to each patient on the basis of the etiology of the AVN, the patient's age, the prognosis, and other associated problems such as nonunion of a femoral neck fracture. The younger patient, with total femoral head involvement from Legg-Calvé-Perthes' disease at age 4, has a better prognosis than the 12-year-old child with segmental collapse but less deformity from AVN caused by a slipped capital femoral epiphysis. The ability to remodel a cartilaginous head and acetabulum makes all the difference.

Certain factors must be considered in designing an individual treatment plan. First, the damage to the growing epiphysis and the epiphyseal growth plate cannot be prevented by present means. Second, the femoral head will shape to the pressures exerted on it through the molding of the acetabulum. Third, the superficial articular cartilage will proliferate and thicken relative to the deeper layers deprived of nutrition by the avascularity. Lastly, the blood supply will return peripherally first and then centrally, producing a widened neck and coxa magna.

Attempts at biologic treatment of AVN have been reported. Nondisplaced proximal femoral osteotomies to enhance venous drainage have been reported in separate studies by Kendig and Evans[38] and Clancy and Steel.[39] No difference in the rate of epiphyseal reconstitution was shown in their studies. There has been one report of an improved rate of healing after extensive synovectomy and drilling of the femoral head.[40]

Containment of the femoral head in the acetabulum remains the cornerstone of treatment for AVN, whether it be accomplished surgically or nonsurgically.[41] The principle behind containment is the equalization of pressures on the diseased epiphysis through acetabular molding to prevent deformity.

Nonsurgical treatment initially includes complete bed rest, traction (usually split Russell's traction), and aspirin. Later, bracing, casting, or crutches may be utilized. When determining whether nonsurgical treatment is best for a particular patient, assessment should include the degree of severity of the AVN, the child's ability to cooperate, the parent's reliability in carrying out the treatment recommendations, and the age of the child.

When Petrie casts are used,[42] the child is generally placed in the cast for six to eight weeks, assuring maintenance of the containment achieved in the operating room, such as after an adductor release. It permits a protected range of motion while the child is less mobile. The cast is not removable.

Crutches may relieve symptoms in some patients.[43] They provide protected weightbearing and the maintenance of range of motion. Frequently, however, patients put more pressure on the femoral head by a nonweightbearing gait pattern.

Abduction bracing, such as the Scottish Rite brace, has become popular and is usually used for a six- to 18-month period.[41,44,45] It allows containment within a protected range of motion. A surprising amount of mobility is possible during most activities, and the brace can be removed at night for non-weightbearing exercises and sleep. It is important to document containment by a standing anteroposterior radiograph. An arthrogram or magnetic resonance imaging should be used to prove containment in questionable cases.

When surgical management is indicated, as in the older patient or the noncompliant brace-wearer, it offers distinct advantages. It provides a limited period of immobilization and produces a lasting effect with the head contained within the acetabulum. It does, however, have the possible side effects of a shortened limb (as from a varus femoral osteotomy), an elevated trochanteric height, or a second procedure for hardware removal. The theoretical advantage of improved femoral venous drainage has not been borne out.[38,39] In those patients with nonunion caused by fractures of the femoral neck, surgery may be indicated to align the fracture site better and to improve healing. Late reconstructive procedures may be necessary in some cases to improve the biomechanics by advancing the trochanter or better aligning the joint surfaces through a valgus osteotomy.

The types of surgery include those on the femoral side with varus, varus with derotation, derotation alone, valgus in the late phases, or reconstructive surgeries such as chilectomy or trochanteric transfers.[41,46–49]

Those who prefer to approach this disease from the pelvic side have used the innominate osteotomy described by Salter or one of its variants. After triradiate cartilage closure, the dial osteotomy has also been used to improve coverage.[28,50] Some surgeons combine these two approaches, doing both femoral and pelvic osteotomies.

Coring methods found to be useful in treating adults with AVN[51,52] have not been used to treat growing children because of the risk of damage to the growth plate. However, in older adolescents with closed physes, early drilling may offer some theoretical advantage by promoting vascular ingrowth into small areas of avascularity.

Arthrodesis remains a good salvage procedure for the young patient with unrelieved pain and a stiff hip from deformity. Fusion in such cases can relieve pain and position the hip more functionally. The method described by Mowery and associates[53] is preferred.

Summary

Two types of AVN occur in childhood. The first is the idiopathic type best characterized by Legg-Calvé-Perthes' disease associated with repeated infarctions that slow the healing process. The second is the traumatic type caused by a direct insult to the blood supply of the developing femoral head. Both can result in profound growth disturbances of the proximal femur and early degenerative changes. They may have little effect on hip function or appearance. The variables affecting these outcomes are the age of the child, the degree of femoral head involvement, the presence of at-risk signs, the ability of the acetabulum to contain the healing head, and whether or not the growth plate closes as a result of the AVN. Bone scans and magnetic resonance imaging offer some potential for improved accuracy in diagnosis and prediction.

The recommended treatment for AVN in children is to treat the synovitis whenever it occurs or recurs. Abduction bracing should be used for the first six months in most young children with idiopathic AVN of the Legg-Calvé-Perthes' type. Protected weightbearing with crutches should suffice for the early phases of traumatic AVN. Within six months, one should be able to determine the classification and whether to continue the treatment being used or to change to another form of treatment. Petrie casts are used rarely but can be very useful in certain patients. Prolonged crutch use may help to prevent collapse while relieving symptoms in the older child. Surgery remains the mainstay of treatment for older children, those with at-risk signs unimproved by bracing or casting, and those requiring improved coverage or reconstructive procedures.

The ultimate goal is the achievement of an almost spherical femoral head that will be congruent to the acetabulum at the completion of growth.

References

1. Ogden JA: Development of hip vascularity, in Katz JF, Siffert RS (eds): *Management of Hip Disorders in Children.* Philadelphia, JB Lippincott, 1983, pp 33–50.
2. Trueta J: The normal vascular anatomy of the human femoral head during growth. *J Bone Joint Surg* 1957;39B:358–394.
3. Ogden JA: Changing patterns of proximal femoral vascularity. *J Bone Joint Surg* 1974;56A:941–950.
4. Chung SMK: The arterial supply of the developing proximal end of the human femur. *J Bone Joint Surg* 1976;58A:961–970.
5. Weinstein SL: Legg-Calvé-Perthes disease, in American Academy of Orthopaedic Surgeons *Instructional Course Lectures, XXXII.* St. Louis, CV Mosby Co, 1983, pp 272–291.
6. Nielsen PT, Thaarup P: An unusual course of femoral head necrosis complicating an intertrochanteric fracture in a child. *Clin Orthop* 1984;183:79–81.
7. Stougård J: Post-traumatic avascular necrosis of the femoral head in children: Report of two cases. *J Bone Joint Surg* 1969;51B:354–355.
8. Canale ST, Bourland WL: Fracture of the neck and intertrochanteric region of the femur in children. *J Bone Joint Surg* 1977;59A:431–443.
9. Pollen AG: *Fractures and Dislocations in Children.* Baltimore, Williams & Wilkins, 1973, pp 148–168.
10. Rang M: *Children's Fractures,* ed 2. Philadelphia, JB Lippincott, 1983, pp 242–263.
11. Glass A, Powell HDW: Traumatic dislocation of the hip in children: An analysis of forty-seven patients. *J Bone Joint Surg* 1961;43B:29–37.
12. Khermosh O, Weissman SL: Coxa vara, avascular necrosis and osteochondritis dissecans complicating solitary bone cysts of the proximal femur. *Clin Orthop* 1977;126:143–146.
13. Gore DR: Iatrogenic avascular necrosis of the hip in young children: A review of six cases. *J Bone Joint Surg* 1974;56A:493–502.
14. Lloyd-Roberts GC, Ratliff AHC: *Hip Disorders in Children.* London, Butterworths, 1978, pp 112–117, 172.
15. Kay SP, Hall JE: Fracture of the femoral neck in children and its complications. *Clin Orthop* 1971;80:53–71.
16. Ishii E, Yoshida N, Miyazaki S: Avascular necrosis of bone in neuroblastoma treated with combination chemotherapy. *Eur J Pediatr* 1984;143:152–153.
17. Cole WG, Neal BW: Corticosteroids and avascular necrosis of the femoral head in childhood. *Aust Paediatr J* 1975;11:243–246.
18. Ferguson AB Jr: Segmental vascular changes in the femoral head in children and adults. *Clin Orthop* 1985;200:291–298.
19. Wynne-Davies R: Some etiologic factors in Perthes' disease. *Clin Orthop* 1980;150:12–15.
20. Hall DJ: Genetic aspects of Perthes' disease. *Clin Orthop* 1986;209:100–114.
21. Tanaka H, Tamura K, Takano K, et al: Serum somatomedin A in Perthes' disease. *Acta Orthop Scand* 1984;55:135–140.
22. Inoue A, Ono K: A histological study of idiopathic avascular necrosis of the head of the femur. *J Bone Joint Surg* 1979;61B:138–143.
23. Inoue A, Freeman MAR, Vernon-Roberts B: The pathogenesis of Perthes' disease. *J Bone Joint Surg* 1976;58B:453–461.
24. McKibbin B, Rális Z: Pathological changes in a case of Perthes' disease. *J Bone Joint Surg* 1974;56B:438–447.
25. Klisic P: Current trends in Legg-Calvé-Perthes disease with special respect to older children. *Bull Hosp Joint Dis* 1985;45:99–110.
26. Ratliff AHC: Fractures of the neck of the femur in children. *J Bone Joint Surg* 1962;44B:528–542.
27. Catterall A: The natural history of Perthes' disease. *J Bone Joint Surg* 1971;53B:37–53.
28. Salter RB: Legg-Perthes disease: The scientific basis for the methods of treatment and their indications. *Clin Orthop* 1980;150:8–11.
29. Fisher RL, Roderique JW, Brown D, et al: The relationship of isotopic bone imaging findings to prognosis in Legg-Perthes disease. *Clin Orthop* 1980;150:23–29.
30. Minikel J, Sty J, Simons G: Sequential radionuclide bone imaging in avascular pediatric hip conditions. *Clin Orthop* 1983;175:202–208.
31. Bleumm RG, Falke THM, Ziedses des Plantes BG Jr, et al: Early Legg-Perthes disease (ischemic necrosis of the femoral head) demonstrated by magnetic resonance imaging. *Skeletal Radiol* 1985;14:95–98.
32. Thickman D, Axel L, Kressel HY, et al: Magnetic resonance imaging of avascular necrosis of the femoral head. *Skeletal Radiol* 1986;15:133–140.
33. Mitchell MD, Kundel HL, Steinberg ME, et al: Avascular necrosis of the hip: Comparison of MR, CT and scintigraphy. *AJR* 1986;147:67–71.
34. Scoles PV, Yoon YS, Makley JT, et al: Nuclear magnetic resonance imaging in Legg-Calvé-Perthes disease. *J Bone Joint Surg* 1984;66A:1357–1363.
35. Schoenecker PL: Legg-Calvé-Perthes disease. *Orthop Rev* 1986;15:19–31.
36. Kelly FB Jr, Canale ST, Jones RR: Legg-Calvé-Perthes disease: Long-term evaluation of non-containment treatment. *J Bone Joint Surg* 1980;62A:400–407.
37. O'Hara JP, Davis ND, Gage JR, et al: Long-term follow-up of Perthes' disease treated nonoperatively. *Clin Orthop* 1977;125:49–56.
38. Kendig RJ, Evans GA: Biologic osteotomy in Perthes' disease. *J Pediatr Orthop* 1986;6:278–284.

39. Clancy M, Steel HH: The effect of an incomplete intertrochanteric osteotomy on Legg-Calvé-Perthes disease. *J Bone Joint Surg* 1985;67A:213–216.

40. Jian-de D, Yu-kui Z, You-cai L, et al: New surgical approach in pediatric femoral head avascular necrosis. *Chin Med J* 1982;95:31–39.

41. Klisic P, Blaževic U, Seferovic O: Approach to treatment of Legg-Calvé-Perthes disease. *Clin Orthop* 1980;150:54–59.

42. Petrie JG, Bitenc I: The abduction weight-bearing treatment in Legg-Perthes' disease. *J Bone Joint Surg* 1971;53B:54–62.

43. Washington ER, Root L: Conservative treatment of sickle cell avascular necrosis of the femoral head. *J Pediatr Orthop* 1985;5:192–194.

44. Purvis JM, Dimon JH III, Meehan PL, et al: Preliminary experience with the Scottish Rite Hospital abduction orthosis for Legg-Perthes disease. *Clin Orthop* 1980;150:49–53.

45. King EW, Fisher RL, Gage JR, et al: Ambulation-abduction treatment in Legg-Calvé-Perthes disease (LCPD). *Clin Orthop* 1980;150:43–48.

46. Wenger DR: Selective surgical containment for Legg-Perthes disease: Recognition and management of complications. *J Pediatr Orthop* 1981;1:153–160.

47. Canario AT, Williams L, Wientroub S, et al: A controlled study of the results of femoral osteotomy in severe Perthes' disease. *J Bone Joint Surg* 1980;62B:438–440.

48. Wagner H, Zeiler G: Idiopathic necrosis of the femoral head, in Weil UH (ed): *Segmental Idiopathic Necrosis of the Femoral Head.* New York, Springer-Verlag, 1981, pp 87–116.

49. Sugioka Y: Transtrochanteric rotational osteotomy in the treatment of idiopathic and steroid-induced femoral head necrosis, Perthes' disease, slipped capital femoral epiphysis and osteoarthritis of the hip: Indications and results. *Clin Orthop* 1984;184:12–23.

50. Stevens PM, Williams P, Menelaus M: Innominate osteotomy for Perthes' disease. *J Pediatr Orthop* 1981;1:47–54.

51. Ficat RP, Arlet J, Hungerford DS: *Ischemia and Necrosis of Bone.* Baltimore, Williams & Wilkins, 1980, pp 172–177.

52. Zizic TM, Marcoux C, Hungerford DS, et al: Core decompression and the course of preradiologic ischemic necrosis of bone. *Arthritis Rheum* 1983;26:537.

53. Mowery CA, Houkom JA, Roach JW, et al: A simple method of hip arthrodesis. *J Pediatr Orthop* 1986;6:7–10.

Long-Term Follow-up of Total Hip Replacement in Patients With Avascular Necrosis

Eduardo A. Salvati, MD

Charles N. Cornell, MD

Introduction

Most cases of osteonecrosis of the femoral head are diagnosed late, after the onset of hip pain, which is usually secondary to microfractures that eventually lead to superior segmental collapse. Once this has occurred, attempts to reconstitute the femoral head are usually unsuccessful, and some form of replacement arthroplasty must be considered. A high degree of suspicion will help identify osteonecrosis early in the contralateral hip, before superior segmental collapse.[1] Both radioisotope technetium scanning and magnetic resonance imaging can provide valuable information in this early stage.

Since avascular necrosis most commonly occurs in the third through the fifth decades of life, affecting young, active patients, treatment in the later stages is challenging in that surgery must produce a painless, functional, and durable hip. Arthroplasty and joint reconstruction techniques fall into four categories: (1) osteotomies that aim to transfer weightbearing to healthy areas of the femoral head[2-5]; (2) bone and osteochondral grafts[6-8]; (3) surface, bipolar, and total hip replacements[9-12]; and (4) arthrodesis.[13] Because of the high incidence of bilateral osteonecrosis (35% to 72% of cases),[14] arthrodesis is indicated only if there is a certainty of monoarticular abnormality, something almost impossible to establish prospectively. Arthrodesis is indicated more clearly in the young patient with severe posttraumatic osteonecrosis, with limited and painful hip motion.

At The Hospital for Special Surgery we use total hip replacement in the later stages of osteonecrosis of the hip, once extensive superior segmental collapse has occurred. We reviewed our experience from 1972 to 1975 to evaluate the long-term results because the early and intermediate results are of questionable value in this population, who require surgery at a young age and who are expected to live for three or four decades after the surgery.

Methods

Thirty-three consecutive patients with osteonecrosis underwent total hip replacement at The Hospital for Special Surgery from 1972 through 1975. Only nontraumatic cases and those in which no previous hip procedure had been performed were included in this review. Data were gathered from hospital and office charts and from review of radiographs. We assessed follow-up hip function by The Hospital for Special Surgery (HSS) Hip Scoring System[15] in which hip pain, walking ability, motion, and muscle power and function are each graded on a scale of zero to 10 points, with zero being the worst and 10 the best grade. The grades for the four categories are then totaled to determine whether the result is poor, fair, good, or excellent.

Of the original 33 patients, four had died (12%) before long-term follow-up could be obtained. There were no deaths in the immediate postoperative period and none of the above deaths could be related to total hip arthroplasty. We excluded five patients for whom complete follow-up data could not be obtained, leaving 24 patients with 28 total hip replacements for review. Up-to-date follow-up evaluations were performed by attending surgeons in private cases and by residents or fellows in service cases.

There were 13 men (16 hips) and 11 women (12 hips) at the time of review. Their mean age was 45 years (range, 21 to 69 years). The mean follow-up was eight years (range, five to ten years). Nine patients (11 hips) had histories of prolonged, systemic steroid use, three patients (three hips) had histories of alcohol abuse, two patients (three hips) had sickle cell anemia, one patient (one hip) had caisson disease, one patient (one hip) had radiation-induced osteonecrosis, and in eight patients (nine hips) no obvious etiologic factor could be identified. This last group of patients was labeled "idiopathic."

Radiographs taken immediately after surgery were available in 22 patients (23 hips). A technical rating was assigned to each arthroplasty using previously described criteria.[16,17] To be graded as satisfactory, the acetabular component had to be surrounded circumferentially by a cement layer at least 2 mm thick. No more than 10 mm of the cup could be uncovered by bone and there had to be good penetration of cement in the fixation holes without significant radiolucent lines. For a satisfactory grading of the femoral component, the stem had to be positioned in valgus or neutral and had to be surrounded completely by a cement mantle without significant radiolucent lines. Cement between the calcar and superomedial aspect of the stem was required to be 4 mm thick. At least 10 mm of cement had to be present below the tip of the prosthesis.

To make the final analysis of this review more meaningful, we grouped the patients by age, sex, weight, etiology, Charnley category, and technical quality of the arthroplasty.

Results

Eleven of the 28 arthroplasties failed during the follow-up period (mean, eight years; range, five to ten years) for an overall failure rate of 37%. The 11 failures included five hips with acetabular loosening, one hip with femoral component loosening, three hips with femoral stem fracture, and two hips with deep, late infections requiring implant removal. Of the remaining 18 total hip replacements, 16 had good to excellent ratings by their HSS hip scores. Two hips received fair ratings in two patients who were severely limited by systemic manifestations of systemic lupus erythematosus.

Factors

Sex Six of the 16 total hip replacements performed in 13 male patients failed, for a failure rate of 38%. Five of the 12 total hip replacements performed in 11 females failed, for a failure rate of 42%. Sex appeared to be unrelated to failure.

Age Age weighed heavily in the outcome of the arthroplasties: in the seven patients under 30 years of age, all seven total hip replacements had unsatisfactory results: two were fair and five were mechanical failures. Time to failure in this group ranged from six to ten years with an average of 8.4 years, suggesting that cemented total hip replacements have a finite life, and in very young patients they may provide only between six and ten years of near-normal hip function.

Patient's Weight Of six patients weighing less than 60 kg, only one (16%) experienced mechanical failure. In those weighing 60 to 100 kg, eight of 22 (36%) experienced mechanical failures. The time to implant failure appeared to decrease in almost linear fashion as the patients' weight increased.

Etiology The hip replacements failed in 40% of those with ethanol-induced avascular necrosis and 30% of those with steroid-induced avascular necrosis. All three total hip replacements in the two patients with sickle cell anemia failed mechanically. In the idiopathic group with no identifiable cause of avascular necrosis, the failure rate was 11%.

Charnley Class The mechanical failure rate appeared to vary significantly with the extent of disease. In Charnley Class A patients with involvement of only one hip, the failure rate was 22%. In Class B patients with both hips involved, the failure rate was 46%. In Class C patients with polyarticular involvement or who were

limited by systemic manifestations of their disease, the failure rate was 25%.

Technical Factors In the technically satisfactory group the failure rate was half that observed in the unsatisfactory group (16% vs 33%).

Discussion

The findings in this study are sobering. The failure rate of total hip replacements in osteonecrosis is markedly higher than that observed in primary surgery for other diagnoses.

Charnley and Cupic[18] in a nine- and ten-year follow-up study of 106 total hip replacements done primarily for osteoarthritis found an overall failure rate of 9.6%. Salvati and associates[15] found a 5% failure rate in the ten-year follow-up of the first 100 consecutive Charnley total hip replacements performed at The Hospital for Special Surgery in a group of patients treated primarily for osteoarthritis, whose average age at the time of surgery was 60 years.

Stauffer[19] of the Mayo Clinic reported an overall revision rate of 9.1% for the ten-year follow-up of their first 231 Charnley total hip replacements. In other studies of Charnley total hip replacements with more than ten years of follow-up, the overall failure rate was below 10% and the failure rate for aseptic loosening was below 5%.[10]

Ranawat and associates[20] reported the five- to ten-year follow-up on a series of 77 total hip replacements, done in younger patients with a mean age of 53 years (range, 40 to 60 years), with degenerative hip disease. The overall revision rate was 10%. This study provides a valuable comparison as the surgery was also performed at The Hospital for Special Surgery, during a similar period of time, with techniques similar to those we analyzed. However, Ranawat and associates' series included only total hip replacements performed by three senior surgeons while our study includes all cases.

The overall failure rate of 37% in our study contrasted with the above results and was consistent with previous reports of a poor prognosis for total hip replacement performed for avascular necrosis. Stauffer[19] reported a 50% rate of femoral loosening in patients with osteonecrosis. This marked difference in failure rate can be attributed to several factors. Youth is clearly a poor prognostic factor for the durability of total hip replacements.[16,21] Young patients with high activity levels overuse their prostheses and, therefore, surpass the stress limits of the bone-cement interface.

A similar mechanism applies in regard to excessive weight. Our findings established a correlation between excessive weight and decreased durability of the artificial joint, supporting previous studies.

One half of the total hip replacements failed in patients with bilateral hip involvement (Charnley Class B), probably because of the added stress imposed on the artifical hip while the contralateral hip was symptomatic. The failure rate in patients with monoarticular hip abnormalities was similar to the failure rate of patients with multiple joint involvement (22% and 25%, respectively), probably because of favoring the artificial hip in the former group and because of restraints in the latter group.

Another factor appears to be the nature of the bone in osteonecrosis. Dutton and associates[9] pointed out that bone stock in patients with osteonecrosis is often inferior to that in patients with osteoarthritis. Hedley and Kim[12] found that hip arthroplasties performed in patients with posttraumatic osteonecrosis have a lower failure rate than those performed in patients with idiopathic avascular necrosis. The Hospital for Special Surgery experience related here suggests that the different etiologic factors leading to idiopathic avascular necrosis carry with them different prognoses regarding the long-term outcome of total hip replacements. Patients with an established etiologic factor for the osteonecrosis (steroids, alcohol, sickle cell, renal transplantation) appear to fare worse than those in whom no inciting cause of osteonecrosis can be found.[22-26]

Arlot and associates[27] reported the iliac bone histologic findings in 77 patients with osteonecrosis and nonapparent bone disease with normal kidney function. They studied in detail several static and dynamic histomorphometric factors. Osteomalacia was found in nine patients; in the remaining 68, marked decreases in osteoblastic appositional rate and bone formation were observed. This profile of osteoporosis could produce a healing defect of microfractures and thus facilitate subchondral fractures. Both corticosteroids and alcohol induce osteoporosis by a depressive effect on osteoblastic activity. In addition, intestinal malabsorption of calcium produces a secondary hyperparathyroidism, which increases the bone loss by resorption.

Because fixation in total hip replacements requires a stable bone-cement interface, it stands to reason that ongoing bone necrosis or progressive associated osteoporosis or osteomalacia will accelerate mechanical failure. Patients with uncontrolled hemoglobinopathy or long-term ethanol or steroid use may continue to lose bone, most critically along the bone-cement interface.

Dutton and associates[9] and Hedley and Kim[12] proposed this as the reason fixation is lost so early when surface replacement is performed for idiopathic avascular necrosis. However, our idiopathic group fared better than any of the other etiologic groups with osteonecrosis. Their lower failure rate of 16% may be attributed to better bone quality and older age (the fourth and fifth decades). These patients may have experienced a single, self-limited episode of avascular necrosis with no further progression of their disease, and no significant bone abnormalities, thereby maintaining

a more stable bone-cement interface and producing a better long-term result.

As osteonecrosis occurs in young adults with normal life expectancy, future revision surgery following total hip replacement is expected. The experience of the 1970s indicates that the results of revision surgery are not as good as those of primary total hip replacement.[17] Only about two thirds of the patients have satisfactory results. The incidence of local complications is increased two to three times. Rerevision is necessary in 5% to 10% percent after an average follow-up of only three years; this increases to about 20% after eight years of follow-up.[28] Thus, revision and rerevision can also be expected in some patients with increasing complexity, progressive bone loss, and larger skeletal defects.

In the future, better preoperative planning and restoration of bone stock to obtain a more anatomic reconstruction, better surgical and cementing techniques (hypotensive anesthesia to reduce bone bleeding and preparation of the bone with a Water-Pik, combined with pressurization of the cement), as well as newer implant designs and materials (superalloys, metal-backed cups, and antibiotic-impregnated cement) may help to reduce failure rates and lengthen the time between revision and failure. The learning curve for the performance of revision surgery is long, as we are still improving and modifying the procedure. In some patients, especially young ones with massive loss of bone stock, a cemented revision may provide only a temporary solution. New solutions to this problem are needed. The use of a prosthesis to replace large skeletal defects should be considered with caution in patients with extended life expectancies, as loosening and prosthetic failure could lead to extreme disability. Massive bone allografts may be preferable in such patients (Fig. 8–1). A Girdlestone procedure may still be the only reasonable option in some extreme circumstances.

Because the number of hips in this study was limited and because more than one of the different factors analyzed occurred in individual hips, we cannot accept our findings as conclusive. Must we conclude that total hip replacement is to be discouraged in young patients with osteonecrosis? Before doing so, we must examine the alternatives. The usefulness and place of osteochondral grafting remains to be seen in long-term follow-up.[7] Surface replacement has less durability than total hip replacement,[9,11] particularly in osteonecrosis, and most surgeons have abandoned it.

Enneking[29] pointed out the problems associated with osteotomies that merely transfer weightbearing to other diseased areas of the femoral head. Although the articular cartilage in these areas may be healthy, if the underlying bone is necrotic, further subchondral fracture and collapse will occur. Sugioka[30] reported encouraging results with rotational osteotomy but his experience has not yet been corroborated elsewhere.

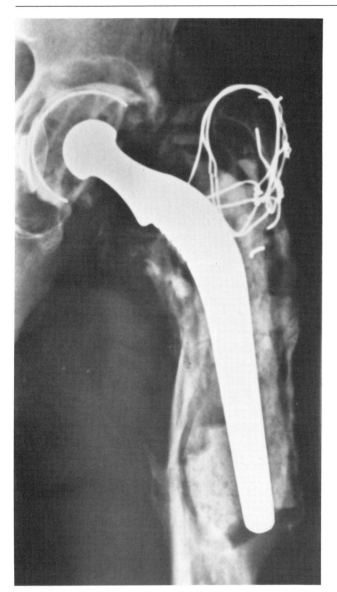 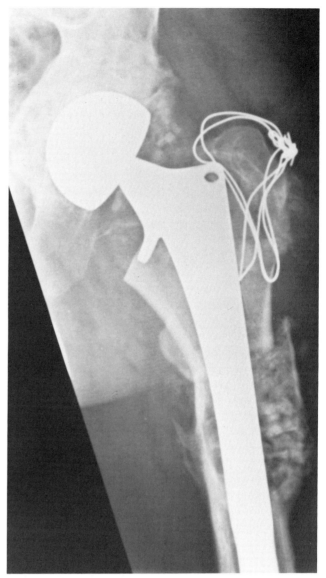

Fig. 8-1 Radiographs of a 36-year-old man with osteonecrosis from alcoholism. **Left:** Anteroposterior view shows a grossly loose total hip replacement with severe acetabular and femoral bone loss. **Right:** View after surgical revision that included a massive bone allograft to the acetabulum and proximal femur.

However, in selected cases, if the area of superior segmental collapse is more limited, involving an arc of less than 180 degrees (adding the anteroposterior and lateral views), a varus and flexion osteotomy can produce satisfactory results (Fig. 8–2). The advantage of preserving the femoral head cannot be overemphasized, particularly in light of the limited long-term success of primary prosthetic and revision arthroplasty in osteonecrosis.[3-5]

Efforts to revascularize the femoral head with microvascular anastomosis and with pulsed electromagnetic fields are being conducted, but it is too early to judge the results.[31,32]

Thus, before abandoning total hip replacement in this condition, one must acknowledge that it provides excellent pain relief while preserving near-normal hip function for a limited period of time.

This study presents the long-term experience of the early and mid 1970s. Since then significant progress has been made, so it is reasonable to expect increased longevity with current improved techniques.[33] In fact, about one fourth of the failures were caused by fractures of the stem, a complication that has already decreased as a result of improved design, metallurgy, and fixation. Most of the advances made have addressed the technologic aspects of the procedure. Future studies concentrating on patient factors and particularly on bone biology are necessary.

In addition to decreasing the patient's weight and activity level, attempts should be made to improve bone

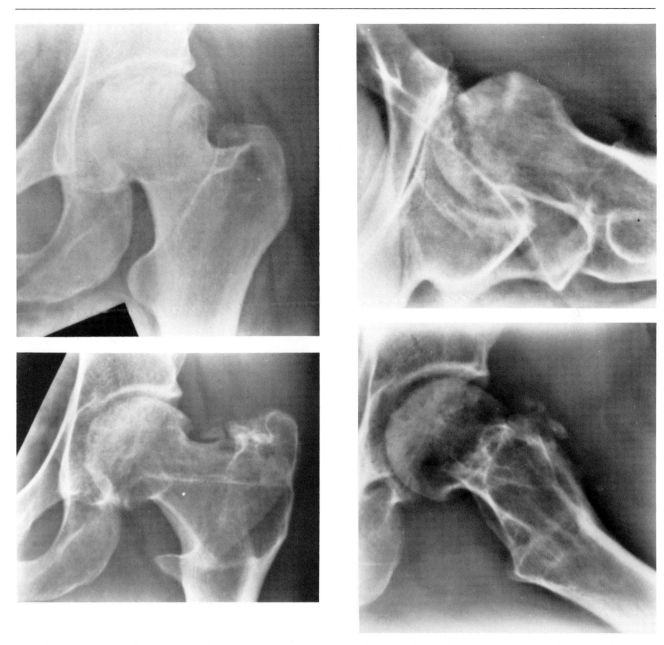

Fig. 8-2   The left hip of a patient who developed osteonecrosis after steroid therapy. **Top left:** Anteroposterior view. **Top right:** A through-the-groin lateral view demonstrates the extent of superior segmental collapse, which extends through most of the superior aspect of the femoral head. **Bottom left and Bottom right:** Four years after varus and flexion osteotomy. The joint is painless and functional with a good range of motion. The superior segmental collapse has not worsened. The patient has unlimited walking ability, does not limp, and does not require an external support.

quality in patients with osteonecrosis secondary to identifiable etiologic factors. Alcoholic patients should be rehabilitated and their osteoporosis treated. Patients who require steroid therapy may also benefit from drug regimens that combat osteoporosis. Drugs that can increase the osteoblastic appositional rate and bone formation, such as fluoride, could be of help to osteoporotic bone.[34] In those patients with osteomalacia, administration of adequate doses of vitamin D should improve calcification.

More research is needed to determine the effect of anti-osteoporosis regimens on steroid-induced osteoporosis. Patients with hemoglobinopathies may benefit from transfusion programs that maintain more normal hematocrit levels with lower levels of abnormal circulating hemoglobins.

Although the first decade of experience with total hip replacement in patients with osteonecrosis has been discouraging, the future should be brighter because of a greater understanding of the principles of cement fixation, improved materials and prosthetic design, and perhaps the development of anatomically designed press-fitted prostheses and/or porous ingrowth fixation.

Summary

Long-term studies show that patients with osteonecrosis who undergo total hip replacement experience an overall failure rate four times greater than those with osteoarthritis. Different etiologic factors associated with osteonecrosis appear to carry different prognoses for the durability of total hip replacements. Important factors, in addition to discouraging total hip replacement in patients under 30 to 40 years of age and making all possible efforts to decrease the patient's weight and activity level, include improvements in bone quality, surgical and cementing techniques, prosthetic design, and materials that will prolong the durability of total hip replacements. Despite the inferior long-term results of total hip replacement performed for advanced osteonecrosis, we feel the procedure should not be abandoned for patients in their fifth decade of life or older because it provides a painless, functional hip more consistently than does any other form of arthroplasty.

These patients should be informed about the importance of protecting the hip replacement by avoiding strenuous activities, impact, and obesity, and about the possibilities of future mechanical failure that may require revision surgery.

Although significant improvements have been made in regard to the technology of total hip replacement, future research in the bone biology of osteonecrosis is necessary.

References

1. Marcus ND, Enneking WF, Massam RA: The silent hip in idiopathic aseptic necrosis. *J Bone Joint Surg* 1973;55A:1351–1366.
2. Merle d'Aubigné RM, Postel M, Magabraud M, et al: Idiopathic necrosis of the hip in the adult. *J Bone Joint Surg* 1965;47B:612–633.
3. Ganz R, Buchler U: Overview of attempts to revitalize the dead head in aseptic necrosis of the femoral head: Osteotomy and revascularization, in *The Hip: Proceedings of the 11th Open Scientific Meeting of the Hip Society.* St. Louis, CV Mosby Co, 1983, pp 296–305.
4. Jacobs MA, Hungerford DS, Krackow KA, et al: Results of intertrochanteric hip osteotomies for avascular necrosis. Presented at the 54th Annual Meeting of the American Academy of Orthopaedic Surgeons, San Francisco, Jan 26, 1987.
5. Maistrelli GL, Fusco U, Avai A, et al: Osteonecrosis of the hip treated by intertrochanteric osteotomy: A four- to 15-year follow-up. Presented at the 54th Annual Meeting of the American Academy of Orthopaedic Surgeons, San Francisco, Jan 26, 1987.
6. Lee CK, Rehmatullah N: Muscle-pedicle bone graft and cancellous bone graft for the "silent hip" of idiopathic ischemic necrosis of the femoral head in adults. *Clin Orthop* 1981;158:185–194.
7. Meyers MH, Jones RE, Bucholz RW, et al: Fresh autogenous grafts and osteochondral allografts for the treatment of segmental collapse in osteonecrosis of the hip. *Clin Orthop* 1983;174:107–112.
8. Smith KR, Bonfiglio M, Montgomery WJ: Non-traumatic necrosis of the femoral head treated with tibial bone-grafting. *J Bone Joint Surg* 1980;62A:845–847.
9. Dutton RO, Amstutz HJ, Thomas BJ, et al: Tharies surface replacement for osteonecrosis of the femoral head. *J Bone Joint Surg* 1982;64A:1225–1237.
10. Eftekhar NS: Editorial. *Clin Orthop* 1986;211.
11. Jolley MN, Salvati EA, Brown GC: Early results and complications of surface replacement of the hip. *J Bone Joint Surg* 1982;64A:366–377.
12. Hedley AK, Kim W: Prosthetic replacement in osteonecrosis of the hip, in American Academy of Orthopaedic Surgeons *Instructional Course Lectures, XXXII.* St. Louis, CV Mosby Co, 1983, pp 265–271.
13. Callaghan JJ, Brand RA, Pedersen DR: Hip arthrodesis: A long-term follow-up. *J Bone Joint Surg* 1985;67A:1328–1335.
14. Kenzora JE: Treatment of idiopathic osteonecrosis: The current philosophy and rationale. *Orthop Clin North Am* 1985;16:717–725.
15. Salvati EA, Wilson PD Jr, Jolley MN, et al: A ten-year follow-up of our first one hundred consecutive Charnley total hip replacements. *J Bone Joint Surg* 1981;63A:753–767.
16. Dorr LD, Takei GK, Conaty JP: Total hip arthroplasties in patients less than forty-five years old. *J Bone Joint Surg* 1983;65A:474–479.
17. Pellicci PM, Salvati EA, Robinson HJ Jr: Mechanical failures in total hip replacement requiring reoperation. *J Bone Joint Surg* 1981;61A:28–39.
18. Charnley J, Cupic Z: The nine and ten year results of the low-friction arthroplasty of the hip. *Clin Orthop* 1973;95:9–25.
19. Stauffer RN: Ten-year follow-up study of total hip replacement. *J Bone Joint Surg* 1982;64A:983–990.
20. Ranawat CS, Atkinson R, Salvati EA: Conventional total hip arthroplasty for degenerative joint disease in patients between the ages of forty and sixty years. *J Bone Joint Surg* 1984;66A:745–753.
21. Chandler HP, Reineck FT, Wixson RL, et al: Total hip replacement in patients younger than thirty years old. *J Bone Joint Surg* 1981;63A:1426–1434.
22. Chmell SJ, Schwartz CM, Giacchino LJ, et al: Total hip replacement in patients with renal transplants. *Arch Surg* 1983;118:489–495.
23. Chung SM, Alavi A, Russell MO: Management of osteonecrosis in sickle cell anemia and its genetic variants. *Clin Orthop* 1978;130:158–174.
24. Hungerford DS, Zizic TM: Alcoholism associated with ischemic necrosis of the femoral head. *Clin Orthop* 1978;130:144–153.
25. Kenzora JE, Sledge CB: Hip arthroplasty and the renal transplant patient, in *The Hip: Proceedings of the Third Open Scientific Meeting of the Hip Society.* St. Louis, CV Mosby Co, 1975, pp 35–59.
26. Prupas HM, Patzakis M, Quismorio FP Jr: Total hip arthroplasty for avascular necrosis of the femur in systemic lupus erythematosus. *Clin Orthop* 1981;161:186–190.
27. Arlot ME, Bonjean M, Chavassieux PM, et al: Bone histology in adults with aseptic necrosis: Histomorphometric evaluation of iliac biopsies in seventy-seven patients. *J Bone Joint Surg* 1983;65A:1319–1327.
28. Pellicci PM, Wilson PD Jr, Sledge CB, et al: Long-term results of revision total hip replacement: A follow-up report. *J Bone Joint Surg* 1985;67A:513–516.

29. Enneking WF: The choice of surgical procedure in idiopathic aseptic necrosis, in *The Hip: Proceedings of the Seventh Open Scientific Meeting of the Hip Society*. St. Louis, CV Mosby Co, 1979, pp 238–243.

30. Sugioka Y: Transtrochanteric anterior rotational osteotomy of the femoral head in the treatment of osteonecrosis affecting the hip. *Clin Orthop* 1978;130:191–201.

31. Eftekhar NS, Schink-Ascani MM, Mitchell SN, et al: Osteonecrosis of the femoral head treated by pulsed electromagnetic fields (PEMFS): A preliminary report, in *The Hip: Proceedings of the 11th Open Scientific Meeting of the Hip Society*. St. Louis, CV Mosby Co, 1983, p 306–330.

32. Gilbert A, Judet H, Judet J, et al: Microvascular transfer of the fibula for necrosis of the femoral head. *Orthopedics* 1986;9:885–890.

33. Harris WH, McCarthy JC Jr, O'Neill DA: Femoral component loosening using contemporary techniques of femoral cement fixation. *J Bone Joint Surg* 1982;64A:1063–1067.

34. Lane JM, Vigorita VJ: Osteoporosis. *J Bone Joint Surg* 1983;65A:274–278.

The Child's Foot

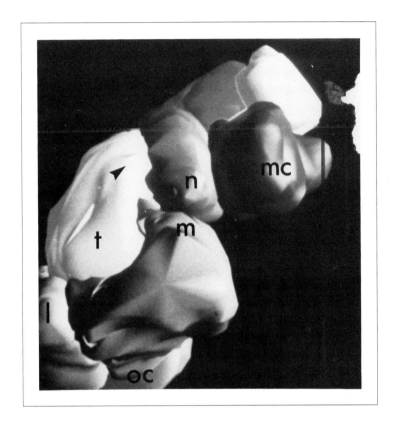

The Painful Foot in the Child

Kaye E. Wilkins, MD

Foot pain in the pediatric patient is, fortunately, rare. Thus, the practicing orthopaedic surgeon seldom has much experience in distinguishing the various conditions that cause painful feet in children. In many cases the diagnosis is obvious. In others, the physical findings and complaints may be less specific. My intent is to outline some of the specific conditions to consider when attempting to find the cause of foot pain in the pediatric age group.

It would be nice if the various conditions that cause pain could be classified by the age groups they affect. In a few cases they can be, but many of the conditions occur in all age groups. A better division of these conditions is to classify them as traumatic, inflammatory, and tumorous (Outline 9–1). I will discuss only those conditions that occur before skeletal maturity.

Traumatic Conditions

Acute Bone and Ligament Injuries

Often these conditions have a definite history of acute onset of pain after a traumatic episode. The diagnosis may be obvious because the location of the injury is specific. Radiographs often show the specific bone or bones that are fractured or injured. The young child's foot is very flexible and fractures are less common. Often the force is transmitted more proximally to the tibia or femur. Injuries to specific ligaments in the foot are difficult to localize. The best that can be done in many cases is to delineate the sprain as to being hindfoot, midfoot, or forefoot, depending on the area of maximum tenderness. The specifics of each of the fracture types that occur in the pediatric foot are beyond the scope of this discussion. The diagnosis and treatment of these individual fractures can be found in the standard textbooks dealing with pediatric fractures.[1-4]

In the small child who has just begun walking, the exact diagnosis of foot pain may be elusive. Often the parents describe a sudden failure to bear weight on the lower extremity. Since the foot has not been bearing weight, it may be swollen and the parents assume that the source of pain is in the foot. In the child who has just begun walking, the most common injury is an undisplaced spiral fracture in the midshaft of the tibia. This has been described as the "toddler's fracture." To make the diagnosis, the physician must carefully examine the child while the child sits in the parent's lap. The extremity needs to be palpated carefully. The foot,

Outline 9–1
Conditions causing foot pain in pediatric patients

I. Traumatic conditions
  A. Acute bone and ligament injuries
  B. Chronic bone-tendon disorders (apophysitis)
    1. Sever's disease (calcaneal apophysis)
    2. Fifth metatarsal apophysitis
    3. Accessory navicular
  C. Neurologic injuries
    1. Acute: reflex sympathetic dystrophy
    2. Chronic: tarsal tunnel syndrome
  D. Circulatory conditions related to trauma
    1. Köhler's disease
    2. Freiberg's infraction
II. Inflammatory conditions
  A. Disorders of the subtalar complex (peroneal spastic disorders)
    1. Tarsal coalition
    2. Degenerative joint disease
    3. Trauma (hidden fractures)
    4. Juvenile rheumatoid arthritis
    5. Infections
    6. Idiopathic disorders
  B. Bone and joint infection
    1. Septic arthritis or osteomyelitis
      a. Primary hematogenous infection
      b. Secondary to puncture wounds
III. Tumorous conditions
  A. Osteoid osteoma
  B. Subungual osteochondroma
  C. Unicameral bone cyst

while swollen, is not painful to deep palpation. The clinical diagnosis is made by percussing lightly along the shaft of the tibia. This usually elicits a consistent painful response, especially when compared with the opposite side. The radiographs may demonstrate a fine spiral fracture line in the midshaft or distal shaft. In some instances there may be only deep soft-tissue swelling and the radiographic evidence may not become apparent until three weeks later when periosteal new bone formation becomes visible (Fig. 9–1).

Chronic Bone-Tendon Disorders

The junction of the tendons with the osseous part of the foot is often less resistant to recurrent stresses in the immature individual. Three major tendon-bone junctions present problems in preadolescents. The first two (calcaneal apophysitis and fifth metatarsal apophysitis) involve junctions of tendons with a growing apophysis where the tendon attaches to the cartilage rather than directly to the bone. The third involves the

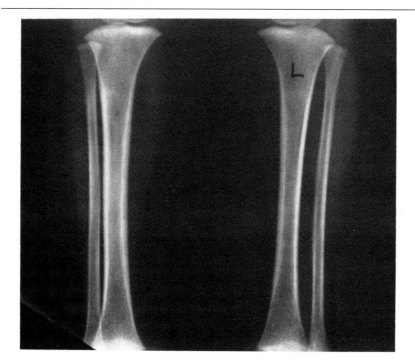
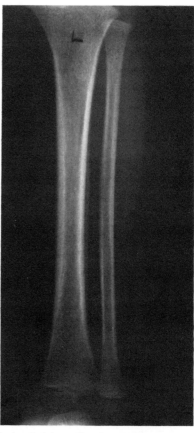

Fig. 9-1 Toddler's fracture. **Left:** A 20-month-old child suddenly stopped walking and had a slightly swollen foot. Radiographs of foot and both tibias were said to be negative. **Right:** A radiograph taken at three weeks shows periosteal new bone formation along the shaft of the tibia.

junction of a tendon with an accessory ossification center (accessory navicular). Why these conditions occur at a later age is not completely clear. It may be that the increased weight of the patient, rapid prepubertal growth, and added physical activity all contribute in part to the development of these conditions just before skeletal maturity.

Calcaneal Apophysitis (Sever's Disease) This condition is common in the young active child who is just beginning to participate in competitive sports. It usually occurs in girls from 8 to 10 years of age and in boys 9 to 10 years of age. The cause is speculative. It was first described by Sever[5] in 1912. For many years it was thought to be an osteochondrosis because of the dense and fragmented appearance of the calcaneal apophysis. This dense radiologic appearance, however, is considered to be normal at this age. The same appearance is often visualized in asymptomatic individuals. This is a disorder of the soft tissue insertion of the Achilles tendon into the calcaneal apophysis. Jahss[6] believed that it was an inflammation of the bursae adjacent to the tendon. No histopathologic descriptions of this disorder can be found in the English orthopaedic literature.

In many cases, the patient localizes the pain to the insertion of the Achilles tendon into the calcaneus. Complaints are often nonspecific as the patient points to the general area of the hindfoot. There is usually tenderness at the specific point where the tendon inserts into the calcaneus. In some individuals with severe pain, the gait may have a calcaneal pattern. Patients usually find it easy to walk on their toes but are reluctant to walk on their heels. There may or may not be heelcord tightness.

Radiographs, although not diagnostic, are helpful in explaining to the patient's parents the location and suspected cause of the problem. Radiographs are also necessary to rule out other rare causes of heel pain such as a unicameral bone cyst or a stress fracture (Fig. 9–2). In these other conditions, the pain is localized over the body of the calcaneus rather than at the tendon insertion.

Treatment is designed to relieve symptoms and reassure the patient and parents that the problem will resolve spontaneously. The parents need to be assured that although the condition "hurts" it will not "harm" the patient and that the child's gait will return to normal when the pain subsides. Treatment with heel-lifts

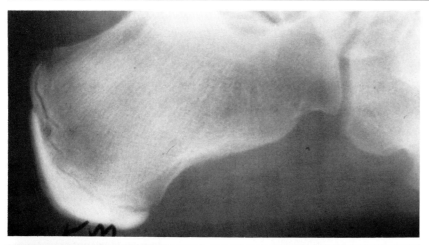

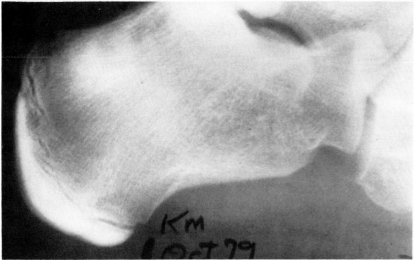

Fig. 9–2 An 11-year-old soccer player with heel pain. **Top:** The original diagnosis was Sever's disease. **Bottom:** A later radiograph demonstrated new bone formation on the dorsal surface and within the body of the calcaneus, indicating that the correct diagnosis was a stress fracture.

and high-top shoes is designed to decrease ankle excursion during running activities. Applying heat to the heel and heelcord stretching before exercise may decrease the severity of the symptoms. Ice applied after exercise may help to decrease the inflammatory response.

Fifth Metatarsal Apophysitis A child 10 to 12 years old may experience a painful swelling at the insertion of the peroneus brevis into the apophysis of the base of the fifth metatarsal. There may or may not be a secondary ossification center in the apophysis. This local prominence can create moderate pain, especially if the patient wears narrow shoes. Treatment should be designed to relieve symptoms and offer reassurance.

Accessory Navicular In many ways the accessory navicular is similar to an apophysis. The accessory navicular usually fuses with the main body of the navicular at skeletal maturity.[7] In about 2% of individuals the ossification center remains separate. An adventitious bursa often develops at the junction of the accessory navicular with the main portion of the navicular. This is not

a true joint but a syndesmosis or fibrous junction. The histopathologic findings are often similar to those seen in the patellar tendon-tibial tubercle junction in Osgood-Schlatter disease. The microscopic changes are those of chronic inflammation.

In the past it was believed that this condition led to pes planus but it is now known that accessory naviculars occur in many individuals who have normal medial metatarsal arches.[8] In some cases of long duration, the function of the posterior tibial tendon may be affected, leading to a relative peroneal overpull with a secondary pes planus.

Treatment should initially consist of a trial of cast immobilization. Relief pads on the medial counters of the shoes may help to decrease mechanical irritation. In most cases the symptoms resolve with time. In those cases in which the symptoms persist, simple excision of the accessory navicular and, in some cases, removal of part of the prominence of the medial aspect of the navicular are all that is necessary. The Kidner procedure, which is an attempt to transfer the insertion of the tibialis posterior to the undersurface of the navicular, does not correct any pes planus that is present.[9]

Neurologic Injuries

Reflex Sympathetic Dystrophy Reflex sympathetic dystrophy, or causalgia as it is sometimes called, is more common in children than is recognized. The diagnosis may be overlooked because it presents a different pattern than it does in adults.[10-13] The condition usually begins after what often was thought to be minimal trauma. The traumatic incident may even have been forgotten. The initial physical findings consist of a painful foot in which the pain is poorly localized and there is relatively little swelling or ecchymosis. The pain usually is out of proportion to the physical findings. The pain is sharp, often burning, and is not relieved by rest. It is often worse at night. Skin changes are inconsistent—the foot may be either pale or somewhat congested. The patient protects the foot and avoids any superficial contact. When the foot is palpated or massaged by the examiner, there is a painful response. Tears are shed and the patient and parents both become quite anxious.

It is important to recognize this entity early, before chronic changes develop. In the pediatric age group, chronic trophic skin changes do not appear until late. Osteoporosis on the radiographs is also a late finding (Fig. 9–3). The key to the diagnosis is pain out of proportion to the physical findings or trauma and which is not relieved by rest. In many instances, the pain increases over a period of time.

Fortunately, if the symptoms are recognized early they can easily be reversed with minimal treatment.

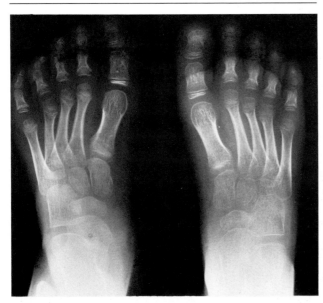

Fig. 9–3 Chronic reflex sympathetic dystrophy in the right foot has produced subtle osteopenia or osteoporosis of the right foot. The changes are more apparent in the tarsal bones.

The patient and the child's anxious parents need to be reassured that the condition can be treated. Often the patient has been examined by many other physicians who may have indicated that the diagnosis was psychogenic in origin. It is important for the physician to communicate to the patient the recognition that the pain is real.

Physical measures are the cornerstone of any therapy program. Narcotic analgesics are not effective and should be avoided. The first goal is to get the patient to reaccept the foot. The patient must be encouraged to stimulate and massage the foot. This will be uncomfortable initially, but with use and stimulation the pain usually decreases. Contrast baths of alternating warm and cold water help to break the pain cycle. The patient is encouraged to start bearing weight on the foot with the assurance that the pain will gradually decrease and that no harm will be done by putting pressure on the foot.

If these simple physical measures fail to reverse the pain cycle, applying a transcutaneous nerve stimulator to the foot is often effective. In very long-standing cases, more aggressive invasive procedures such as perineural catheters, sympathetic nerve blocks, or regional anesthesia using sympatholytic agents may be necessary. In my experience, however, early treatment usually makes these aggressive measures unnecessary.

Tarsal Tunnel Syndrome The classic tarsal tunnel syndrome is extremely rare in children. In fact, it is not even mentioned in two recent texts dealing with foot disorders in children.[14,15] Only two published reports discuss it as occurring in children.[16,17] All 11 patients described in these two articles were girls. None had any systemic or joint diseases. In none were the clinical findings confirmed with electrodiagnostic studies. I have discussed this entity with many orthopaedic surgeons who limit their practice to pediatric patients and none could remember having seen such cases.

Mann[18] stated that three criteria must be present to confirm the diagnosis of tarsal tunnel syndrome: (1) There must be a history of burning pain on the plantar aspect of the foot. It usually increases with activity and decreases with rest. The pain may be worse at night. (2) On the physical examination there must be a positive Tinel's sign along the posterior tibial nerve in the tarsal tunnel. There may also be decreased sensation on the plantar aspect of the foot. (3) The clinical pattern must be confirmed by electrodiagnostic studies such as decreased nerve conduction velocities in the foot or fibrillation potentials in the intrinsic muscles.

If these three criteria are met, then surgical decompression of the tarsal tunnel is probably indicated and usually provides good relief of the symptoms. Surgical intervention in those patients who do not meet all three criteria may not produce uniformly good results.

Circulatory Conditions Related to Trauma

Köhler's Disease Avascular necrosis of the tarsal navicular, or Köhler's disease, occurs in boys 5 to 6 years of age and in girls about a year earlier. These children show the insidious onset of local tenderness and some swelling over the tarsal navicular. They tend to walk with the forefoot supinated. They are able to walk and carry on normal activities, but often complain of increased discomfort with increased activity. The diagnosis is confirmed by the classic pancake condensation of the ossific center of the navicular (Fig. 9–4, *top*).

The ossification process of the navicular is nor-

mally delayed. The navicular lies at the apex of the arch of the foot, which is at the area of maximum compression during weightbearing and the push-off portion of the gait cycle. This combination of a soft cartilaginous structure and increased pressure is thought to contribute to the injury of the vessels supplying the ossific nucleus, producing a temporary avascular necrosis. Fortunately, the bone spontaneously reossifies rapidly and reconstitutes to a normal size and shape within one to two years (Fig. 9–4, *bottom*). Treatment is always conservative with reassurance to the parents that the bone will heal. Temporary immobilization with a cast may decrease the severity of the symptoms.

Freiberg's Infraction Avascular necrosis of the metatar-

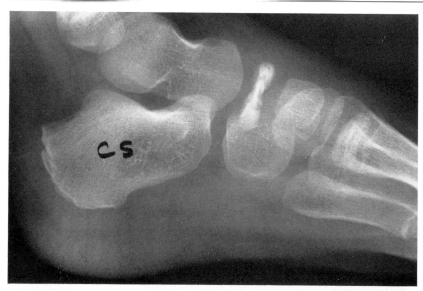

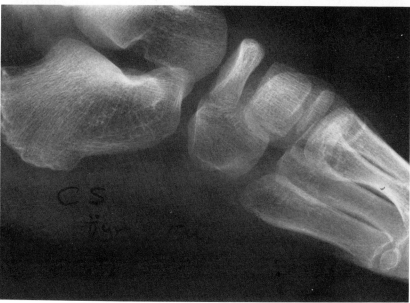

Fig. 9–4 A 5-year-old boy with Köhler's disease. **Top:** The typical pancake condensation of the navicular. **Bottom:** Two years later the navicular ossification center has been reconstituted to a normal appearance.

sal head was first described by Freiberg in 1914.[19] The symptoms develop in adolescence, preponderantly in girls. The head of the second metatarsal is most commonly involved. The condition may be bilateral in some cases.[14]

Braddock's[20] experimental studies demonstrated that the physeal plate of the metatarsal bone is weakened just before skeletal maturity. The second metatarsal, because of its lack of mobility and increased length, is especially vulnerable to repeated stress. These two factors in combination are thought to contribute to the development of avascular necrosis of the metatarsal head during early adolescence.

Radiographs demonstrate a collapse of the subchondral surface of the metatarsal head (Fig. 9–5, *top left* and *bottom left*). There may be an area of sclerosis around the central necrotic area. The metatarsal head may then develop varying degrees of collapse. A tech-

netium bone scan will demonstrate increased uptake in the individual metatarsal. Changes in the bone scan may precede the radiographic changes (Fig. 9–5, *bottom right*). The patient complains of local pain over the involved metatarsal head. Swelling is usually minimal. Treatment is initially supportive with shoe modifications designed to relieve the pressure under the head of the involved metatarsal. In some long-standing cases surgical debridement or arthroplasty may be necessary.[21]

Inflammatory Conditions

Subtalar Complex Problems

The most common conditions creating pain in the hindfoot in children are disorders of the subtalar complex. These usually involve some type of acute inflam-

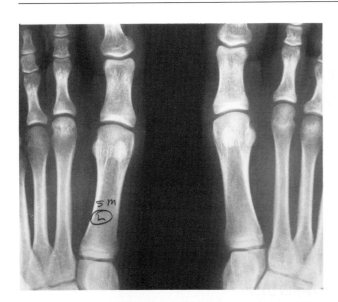

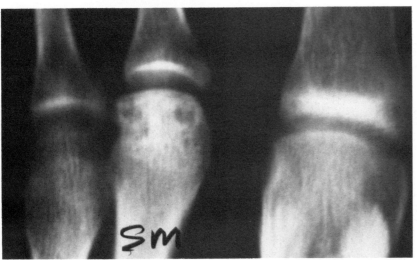

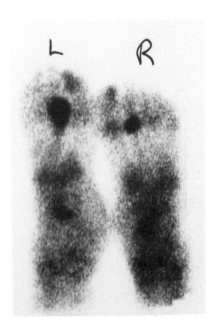

Fig. 9–5 A 13-year-old girl with pain only in the area of the left second metatarsal head. **Top left:** Anteroposterior radiograph. **Bottom left:** Tomograms of the left foot better demonstrate the lytic areas with a sclerotic margin with the metatarsal head. **Bottom right:** A technetium bone scan demonstrated that there was increased uptake in the right second metatarsal head although there were no symptoms or radiologic abnormalities.

matory process or a chronic degenerative condition in the subtalar joint. These individuals are often described as having a peroneal spastic flatfoot because chronic peroneal spasticity produces a valgus hindfoot and a pronated and abducted forefoot.

Kyne and Mankin[22] demonstrated that there is increased pressure in the subtalar joint when the foot is in inversion. They theorized that the peroneal spasm may be a protective reflex to decrease subtalar pressure and, thus, the pain.

The most common cause of peroneal spasm is tarsal coalition. Usually a talocalcaneal coalition produces more severe symptoms. The pain may precede the radiographic changes. In some instances, minor trauma may aggravate the symptoms. There is usually a rigid hindfoot with little or no true subtalar motion.

Radiographic changes include beaking of the talus and obliteration of the middle facet of the subtalar joint (Fig. 9–6, *top left* and *bottom left*). A subtalar arthrogram can be useful in evaluating the patency of the middle facet.[23] More recently, computed tomography has been found to be extremely useful in determining the presence of early coalitions (Fig. 9–6, *bottom right*).[24] The treatment of tarsal coalition is beyond the scope of this discussion. Such information is available elsewhere.[25-27]

In the absence of a defined coalition, other possible causes need to be considered. Juvenile rheumatoid arthritis may start in the subtalar joint. In severe pes planus there may be secondary degenerative disease of the subtalar joint. Undetected fractures of the subtalar complex or even the navicular may cause peroneal spasm. Rarely, infections of the subtalar complex may also be culprits. In some cases no specific cause can be found for the peroneal spasm.

Infections of the Foot

Primary septic arthritis of the ankle or one of the midfoot joints is not uncommon. It has been my ex-

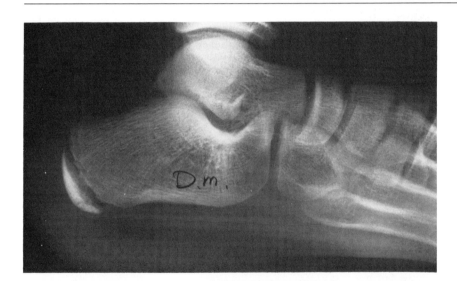

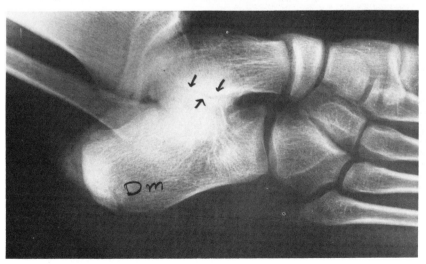

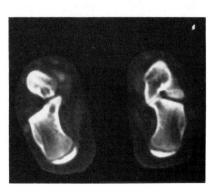

Fig. 9–6 A 9-year-old child with subtalar pain. **Top left:** Initial lateral radiograph appears normal. **Bottom left:** An oblique view demonstrates some narrowing of the middle facet (arrows). **Bottom right:** Computed tomography demonstrates almost complete obliteration of the middle facet of the left foot.

perience that most ankle infections occur in younger children (less than 3 years old) with the primary organism being *Hemophilus influenzae*. One must always remember that septic arthritis in the ankle may be secondary to a primary osteomyelitis of the talus.

Primary hematogenous osteomyelitis usually involves the calcaneus or one of the metatarsals. Swelling, tenderness, and warmth, along with systemic manifestations such as increased temperature and erythrocyte sedimentation rate, should alert the physician to the correct diagnosis. Treatment consists of high levels of antibiotics with or without surgical drainage, depending on the presence of purulent material outside the bony cortex.

One problem that is not often fully appreciated is the morbidity associated with puncture wounds of the foot. This is especially true if they occur next to one of the metatarsophalangeal joints. Often these patients are seen initially in an emergency room where minimal surgical debridement is performed. The patient is then treated with oral antistaphylococcus antibiotic. Early in the course there are few clinical symptoms. After two to three weeks the local signs have progressed so that it is apparent that surgical drainage is necessary. This delay, however, may result in loss of joint space with permanent destruction of the joint (Fig. 9–7). The offending organism is almost always a *Pseudomonas* species that requires prolonged administration of parenteral antibiotics.[28,29] The orthopaedic surgeon must alert colleagues to the fact that puncture wounds of the foot,

especially near joints, can have serious consequences. These puncture wounds should be adequately debrided surgically and appropriate cultures obtained before antibiotic treatment is started.

Tumors

Osseous Tumors

Soft-tissue tumors are usually clinically apparent and are rarely painful. Primary osseous tumors of the child's foot are also rare and usually benign.

Osteoid Osteoma An osteoid osteoma in the foot produces the same symptoms as it does in other parts of the body. The chronic pain, which increases in intensity at night, can be relieved by aspirin. If it involves the surface, there may be some palpable enlargement of the bone. The radiographs show a peripheral sclerotic margin with a radiolucent nidus. Treatment consists of excision of the nidus with or without bone grafting.

Osteochondroma (Subungual Exostosis) An osteochondroma may occur as an isolated lesion under the great toe.[30] The mass distorts the nail and develops local tenderness. Oblique radiographs of the toe show the typical sessile lesion (Fig. 9–8). Local excision usually relieves the pain.

Unicameral Bone Cyst This can occur in the body of the

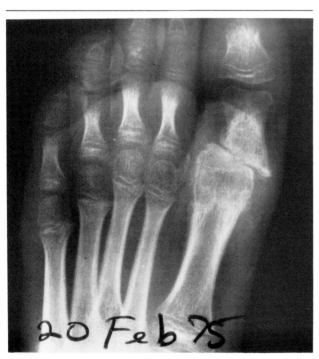

Fig. 9–7 Radiograph of a foot four weeks after an untreated puncture wound contaminated with *Pseudomonas* sp. demonstrates destruction of the metatarsal phalangeal joint of the great toe.

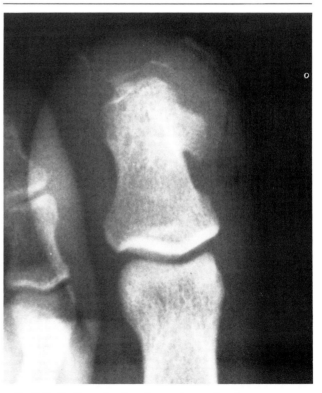

Fig. 9–8 Radiograph of a subungual osteochondroma.

calcaneus. Microfractures may create local tenderness. The radiographs show a large lucent area with a well-defined sclerotic margin. Treatment consists of either local irrigation with steroids or curettement and bone grafting.

Nonossifying Fibromas This lesion can also develop in the calcaneus and be large enough to cause a fracture. Again, curettement and bone grafting usually obliterate the lesion.

References

1. Ogden J: *Skeletal Injury in the Child.* Philadelphia, Lea & Febiger, 1982, pp 621–641.
2. Rang M: *Children's Fractures,* ed 2. Philadelphia, JB Lippincott, 1983, pp 223–330.
3. Rockwood CA Jr, Wilkins KE, King RE (eds): *Fractures: Vol III. Fractures in Children.* Philadelphia, JB Lippincott, 1984, pp 1043–1103.
4. Weber BG, Brumer C, Freuler F: *Treatment of Fractures in Children and Adolescents.* New York, Springer-Verlag, 1980, 385–393.
5. Sever JG: Apophysitis of the os calcis. *NY J Med* 1912;95:1025.
6. Jahss MH: *Disorders of the Foot.* Philadelphia, WB Saunders, 1983, vol 1, pp 203 and 204.
7. Zadek I, Gold AM: The accessory tarsal scaphoid. *J Bone Joint Surg* 1948;30A:957–968.
8. Sullivan JA, Miller WA: The relationship of the accessory navicular to the development of the flat foot. *Clin Orthop* 1979;144:233–237.
9. Veitch JM: Evaluation of the Kidner procedure in treatment of symptomatic accessory tarsal scaphoid. *Clin Orthop* 1978;131:210–213.
10. Forster RS: Reflex sympathetic dystrophy in children. *Orthopedics* 1985;8:475–477.
11. Ruggeri SB, Athreya BH, Doughty R, et al: Reflex sympathetic dystrophy in children. *Clin Orthop* 1982;163:225–230.
12. Bernstein BH, Singsen BH, Kent JT, et al: Reflex neurovascular dystrophy in childhood. *J Pediatr* 1978;93:211–215.
13. Fermoglich DR: Reflex sympathetic dystrophy in children. *Pediatrics* 1977;60:881–883.
14. Tachdjian MO: *The Child's Foot.* Philadelphia, WB Saunders, 1985.
15. Coleman SS: *Complex Foot Deformities in Children.* Philadelphia, Lea & Febiger, l983.
16. Albrektsson B, Rydholm A, Rydholm U: The tarsal tunnel syndrome in children. *J Bone Joint Surg* 1982;64B:215–217.
17. Langan P, Weiss CA: Subluxation of the tibialis posterior, a complication of tarsal tunnel decompression: A case report. *Clin Orthop* 1980;146:226–227.
18. Mann RA: Tarsal tunnel syndrome, in Evart CM (ed): *Surgery of the Musculoskeletal System.* New York, Churchill Livingstone, l983, vol 9, pp 79–84.
19. Freiberg AH: Infraction of the second metatarsal bone. *Surg Gynecol Obstet* 1914;19:191–193.
20. Braddock GTF: Experimental epiphysial injury and Freiberg's disease. *J Bone Joint Surg* 1959;41B:154–159.
21. Bordelon RL: Silicone implant for Freiberg's disease. *South Med J* 1977;70:1002–1004.
22. Kyne PJ, Mankin HJ: Changes in intra-articular pressure with subtalar motion with special reference to the etiology of peroneal spastic flat foot. *Bull Hosp Joint Dis* 1965;26:181–185.
23. Kaye JJ, Ghelman B, Schneider B: Talocalcaneal navicular joint arthrography for sustentacular-talar tarsal coalitions. *Radiology* 1975;115:730–731.
24. Stoskopf CA, Hernandez RJ, Kelikian A, et al: Evaluation of tarsal coalition by computed tomography. *J Pediatr Orthop* 1984;4:365–369.
25. Mosier KM, Asher M: Tarsal coalitions and peroneal spastic flat foot: A review. *J Bone Joint Surg* 1984;66A:976–984.
26. Cowell HR, Elener V: Rigid painful flatfoot secondary to tarsal coalition. *Clin Orthop* 1983;177:54–60.
27. Russo V, Means DC: Fat graft interposition: An adjunct to resection of calcaneonavicular bar. *Orthopedics* 1980;3:407–409.
28. Brand RA, Black H: Pseudomonas osteomyelitis following puncture wounds in children. *J Bone Joint Surg* 1974;56A:1637–1642.
29. Miller EH, Semian DW: Gram-negative osteomyelitis following puncture wounds of the foot. *J Bone Joint Surg* 1975;57A:535–537.
30. Landon GC, Johnson KA, Dahlin DC: Subungual exostoses. *J Bone Joint Surg* 1979;61A:256–259.

Surgical Correction of Clubfoot

Douglas W. McKay, MD

The major deformity in clubfeet is in the subtalar complex. The navicular is displaced medially around the head of the talus and articulates with the medial malleolus. The calcaneocuboid joint is deformed because of internal rotation and adduction. The internal rotation that causes the subtalar complex deformity and the progressive medial plantar angulation of the talar neck is in the talocalcaneal (subtalar) joint (Fig. 10–1). The rotation in the subtalar joint causes the calcaneus to be displaced medially under the head and neck of the talus anterior to the ankle joint. The calcaneus pivots on the interosseous ligament and is displaced laterally toward the lateral malleolus posterior to the ankle joint. Thus, when correcting the deformity, the surgeon has to realign the talonavicular and calcaneocuboid joint and push the calcaneus anterior to the calcaneocuboid joint laterally. Posterior to the ankle joint, the calcaneus has to be pushed medially toward the medial malleolus. Pushing the calcaneus medially posterior to the ankle contradicts established principles.

There are two indications for surgical correction of clubfoot: (1) failure to obtain correction in six to eight weeks with casts, and (2) two recurrences after correction.

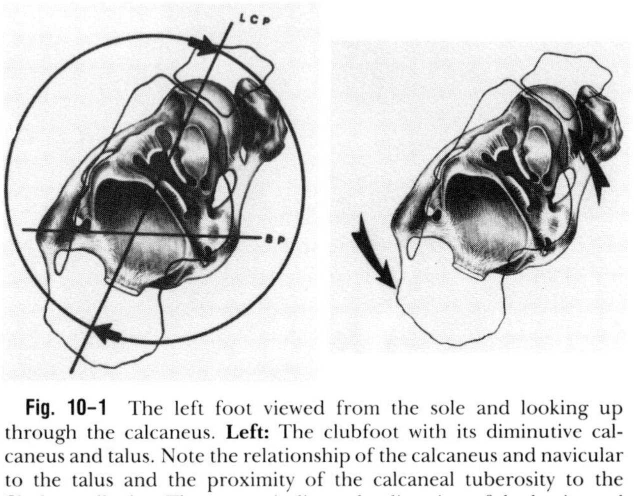

Criteria for Surgical Correction

How is surgical correction determined? The more rigid the criteria for correction, the higher the percentage of cases that come to surgery. Ninety-five percent of the clubfeet that I treat come to surgery because they do not meet the following criteria for correction: (1) an 85 to 90 degree angle between the bimalleolar plane and longitudinal axis of the foot (Fig. 10–2); (2) foot dorsiflexion 10 to 15 degrees above neutral; (3) walking with normal foot strike and without internal rotation, the heel and forefoot in neutral position; and (4) anteroposterior and lateral radiographs showing a normal relationship and placement of the talus to calcaneus and of the navicular to talus and cuboid to calcaneus. That is, an anteroposterior radiograph that shows a divergent angle of 20 degrees between the calcaneus and talus and a lateral radiograph that shows the head of the talus overlapping the calcaneus by 0.25 inch.

Fig. 10-1 The left foot viewed from the sole and looking up through the calcaneus. **Left:** The clubfoot with its diminutive calcaneus and talus. Note the relationship of the calcaneus and navicular to the talus and the proximity of the calcaneal tuberosity to the fibular malleolus. The arrows indicate the direction of the horizontal talocalcaneal rotation. BP, bimalleolar plane; LCP, longitudinal calcaneal plane or axis of the calcaneus and cuboid. **Right:** Placement of force to correct horizontal talocalcaneal rotation in the clubfoot. As shown by the arrows, force should be exerted toward the tibial malleolus anterior to the ankle joint on the medial side of the calcaneocuboid joint and posterior to the ankle on the lateral side of the calcaneal tuberosity. (Reproduced with permission from McKay DW: New concept of and approach to clubfoot treatment: Section I. Principles and morbid anatomy. *J Pediatr Orthop* 1982;2:347–356.)

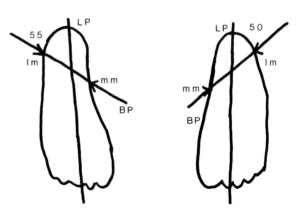

Fig. 10-2 Simple way to determine the relationship of the bimalleolar plane (BP) to the longitudinal plane (LP) of the foot. Have the patient stand or sit while pressing the foot against a sheet of paper. Draw an outline of the foot, marking the lateral malleolus (lm) and the medial malleolus (mm). (The medial malleolus may be difficult to identify if it is located anteriorly.) Draw lines BP and LP and measure the resulting angle. The angles shown here are 55 and 50 degrees. The normal angle is 80 to 90 degrees. (Adapted with permission from McKay DW: New concept of and approach to clubfoot treatment: Section II. Correction of the clubfoot. *J Pediatr Orthop* 1983;3:10–21.)

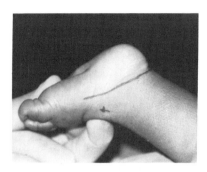
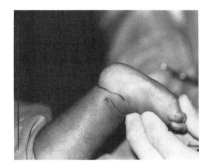
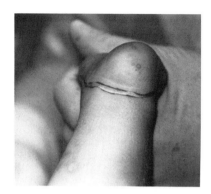
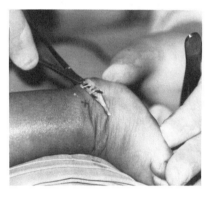

Fig. 10-3 Three photographs showing a transverse skin incision. The medial and lateral malleolus are marked (X). **Top left:** Medial side of left foot. **Top center:** Lateral side of left foot. **Top right:** Posterior view of left foot. **Bottom:** Lateral view showing preservation of the veins and sural nerve. (Reproduced with permission from McKay DW: New concept of and approach to clubfoot treatment: Section II. Correction of the clubfoot. *J Pediatr Orthop* 1983;3:10–21.)

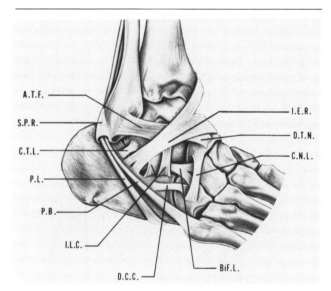

Fig. 10-4 The clubfoot from the lateral aspect. A.T.F., anterior talofibular ligament; S.P.R., superior peroneal retinaculum; C.T.L., lateral talocalcaneal ligament; P.L., peroneus longus tendon; P.B., peroneus brevis tendon; I.L.C., interosseous ligament (cervical ligament); D.C.C., dorsal calcaneocuboid ligament; BiF.L., bifurcated ligament; C.N.L., cubonavicular oblique ligament; D.T.N., dorsal talonavicular ligament; I.E.R., inferior extensor retinaculum (cruciate crural ligament). (Reproduced with permission from McKay DW: New concept of and approach to clubfoot treatment: Section I. Principles and morbid anatomy. *J Pediatr Orthop* 1982;2:347–356.)

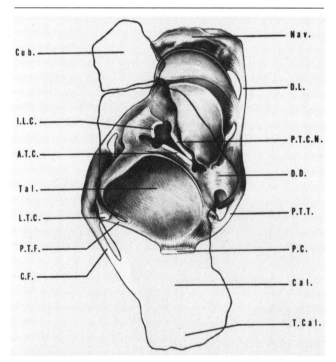

Fig. 10-5 The normal foot. The relationship of the subtalar complex. Cub., cuboid; I.L.C., interosseous ligament (cervical ligament); A.T.C., anterior ligament of subtalar joint (posterior talocalcaneal joint); Tal., talus; L.T.C., lateral talocalcaneal ligament; P.T.F., posterior talofibular ligament; C.F., calcaneofibular ligament; Nav., navicular; D.L., deltoid ligament (tibial talonavicular ligament); P.T.C.N., posterior ligament of the talocalcaneonavicular joint; D.D., deep deltoid (tibiotalar ligament); P.T.T., posterior talotibial ligament; P.C., posterior talocalcaneal ligament and capsule; Cal., calcaneus; T. Cal., calcaneal tuberosity. (Reproduced with permission from McKay DW: New concept of and approach to clubfoot treatment: Section I. Principles and morbid anatomy. *J Pediatr Orthop* 1982;2:347–356.)

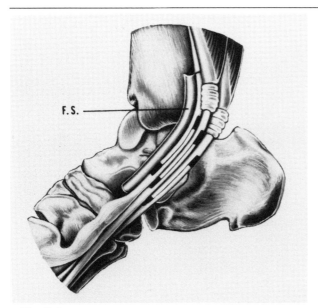

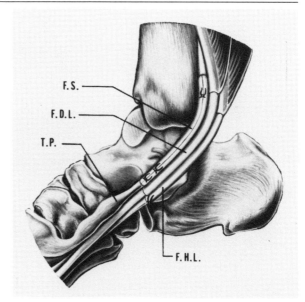

Fig. 10-6 Left: Lengthened tibialis posterior, flexor digitorum longus, and flexor hallucis longus tendons. The sheaths of the toe flexor tendons are freed and recessed above the ankle, and the sheath of the tibialis posterior is opened. **Right:** The tendons are repaired with the sheaths covering the tendons and the ankle joint. (Reproduced with permission from McKay DW: New concept of and approach to clubfoot treatment. Section II. Correction of the clubfoot. *J Pediatr Orthop* 1983;3:10–21.)

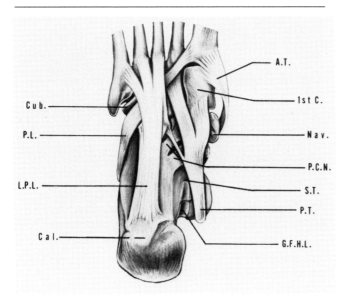

Fig. 10-7 The clubfoot from the interior direction with the deep ligaments and tendons of the hindfoot shown. Cub., cuboid; P.L., peroneus longus tendon; L.P.L., long plantar ligament; Cal., calcaneus; A.T., tibialis anterior tendon; 1st C., first or medial cuneiform; Nav., navicular; P.C.N., plantar calcaneonavicular ligament (spring ligament); S.T., sustentaculum tali; P.T., tibialis posterior tendon; G.F.H.L., groove of the flexor hallucis longus tendon. (Reproduced with permission from McKay DW: New concept of and approach to clubfoot treatment: Section I. Principles and morbid anatomy. *J Pediatr Orthop* 1982;2:347–356.)

Fig. 10-8 Checking the foot position with the surgeon's thumb and index finger holding the tibial and fibular malleolus. Note the pin between the first and second toes. The angle between the longitudinal plane and the bimalleolar plane of the foot is 85 to 90 degrees, as shown by the surgeon's fingers. (Reproduced with permission from McKay DW: New concept of and approach to clubfoot treatment: Section II. Correction of the clubfoot. *J Pediatr Orthop* 1983;3:10–21.)

Surgical Procedure

Operating with the patient in a prone position using a Cincinnati incision gives excellent exposure and is an excellent position for teaching. The Cincinnati incision should be done with care in a severe deformity, especially severe equinus. The incision can be dangerous if the operation must be repeated after the more traditional posterior medial release. Complete slough of the heel pad can occur in children with myelodysplasia.

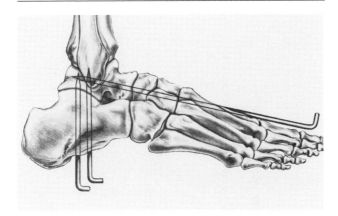

Fig. 10-9 Placement of pins in the foot following surgical correction. Pins passed up through the heel do not cross the ankle joint. (Reproduced with permission from McKay DW: New concept of and approach to clubfoot treatment: Section II. Correction of the clubfoot. *J Pediatr Orthop* 1983;3:10–21.)

Figure 10–3 shows medial, lateral, and posterior views of a transverse skin incision.

Start the Cincinnati incision laterally and continue medially to release the deformity of the foot. Elevate the origin of the extensor digitorum brevis to expose the inferior extensor retinaculum and cervical portion of the interosseous ligament and incise them off the calcaneus. This incision of the extensor retinaculum and interosseous ligament exposes the calcaneocuboid joint and the capsule over the head of the talus. Open the calcaneocuboid joint dorsally and the capsule over the talus laterally (Fig. 10–4) protecting the sural nerve and vein (Fig. 10–3, *bottom*).

Elevate the peroneal tendons and sheath by a sharp dissection off the calcaneus that includes the superior peroneal retinaculum and exposes the fibulocalcaneal ligament. Take the fibulocalcaneal ligament off of the calcaneus by a sharp dissection that leaves as much length as possible so that it can be resutured to the calcaneus. Elevate the skin and subcutaneous tissue over the Achilles tendon and medial malleolus dorsally to lengthen the Achilles tendon. Then lengthen the Achilles tendon in a coronal direction and preserve the fat pad anterior to the Achilles tendon. This fat pad is left attached to the calcaneus to cover the ankle joint later (Fig. 10–5).

Skin and subcutaneous dissection is started medially to expose the medial malleolus and distally to expose the medial cuneiform. Inferior dissection is then performed to expose the abductor hallucis and calcaneal branch of the lateral plantar nerve. The abductor hallucis is elevated from its origin distally and about half of the muscle is excised and removed. Open the sheath of the posterior tibial tendon over the medial malleolus and note how far anterior the medial malleolus appears in relation to the foot (Fig. 10–6, *left*). The posterior tibial tendon also appears more anteriorly located from

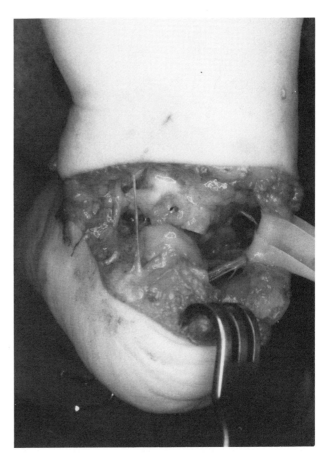

Fig. 10-10 Corrected clubfoot without the posteromedial portion of the talus. The heel is in a neutral position and the talocalcaneal joint is distorted. (Reproduced with permission from McKay DW: New concept of and approach to clubfoot treatment: Section I. Principles and morbid anatomy. *J Pediatr Orthop* 1982;2:347–356.)

this perspective. The sheath is opened down the foot until its insertion in the navicular and its attachment to the sustentaculum tali is found. The tendon is then "z" lengthened and the insertion into the sustentaculum tali is incised (Fig. 10–6).

Both the medial and lateral plantar nerves and then the neurovascular bundle are freed. To free the lateral plantar nerve, incise the medial flexor retinaculum, plantar fascia, flexor digitorum brevis, and abductor digiti quinti from the calcaneus. In order for these structures to slide distally, the surgeon has to incise attachments of skin and subcutaneous fat from plantar fascia distally and incise a piece of fascia between the medial and lateral plantar nerves that are attached to the sustentaculum tali. A master knot under the navicular is incised, exposing the flexor hallucis longus (FHL) and flexor digitorum longus (FDL). The sheath and fibrous attachments are incised from the tendons. The sheath of the FHL and FDL is recessed by a sharp dissection from the calcaneus and talus that starts distally and progresses proximally to just above the ankle

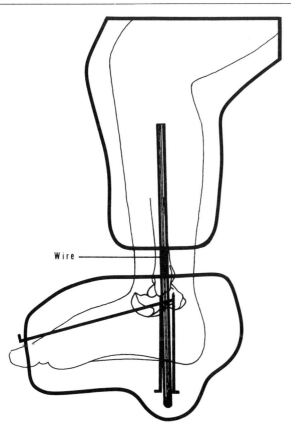

Wire

Fig. 10-11 The hinge cast. Note the ankle joint with the three pins in place and the 90-degree angle of the knee. The cast boot incorporates the foot and pins and is connected to the long-leg cylinder with 14- or 16-gauge stranded wire. (Reproduced with permission from McKay DW: New concept of and approach to clubfoot treatment: Section II. Correction of the clubfoot. *J Pediatr Orthop* 1983;3:10–21.)

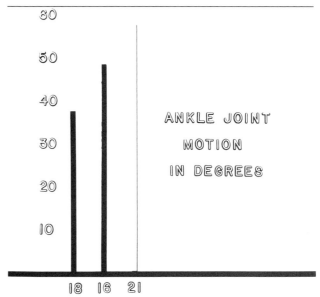

ANKLE JOINT
MOTION
IN DEGREES

18 16 21

Fig. 10-12 Graph shows progressively improved ankle motion with changes in procedure in 18 cases treated with correction of subtalar rotation alone, 16 treated with correction of subtalar rotation and sheath recession, and 21 treated with correction of subtalar recession, sheath recession, and a hinge cast.

joint. This dissection is achieved by entering the opened sheath of the posterior tibialis under the quadratus planti posteriorly. It is difficult to get the sheath off the talus under the FHL because of the FHL grooves. The purpose of this procedure is to preserve function in the FHL and gain ankle joint motion.

Using the posterior tendon as a guide to the talonavicular joint, open the talonavicular joint with a sharp dissection cutting all the way around the capsule, spring ligament, and deltoid ligament to the navicular (Fig. 10–7). Be careful not to destroy any of the articular cartilage of the joints. Elevate the quadratus planti with a blunt dissection off the calcaneus and expose the long plantar ligament. Elevate the long plantar ligament from the calcaneus with a sharp dissection. Free the talonavicular and calcaneocuboid joints by completely incising the capsule and bifid ligament. Be careful not to cut the peroneus longus tendon, which is just lateral to the calcaneocuboid joint. The FHL and FDL are not lengthened unless it is absolutely necessary.

Next, open the ankle posteriorly by capsulotomy. Incise a little of the posterior deltoid ligament and lengthen the posterior fibulotalar ligament. Some-

times, the fibulotalar ligament may have to be incised to enable the talus to roll back into the ankle joint. Open the subtalar joint all the way around, and cut the deep anterior and posterior talocalcaneal ligaments if they do not allow easy correction.

Positioning the foot is the most important and difficult thing to do (Fig. 10–8). First, look at the amount of medial deviation of the talus neck. If there is a lot of deviation, pass a pin through the talus from the posterior to the anterior direction so that the pin comes out laterally on the head of the talus. Place the navicular in front of the head of the talus in relation to dorsal and plantar directions. The navicular and cuneiform should be in line with the body of the talus, not the head of the talus. Therefore, after positioning, a fair amount of cartilage from the head of the talus is showing. Position the calcaneus under the talus and note the severe subtalar joint incongruity. Determine the correct rotation of the calcaneus by lining up the axis of the foot 90 degrees to the bimalleolar plane (Fig. 10–8). The calcaneus has to be pushed medially toward the medial malleolus, causing severe subtalar joint incongruity, and then pinned with two pins to maintain the correct rotation (Fig. 10–9). Do not cross the ankle joint with pins. Be careful not to push the calcaneus posteriorly. In some feet, the calcaneal cuboid joint is so severely deformed that pin placement is necessary to prevent forefoot adduction (Fig. 10–10).

Examine the foot and move the ankle joint for normal appearance and motion. The Achilles tendon, tibialis posterior tendon, flexor sheath, calcaneofibular ligament, and posterior fibulotalar ligament are repaired with 4-0 nylon suture thread. Decrease the tourniquet pressure and control major bleeding. Note the blood supply to the heel. Suture the skin and, with the knee bent at a 90-degree angle, place the leg in a Jones pressure dressing covered by a layer of plaster.

Postoperative Care

Apply a hinge cast seven to ten days postoperatively (Fig. 10–11). A hinge cast is applied using a long-leg cylinder with the knee at a 90-degree angle. Place a boot cast over the pins and foot and loop a multifilament 16- to 19-gauge wire around the heel. Run the wire along the side of the leg in the same plane as the bimalleolar plane of the foot. Roll plaster over the wire leaving the ankle free for motion. The child's caretaker should move the ankle, particularly in plantar flexion, with each diaper change for five weeks.

The cast and pins are removed six weeks after surgery. A child who is not walking is placed in a short-leg cast for two weeks. A walking child is placed in a walking cast for four weeks. After removing the short-leg cast, parents should stretch the ankle and encourage the child to walk on the toes. Special shoes should not be needed. Figure 10–12 shows the improvement in ankle motion with progressive changes in procedure.

Pathoanatomy and Surgical Treatment of the Resistant Clubfoot

Norris C. Carroll, MD, FRCS(C)

Introduction

Anatomists and surgeons have been studying clubfoot since Hippocrates' first written description.[1] "Idiopathic clubfoot is the result of a multifactorial inheritance system modified by environmental factors. Male risk is greater because of a lowered gene threshold number."[2] The etiology of clubfoot is unknown. Numerous hypotheses have been proposed implicating such causes as arrested embryologic development, intrauterine mechanical forces, myodysplasia, muscle imbalance, local dysplasia in the foot, nutrition, hormones, and infection.[3-6]

In idiopathic congenital clubfoot, the ankle is in equinus and the forefoot is adducted and supinated. Other morphologic features, such as tibial torsion, rotation of the talus within the ankle mortice, subluxation of the talonavicular joint, shortening of the deltoid ligament, and abnormal tendon insertions have been described.[7-11] Medial and plantar deviation of the talus neck is the structural deformity that has been demonstrated consistently in anatomic dissections (Fig. 11-1).[12-20] Treatment of congenital clubfoot varies from manipulation alone to a posterior, medial, plantar, and lateral release, or a triple arthrodesis.[21-39]

In 1971, we studied a group of patients in their second and third decades who had required surgery to correct their resistant clubfoot deformity.[40] Our initial treatment was manipulation of the deformed foot, and then the application of a plaster cast to maintain the position obtained by the manipulation. We assumed that forefoot supination and adduction

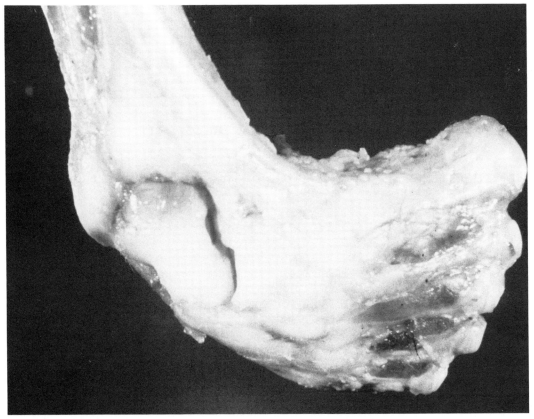

Fig. 11-1 Superior lateral view of the right clubfoot from a stillborn fetus. Note the anterior extrusion of the talus; the talar body pointing laterally; the talar neck curved medially; and the navicular subluxated against the medial malleolus.

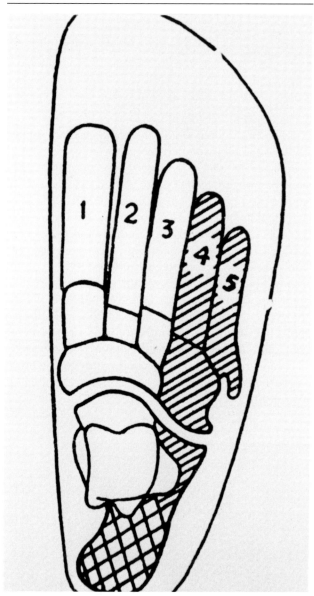

Fig. 11-2 The two columns of the foot. The os calcis, cuboid, and fourth and fifth metatarsals make up the lateral column. The talus, navicular, cuneiforms, and the first three metatarsals make up the medial column.

could be satisfactorily corrected, even though ankle equinus persisted. Each foot with persistent ankle equinus was then treated by Achilles tendon lengthening and a posterior capsulotomy.

We found that patients with a residual clubfoot deformity often functioned well in their second and third decades in spite of the deformity.[40] The patient's ability to function with a clubfoot varied inversely with the number of surgical procedures on the foot. When forefoot adduction and supination persisted, the lateral malleolus was in a far posterior position, the neck of the talus was directed laterally and the navicular was subluxated medially. Other studies showed that the bony architecture was abnormal in all resistant

clubfeet.[41–43] Because the appearance and function of the clubfoot varied inversely with the number of operations on it, we considered correcting all the components of the resistant clubfoot deformity at the same time. To determine the validity of this approach, it was first necessary to identify the pathoanatomy of the resistant clubfoot and then study ways to correct it.

Initial Anatomic Studies

When we first began studying the pathoanatomy of resistant clubfeet, we were reminded of the nursery tale of the three blind men and the elephant; each time we looked at a deformed foot, we seemed to recognize something different.

We dissected 17 normal embryologic and fetal feet from 8 to 20 weeks of gestational age. These feet were examined with a dissecting microscope and sections of some feet were made. Even in the youngest feet we studied, the mesenchymal condensation of the early cartilage model of the navicular had a normal relationship with the head of the talus, although the first metatarsal in the younger feet tended to be in varus. The feet of the 8-week embryo showed no clubfoot deformity. It was difficult to draw conclusions from examining younger embryos since the foot could be manipulated into almost any position.[44]

Next, we studied the untreated clubfeet in a premature stillborn infant, the untreated clubfeet in a full-term stillborn infant, and the recurrent clubfoot of a baby who had expired. In addition to tight tendons, capsules, and ligaments, these dissections demonstrated that the lateral malleolus was directed posteriorly, the neck of the talus pointed laterally, and the navicular was subluxated medially toward the medial malleolus. The body of the talus was externally rotated in the ankle mortice.[40] Beatson and Pearson[41] showed that on the lateral radiograph, the ossific nuclei of the talus and os calcis were parallel. It was clear that the equinus of the os calcis could not be corrected until there was restoration of the normal divergence between the talus and os calcis. We found that a clubfoot assumed a normal appearance if, after releasing the tight posterior calcaneofibular and talofibular ligaments, we medially rotated the body of the talus in the ankle mortice and reduced the navicular onto the head of the talus.

Dissection of a recurrent clubfoot in a 1-year-old child demonstrated the same anatomic relationships.[40] Dissection of an amputation specimen from an 8-year-old boy showed that if the talus was rotated laterally in the ankle mortice and the navicular was displaced medially against the medial malleolus, the foot assumed a clubfoot appearance.[40]

As a result of these studies, we concluded that if the clubfoot deformity persisted after eight to 12 weeks

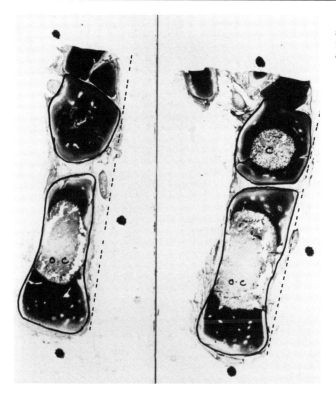

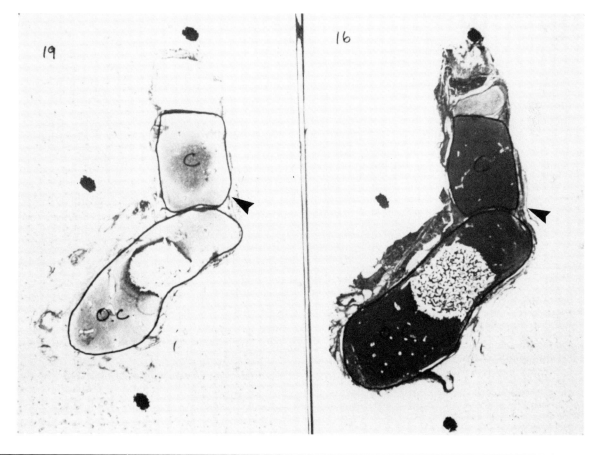

Fig. 11–3 Horizontal sections through a normal foot (**top**) and a clubfoot (**bottom**). Note the straight lateral border in the normal foot (dotted line). The clubfoot shows medial displacement (arrow) of the cuboid (c) in relation to the long axis of the os calcis (oc).

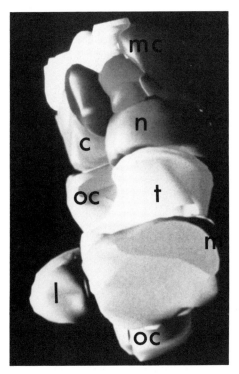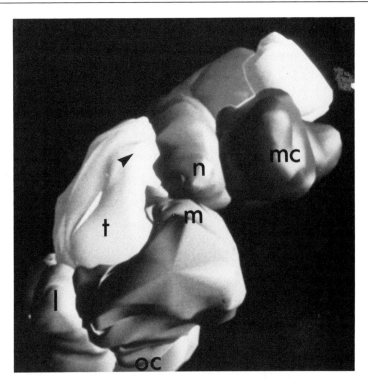

Fig. 11–4   Three-dimensional reconstruction of a normal foot, superior view (**left**). Three-dimensional reconstruction of a clubfoot, superior view (**right**). In the clubfoot, note the medial displacement of the navicular (n); the anterior extrusion of the talus (t) with the body pointing laterally and an increased declination of the talar neck (arrow); the medial rotation of the os calcis (oc); and the supination of the forefoot. m, medial malleolus; l, lateral malleolus; c, cuboid; mc, medial cuneiform.

of manipulations and cast applications, a surgical correction should be performed.

Our initial surgical procedure was a medial and posterior release.[40] A Z-lengthening of the tendo Achillis and tibialis posterior tendons was done, and the flexor hallucis longus was treated either by a tenotomy or recession. The body of the talus was internally rotated in the ankle mortice by placing a K-wire through the long axis of the body from the posterior approach. This K-wire was advanced through the head of the talus and across the navicular after the adductus and supination of the forefoot had been corrected. After several years, it became apparent that we were not giving enough consideration to the tight plantar structures and the lateral side of the foot. In addition to a medial and posterior release, a plantar and lateral release was often necessary.

There are two columns to the foot, a medial column and a lateral column.[45] The lateral column consists of the os calcis, cuboid, and fourth and fifth metatarsals. The medial column consists of the talus, navicular, three cuneiforms, and the first, second, and third metatarsals (Fig. 11–2). For years clubfoot surgeons have discussed the medial displacement of the navicular in relation to the talus head. If the distal portion of the medial column is displaced medially, the distal portion of the lateral column must be displaced medially as

well, since the medial and lateral columns are joined together. This means that in a severely resistant clubfoot, the cuboid is displaced medially (Fig. 11–3).

New Anatomic Studies

Until recently, there were still wide differences in opinion about the positional relationships between the various bones of the hindfoot complex. It was easier for investigators to describe the gross morphology of individual bones than to describe the relationship between the talus and os calcis, the talus and navicular, and the os calcis and cuboid. When the restraining ligaments are removed to expose these bones, their exact positional relationships are disturbed.

When doing a radiographic assessment of clubfoot, it is difficult to draw valid conclusions about anatomic relationships, because a great portion of the "bony architecture" is still cartilaginous. However, the talocalcaneal angles, as seen in the anteroposterior and lateral radiographic projections, have been used to assess the severity of a clubfoot deformity and the results of treatment.[41,43,46–48]

A normal talus has a body, a head, and a neck. The axis of the body does not correspond to the axis of the head and neck.[13–15,18,49] Shapiro and Glimcher have

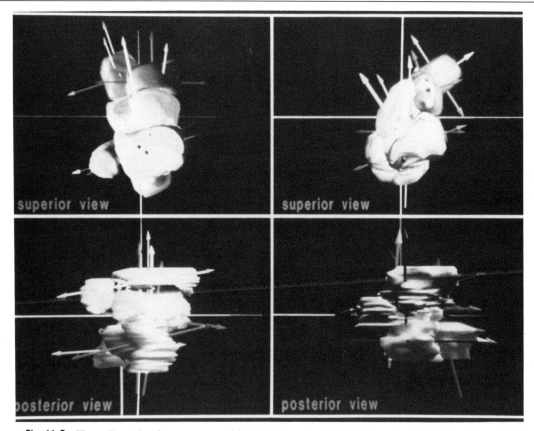

Fig. 11–5 Three-dimensional computer models. Models on the left show the axes of the bones in a normal foot. Models on the right show the axes of the bones in a clubfoot.

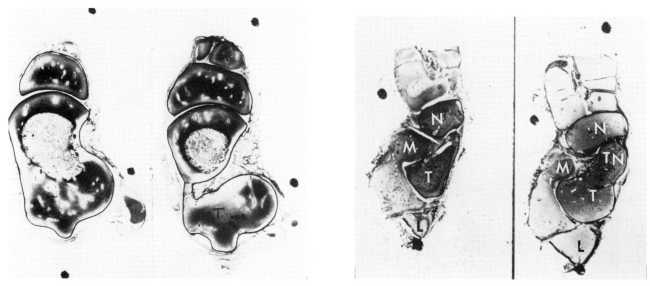

Fig. 11–6 Horizontal sections through the talus (T) and navicular (N) of a normal foot (**left**) and a clubfoot (**right**). Note the anterior extrusion of the talar body in the clubfoot as well as the increased declination of the talar neck (TN) and the medial displacement of the navicular. M, medial malleolus; L, lateral malleolus.

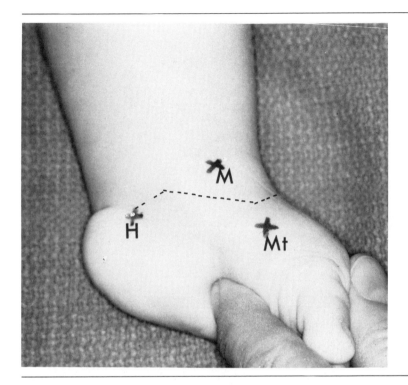

Fig. 11-7 Medial view of the left foot. H, center of heel; M, front of medial malleolus; Mt, base of first metatarsal. The dotted line outlines the skin incision. The central portion of the line is parallel to the sole of the foot and bisects the H-M-Mt triangle.

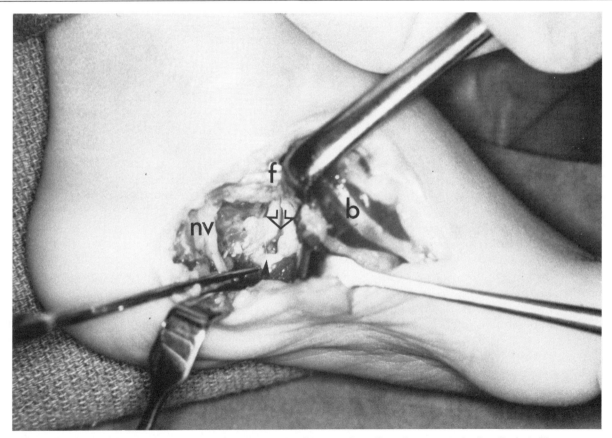

Fig. 11-8 Medial incision exposes the abductor hallucis (b), flexor tendons (f), and neurovascular bundle (nv). The peroneus longus tendon elevated on the nerve hook (black arrow) is the guide to the calcaneocuboid joint (open arrow).

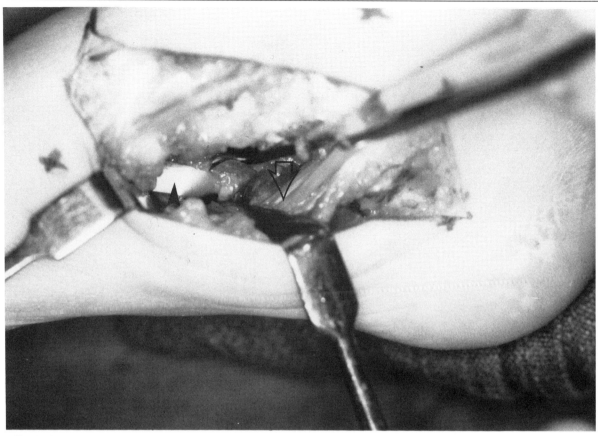

Fig. 11-9 Medial incision of the right foot. The solid arrow points to the peroneus longus tendon. The flexor hallucis longus and flexor digitorum tendons are retracted toward the sole (open arrow).

demonstrated that the ossific nucleus of a clubfoot talus is positioned eccentrically in the neck of the talus.[20] Therefore, it is difficult to draw conclusions based on one line drawn through an eccentric ossific nucleus in a clubfoot when we know that one line cannot be used to describe a normal talus axis.

Arthrography has been proposed as a method of improving the radiographic interpretation of interpositional bony relationships in a clubfoot, but these studies are difficult.[50,51] Computed tomography (CT) is of value in studying residual deformity in the foot of an older child,[52] but CT does not accurately define the positional relationships of the bones in an infant, since it is almost impossible to know where the cartilaginous "bone" ends and the ligaments begin.

In spite of numerous dissections, histologic sections, radiographs, and CT scans, it was still not possible to resolve even the simple question of how the body of the talus was oriented in the ankle mortice.[9] McKay thought that there was neutral alignment,[53,54] Goldner that there was internal rotation,[55] and I thought that there was external rotation.[40] What was needed to measure positional relationships was a method of removing individual bones from a clubfoot, analyzing them for shape, defining their position in space by an X, Y, and Z axis, and then replacing them in their original anatomic position. A three-dimensional computer modeling technique was one way of accomplishing a positional analysis of this kind.

Two feet were studied by three-dimensional computer modeling.[56] One was a left clubfoot from an otherwise normal stillborn baby. The second foot was a normal left foot from a 3-week-old term infant who died of congenital heart disease. The feet were suspended and fixed in 10% neutral-buffered formalin, decalcified in 25% formic acid, and embedded in paraffin. Embedding three reference markers in the paraffin prior to sectioning ensured accurate stacking of the sections for digitization. The feet were sliced into 250 sections, stained with safranin O, mounted on glass slides, and projected on a screen for digitization. Each bone was assigned its own color. The information was processed and three-dimensional images were reconstructed (Fig. 11-4). A graphic computer representation of the clubfoot demonstrates posterior positioning of the lateral malleolus, anterior extrusion of the talus with medial curvature of the talus neck, and medial displacement of the navicular against the medial malleolus. The posterior part of the os calcis is adjacent to the lateral malleolus and the front of

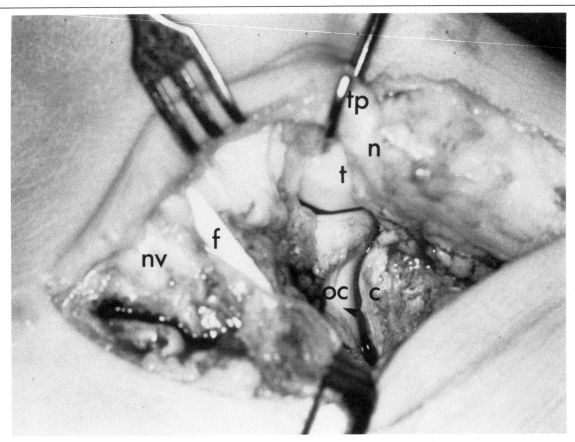

Fig. 11-10   Medial incision of the left foot exposes the neurovascular bundle (nv), flexor digitorum longus (f), os calcis (oc), cuboid (c), talus (t), navicular (n), and tibialis posterior (tp). Note that during the correction, the navicular has moved away from the medial malleolus exposing articular cartilage on the medial side of the head of the talus. (The tendon of the tibialis posterior is being retracted superiorly.) The cuboid is moved laterally, exposing articular cartilage on the distal os calcis (arrow).

the os calcis is rotated medially. The cuboid is displaced medially in relation to the long axis of the os calcis. The forefoot is adducted and supinated as demonstrated by the stacking of the cuneiforms and metatarsal bases. This forefoot position is easily visualized in the superior view of the reconstructed foot (Fig. 11–4, *right*). The posterior view of the normal foot allows a view through the ankle mortice, whereas in the clubfoot the os calcis is rotated toward the lateral malleolus. With the anterior extrusion of the talus in the clubfoot, very little of the talus is visible posteriorly. In addition, the posterior view also demonstrates the medial displacement of the cuboid in relation to the long axis of the os calcis. The medial view also demonstrates the supination and adductus of the forefoot and the medial displacement of the cuboid.

Computer technology also enables us to draw vectors that represent the ankle mortice, the axes of the talus body and neck, and the axes of the os calcis, navicular, and cuboid. These axes demonstrate the increased inclination of the talus neck in the clubfoot, the medial displacement of the navicular toward the

medial malleolus, the medial displacement of the cuboid in relation to the long axis of the os calcis, and the medial rotation of the os calcis. In addition, three-dimensional computer modeling shows that the body of the talus is externally rotated in the ankle mortice (Fig. 11–5).

From dissections, CT examinations, surgical experience, and three-dimensional computer analysis of a severe clubfoot, I conclude that: (1) When the patella points forward, the lateral malleolus is posterior. There is not an internal tibial torsion in congenital clubfoot. (This can be proven by CT scan when one makes a cut through the femoral condyles and a second cut through the ankle mortice.) (2) There is a cavus component to a clubfoot deformity[34] that can be corrected only by lengthening the plantar fascia and intrinsic muscles. (3) There are two columns to the foot, a medial column and a lateral column.[44] If there is medial displacement of the distal portion of the medial column, there must be medial displacement of the distal portion of the lateral column. This means that the cuboid is displaced medially. (4) With the cavus and medial displacement of the cuboid, there is a

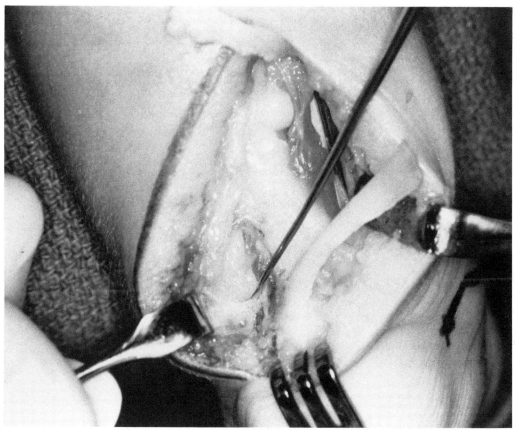

Fig. 11-11 Posterior view of the left foot. The nerve hook demonstrates the posterior calcaneofibular ligament.

contracture of the long and short plantar ligaments and the spring ligament. (5) When the os calcis and talus are ossified, the long axis of the os calcis and the body of the talus are parallel as viewed in the anteroposterior and lateral radiographs of the hindfoot.[41,43] (6) The os calcis is in equinus. (7) The talus is in equinus. (8) The triceps surae, tibialis posterior, flexor hallucis, and flexor digitorum longus are all short. (9) There is a contracture of the posterior capsule and the collateral ligaments of the ankle. (10) When one does a Z-plasty of the tendo Achillis and pushes up on the foot, the equinus does not correct until the tight posterior capsule of the ankle joint is released. This release must include division of the tight posterolateral structures, namely, the posterior calcaneofibular ligament and the posterior talofibular ligament.[57] (11) The navicular is subluxated medially against the medial malleolus (Fig. 11–6).[21] There is medial and plantar deviation of the talus neck and external rotation of the talus body in the ankle mortice (Fig. 11–6, *right*).[40] (12) During the correction of a clubfoot deformity, the body of the talus should be internally rotated in the ankle mortice. (13) When the body of the talus is internally rotated in the ankle

mortice, the os calcis must move down and away from the lateral malleolus. That is, the back of the os calcis moves medially while the front of the os calcis moves laterally. When this divergence is accomplished, the hypoplastic posterior facet of the subtalar joint is easily visualized and there is not a congruous fit of the talus and os calcis.

Surgical Treatment

A clubfoot that cannot be corrected with three months of serial manipulations and cast applications should be treated surgically.

Two incisions are used, a curvilinear medial incision and a posterior lateral incision. The landmarks for the medial incision are the center of the os calcis, the front of the medial malleolus, and the base of the first metatarsal. These three points define a triangle (Fig. 11–7). The incision is parallel with the base of the triangle, but curved in the plantar direction proximally, and curved in the anterior direction distally. The posterior lateral incision runs obliquely from the midline of the distal calf posteriorly to a point midway between the tendo Achillis and the lateral malleolus.

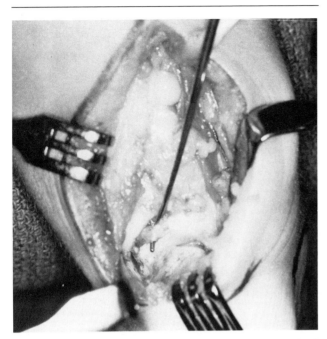

Fig. 11–12 Posterior incision of the left clubfoot. The nerve hook exposes the tight posterior talofibular ligament.

The medial incision exposes the abductor hallucis and frees it proximally from the os calcis (Fig. 11–8). The deep fascia is opened to expose the medial plantar artery and nerve and the lateral plantar artery and nerve. A plane is formed between the plantar fascia and the fat beneath the sole of the foot. The lateral plantar nerve and artery form a tunnel that passes toward the lateral side of the foot. Once the lateral plantar nerve and artery are visualized, it is possible to free the plantar fascia, flexor digitorum brevis, and abductor digiti minimi pedis from the os calcis by placing one blade of the scissors in the tunnel and one blade superficial to the plantar fascia.

At the back of the medial malleolus, the sheath of the flexor digitorum longus is opened and followed distally to Henry's knot where the flexor hallucis longus is identified. Both of these tendons are protected while the dissection is continued distally (Fig. 11–9). The tibialis anterior is identified on the dorsum of the foot and traced to the base of the first metatarsal. The flexor hallucis and flexor digitorum together with the neurovascular bundles are retracted in the plantar direction. The sheath of the peroneus longus tendon is identified and opened, and the tendon is traced proximally to the point where it curves around to the lateral border of the foot. The peroneus longus tendon is protected while the long and short plantar ligaments are divided (Fig. 11–9). This exposes the calcaneocuboid joint (Fig. 11–10).

Through the posterior incision, the sural nerve and short saphenous system are identified and protected by retraction in a lateral direction. The tendo Achillis

is exposed and divided in a sagittal plane separating the distal, medial half from the os calcis and the proximal, lateral half from the triceps surae. The deep fascia overlying the flexor hallucis longus and neurovascular bundle is opened, the bundle is freed distally and the flexor hallucis longus tendon is exposed distally to the level of the subtalar joint. In the lateral part of the wound, the peroneus longus and brevis tendons are identified and retracted laterally to expose the posterior calcaneofibular ligament (Fig. 11–11). Dissection is then continued medially and the fascia overlying the flexor digitorum longus and tibialis posterior is opened. The tibialis posterior tendon is identified and divided by means of a Z-plasty and a suture is attached to the distal portion of the tendon. A narrow retractor is placed underneath the flexor hallucis longus, neurovascular bundle, and flexor digitorum longus. The tip of the long, narrow retractor is brought out through the medial incision. The posterior capsule of the ankle and subtalar joint is opened and the tight posterior calcaneofibular and talofibular ligaments are divided (Fig. 11–12). The posterior portion of the deltoid ligament is divided posterior to the flexor digitorum longus. The back of the subtalar joint is opened. At this point, it should be possible to reduce the body of the talus into the ankle mortice.

Attention is then directed to the medial incision. The distal portion of the tibialis posterior tendon is pulled down through the sheath. The navicular is dissected away from the medial malleolus, and the talonavicular joint is opened medially and inferiorly by dividing the extensions of the tibialis posterior tendon and the spring ligament. A small, curved, blunt elevator is placed in both the talonavicular and calcaneocuboid joints, and the joints are opened so that any residual restricting soft tissue between the anteromedial portion of the os calcis and navicular can be divided.

The body of the talus is externally rotated in the ankle mortice. This can be seen through the posterior wound. A K-wire is placed in the long axis of the body posteriorly, and the body of the talus is internally rotated in the ankle mortice (Fig. 11–13). When the body of the talus is internally rotated in the ankle mortice, the back of the os calcis must move down and medially away from the fibula, while the front of the os calcis moves laterally away from the head of the talus. When the body of the talus has been reduced into the ankle mortice and divergence has been restored between the long axis of the talus body and os calcis, the supination and adduction of the forefoot is corrected. Then, the K-wire that was placed in the back of the talus body is advanced across the reduced mid-tarsal joint and through the skin on the dorsum of the forefoot proximal to the bases of the phalanges.

It is important to assess the quality of the clubfoot correction. The cavus component must be corrected.

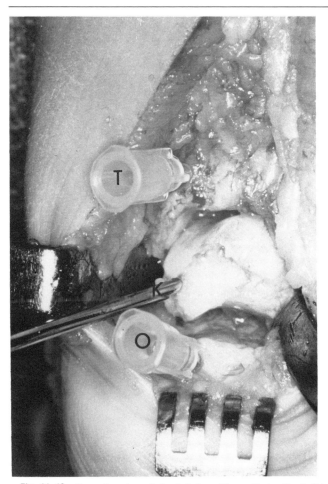 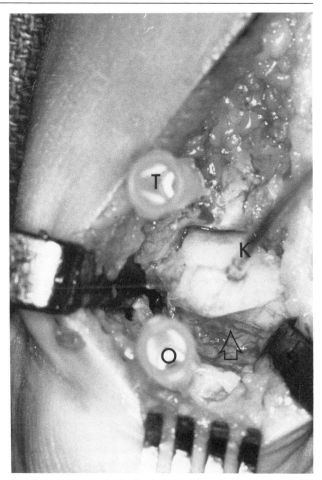

Fig. 11-13 Posterior view of the left foot. T, needle in distal tibia; O, needle in os calcis; K, K-wire in body of talus. The K-wire (**right**) in the body of the talus is used to correct the anterior extrusion and lateral rotation. Note the incongruity of the subtalar joint (arrow).

The heel must align with the long axis of the tibia, the lateral border of the foot must be straight, and the talonavicular and calcaneocuboid joints must be accurately reduced. If an inadequate plantar release is done, the navicular will tend to ride up onto the head of the talus, which will lead to cavus and a recurrent deformity. Displacing the navicular too far laterally will lead to an overcorrected, valgus foot.

The K-wire is advanced so that the back of the wire is flush with the cartilage at the back of the talus. The distal portion of the K-wire is cut against the retracted skin so that the wire is covered when the skin is pulled back into position. At this point, with the foot in a plantigrade position, the great toe has usually been pulled into flexion.

A two-level recession of the intramuscular portion of the flexor hallucis longus tendon is done. With the foot held in a plantigrade position, the tendo Achillis is repaired and the tibialis posterior is pulled back through its sheath and repaired (a small Hemovac drain should be placed in feet of older children when there is gross distortion of anatomic relationships).

The wounds are closed and a compressive dressing is applied that extends from the toes to the hip. Keeping the knee extended in the immediate postoperative period facilitates venous drainage.

The child goes home on the second postoperative day and is brought back to surgery one week later for cast application. The limb is treated in a below-knee cast for a period of twelve weeks. The casts are changed every three to four weeks. When the casts are removed, the feet are treated in an orthosis. This treatment is continued until the child is walking and there is clinical and radiographic evidence that the foot is remaining plantigrade.

The two principles of this technique are (1) to restore the bony architecture to a normal position, and (2) to balance the muscle forces to maintain the corrected position. This is an aggressive surgical approach. Overcorrection of the deformity can be avoided by preserving the anterior portion of the deltoid ligament, being careful not to overdisplace the navicular in a lateral direction, and by not overlengthening the tibialis posterior and tendo Achillis. Finally, the foot must not be placed in a cast in an overcorrected position.

In summary, the steps in the surgical procedure are as follows: (1) a plantar release, (2) a release of Henry's knot, (3) identification of the tibialis anterior, which will facilitate the identification of the peroneus longus tendon, (4) protection of the peroneus longus tendon while the long and short plantar ligaments are divided to expose the calcaneocuboid joint, (5) a Z-plasty of the tendo Achillis, (6) a Z-plasty of the tibialis posterior tendon, (7) a posterior capsulotomy, including the posterior calcaneofibular and posterior talofibular ligaments, (8) an open reduction of the talonavicular joint, (9) placement of a K-wire through the back of the talus body, and correction of the anterior extrusion and external rotation, (10) correction of the forefoot adductus and supination, (11) K-wire fixation of the midtarsal joint, and (12) repair of tendons with the foot held in a plantigrade position.

In 1983, Yoneda and I reported the results of surgical correction of 84 severe cases of clubfeet.[39] The minimum follow-up was five years. Nineteen percent of these feet required further surgery in the form of a plantar and lateral release. Since 1976, I have advocated the full release described in this chapter for a severe case of resistant clubfoot.

Discussion

There are still some differences in clubfoot management, and the exact cause of clubfoot remains unknown.

The three-dimensional computer model shows that the morphologic changes in a severe case of resistant clubfoot are increased declination of the talus neck, a small calcaneus with a hypoplastic sustentaculum and posterior facet, and a medial tilt of the calcaneocuboid joint. The computer model shows that the abnormal relationships are (1) anterior extrusion of the talus in the ankle mortice with the talus body uncovered anteriorly and laterally, and external rotation of the talus body in the ankle mortice; (2) internal rotation of the calcaneus together with some supination; (3) medial displacement of the navicular; and (4) medial displacement of the cuboid.

These studies confirm earlier findings[40] that in a severe clubfoot, there is external rotation of the body of the talus in the ankle mortice; and they confirm McKay's findings[53,54,58] that there is internal rotation of the calcaneus so that the back of the calcaneus comes to lie close to the fibula. Goldner describes "medial spin" in his 1969 study.[55] There is a medial spin in the head and neck of the talus, but not in the body of the talus.

These studies demonstrate that a surgical clubfoot correction must include external rotation of the calcaneus, reduction of the talus in the ankle mortice, internal rotation in the talus body, and external rotation of the talus neck. One way to rotate the body of the talus internally and rotate the neck of the talus externally at the same time is to do a talar neck osteotomy.[49,51,59,60] The alternative is to perform the operation early, when the "bony architecture" is still cartilaginous for the most part. In the correction, one should apply forces that will lead to remodeling of the talus neck.

The concept of applying forces to aid remodeling is routine in the treatment of congenital dislocation of the hip. When the hip is reduced, it is anticipated that the acetabulum will remodel. In surgical correction of clubfoot, there is a coupled motion in the talocalcaneal complex. After the ligamentous release, a pin is placed in the talus body posteriorly and used as a lever to dorsiflex and internally rotate the talus in the mortice to correct the anterior extrusion and the external rotation of the talus body. As the body of the talus comes back into the ankle mortice and is internally rotated, the back of the calcaneus must move down and away from the fibula. During the maneuver of talar reduction and rotation, the medial aspect of the talus neck impinges on the medial malleolus. In the young foot, this should aid in the remodeling process of the cartilaginous anlage so that the declination of the talar neck is reduced.

Surgery should be performed on an infant if repeated manipulations and cast applications have not resulted in a completely corrected clubfoot by the age of 3 months, provided the baby weighs at least 12 lb and is in good health.

Clubfoot should be considered a generic term that represents a spectrum of pathoanatomy. Sufficient surgery should be done to correct the bony architecture to normal and to balance the muscle forces. Some ankle dorsiflexion can be sacrificed if doing so will give the child more calf strength.

Postoperative care involves holding the corrected foot in a plaster cast for 12 weeks. The plaster casts are changed often to allow for growth. The child's foot is then put into an orthosis. The orthosis should be designed to maintain the forefoot in a plantigrade position, to keep the heel aligned with the long axis of the tibia, and to keep the lateral border of the foot at a right angle to the leg. The child is allowed out of the orthosis for a sufficient period of time each day to allow for ankle and tarsal motion. It is likely that severe cases of resistant clubfeet will require keeping the feet protected in an orthosis until the age of 2 years.

Improved results in the treatment of resistant clubfoot should be possible with a better understanding of the pathoanatomy of clubfoot, meticulous attention to detail during surgery, and orthotic maintenance of correction to facilitate remodeling.

References

1. Hippocrates: *Oeuvres Completes D'Hippocrate*, Lettre E (trans). Paris, JB Balliere, 1844, pp 263–269.
2. Cowell HR, Wein BK: Genetic aspects of club foot. *J Bone Joint Surg* 1980;62A:1381–1384.
3. Gray DH, Katz JM: A histochemical study of muscle in club foot. *J Bone Joint Surg* 1981;63B:417–423.
4. Handelsman JE, Badalamente MA: Neuromuscular studies in club foot. *J Pediatr Orthop* 1981;1:23.
5. Isaacs H, Handelsman JE, Badenhorst M, et al: The muscles in club foot: A histological, histochemical and electron microscopic study. *J Bone Joint Surg* 1977;59B:465–472.
6. Reimann I: *Congenital Idiopathic Clubfoot*, la Cour A (trans). Copenhagen, Munksgaard, 1967.
7. Hirsch C: Observationer vid tidig operation av ped equinovarus congenitus. *Nord Med* 1960;63:425–427.
8. Inclán A: Anomalous tendinous insertions in the pathogenesis of club foot. *J Bone Joint Surg* 1958;40B:159.
9. Swann M, Lloyd-Roberts GC, Catterall A: The anatomy of uncorrected club feet: A study of rotation deformity. *J Bone Joint Surg* 1969;51B:263–269.
10. Waisbrod H: Congenital club foot: An anatomical study. *J Bone Joint Surg* 1973;55B:796–801.
11. Wynne-Davies R: Talipes equinovarus: A review of eighty-four cases after completion of treatment. *J Bone Joint Surg* 1964;46B:464–476.
12. Bechtol CO, Mossman HW: Club foot: An embryological study of associated muscle abnormalities. *J Bone Joint Surg* 1950;32A:827–838.
13. Hjelmstedt A, Sahlstedt B: Talar deformity in congenital clubfeet: An anatomical and functional study with special reference to the ankle joint mobility. *Acta Orthop Scand* 1974;45:628–640.
14. Ippolito E, Ponseti IV: Congenital club foot in the human fetus: A histological study. *J Bone Joint Surg* 1980;62A:8–22.
15. Irani RN, Sherman MS: The pathological anatomy of club foot. *J Bone Joint Surg* 1963;45A:45–52.
16. Nichols EH: Anatomy of congenital equino-varus. *Boston Med Surg J* 1897;36:150–153.
17. Parker RW, Shattuck SG: The pathology and etiology of congenital club foot. *Trans Pathol Soc Lond* 1884;35:423–444.
18. Scudder CL: Congenital talipes equinovarus. *Boston Med Surg J* 1887;117:397–399.
19. Settle GW: The anatomy of congenital talipes equinovarus: Sixteen dissected specimens. *J Bone Joint Surg* 1963;45A:1341–1354.
20. Shapiro F, Glimcher MJ: Gross and histological abnormalities of the talus in congenital club foot. *J Bone Joint Surg* 1979;61A:522–530.
21. Addison A, Fixsen JA, Lloyd-Roberts GC: A review of the Dillwyn Evans type collateral operation in severe club feet. *J Bone Joint Surg* 1983;65B:12–14.
22. Adelaar RS, Dannelly EA, Meunier PA, et al: A long term study of triple arthrodesis in children. *Orthop Clin North Am* 1976;7:895–908.
23. Bleck EE: Congenital clubfoot: Pathomechanics, radiographic analysis, and results of surgical treatment. *Clin Orthop* 1977;125:119–130.
24. Crawford AH, Marxen JL, Osterfeld DL: The Cincinnati incision: A comprehensive approach for surgical procedures of the foot and ankle in childhood. *J Bone Joint Surg* 1982:64A:1355–1358.
25. Drummond DS, Cruess RL: The management of the foot and ankle in arthrogryposis multiplex congenita. *J Bone Joint Surg* 1978;60B:96–99.
26. Evans D: Relapsed club foot. *J Bone Joint Surg* 1961;43B:722–733.
27. Garceau GJ, Manning KR: Transposition of the anterior tibial tendon in the treatment of recurrent congenital club foot. *J Bone Joint Surg* 1947;29:1044–1048.
28. Heyman CH, Herndon CH, Strong JM: Mobilization of the tarsometatarsal and intermetatarsal joints for the correction of resistant adduction of the fore part of the foot in congenital club-foot or congenital metatarsus varus. *J Bone Joint Surg* 1958;40A:299–310.
29. Kite JH: Conservative treatment of the resistant recurrent clubfoot. *Clin Orthop* 1970;70:93–110.
30. Laaveg SJ, Ponseti IV: Long-term results of treatment of congenital club foot. *J Bone Joint Surg* 1980;62A:23–31.
31. Lichtblau S: A medial and lateral release operation for club foot: A preliminary report. *J Bone Joint Surg* 1973;55A:1377–1384.
32. Patterson RL Jr, Parrish FF, Hathaway EN: Stabilizing operations on the foot: A study of the indications, techniques used, and end results. *J Bone Joint Surg* 1950;32A:1–26.
33. Ryoppy S, Sairanen H: Neonatal operative treatment of club foot: A preliminary report. *J Bone Joint Surg* 1983;65B:320–325.
34. Sherman FC, Westin GW: Plantar release in the correction of deformities of the foot in childhood. *J Bone Joint Surg* 1981;63A:1382–1389.
35. Spires TD, Gross RH, Low W, et al: Management of the resistant myelodysplastic or arthrogrypotic clubfoot with the Verebelyi-Ogston procedure. *J Pediatr Orthop* 1984;4:705–710.
36. Thompson GH, Richardson AB, Westin GW: Surgical management of resistant congenital talipes equinovarus deformities. *J Bone Joint Surg* 1982;64A:652–665.
37. Turco VJ: Surgical correction of the resistant club foot: One-stage posteromedial release with internal fixation: A preliminary report. *J Bone Joint Surg* 1971;53A:477–497.
38. Turco VJ: Resistant congenital club foot—one-stage posteromedial release with internal fixation: A follow-up report of a fifteen-year experience. *J Bone Joint Surg* 1979;61A:805–814.
39. Yoneda B, Carroll NC: One-stage surgical management of resistant club foot. *J Bone Joint Surg* 1984;66B:302.
40. Carroll NC, McMurtry R, Leete SF: The pathoanatomy of congenital clubfoot. *Orthop Clin North Am* 1978;9:225–232.
41. Beatson TR, Pearson JR: A method of assessing correction in club feet. *J Bone Joint Surg* 1966;48B:40–50.
42. Ponseti IV, El-Khoury GY, Ippolito E, et al: A radiographic study of skeletal deformities in treated clubfeet. *Clin Orthop* 1981;160:30–42.
43. Simons GW: A standardized method for the radiographic evaluation of clubfeet. *Clin Orthop* 1978;135:107–118.
44. Carroll NC, McMurtry R, Leet S: The patho-anatomy of congenital club foot. *J Bone Joint Surg* 1975;57B:530.
45. Grant JCB: *Method of Anatomy*. Baltimore, Williams & Wilkins, 1952.
46. Heywood AWB: The mechanics of the hind foot in club foot as demonstrated radiographically. *J Bone Joint Surg* 1964;46B:102–107.
47. Kite JH: Principles involved in the treatment of congenital club foot: The results of treatment. *J Bone Joint Surg* 1939;21:595–606.
48. Main BJ, Crider RJ: An analysis of residual deformity in club feet submitted to early operation. *J Bone Joint Surg* 1978;60B:536–543.
49. DeHaan JT, Wilkins KE: Talar osteotomy in the treatment of resistant equinovarus deformities. *Orthop Trans* 1987;11:35.
50. Hjelmstedt A, Sahlstedt B: Simultaneous arthrography of the talocrural and talonavicular joints in children: IV. Measurements on congenital clubfeet. *Acta Radiol Diagn* 1978;19:223–236.
51. Matsuno S, Kaneda T, Katoh T, et al: The treatment of congenital club foot. *J Jpn Orthop Assoc* 1978;52:101–103.

52. Fahrenbach GJ, Kuehn DN, Tachdjian MO: Occult subluxation of the subtalar joint in clubfoot (using computerized tomography). *J Pediatr Orthop* 1986;6:334–339.

53. McKay DW: New concept of and approach to clubfoot treatment: Section I. Principles and morbid anatomy. *J Pediatr Orthop* 1982;2:347–356.

54. McKay DW: New concept of and approach to clubfoot treatment: Section II. Correction of the clubfoot. *J Pediatr Orthop* 1983;3:10–21.

55. Goldner JL: Congenital talipes equinovarus: Fifteen years of surgical treatment. *Curr Pract Orthop Surg* 1969;4:61–123.

56. Carroll NC: Congenital clubfoot: Pathoanatomy and treatment, in Griffin PP (ed): American Academy of Orthopaedic Surgeons *Instructional Course Lectures, XXXVI.* Park Ridge, American Academy of Orthopaedic Surgeons, 1987, pp 117–121.

57. Scott WA, Hosking SW, Catterall A: Club foot: Observations on the surgical anatomy of dorsiflexion. *J Bone Joint Surg* 1984;66B:71–76.

58. McKay DW: New concept of and approach to clubfoot treatment: Section III. Evaluation and results. *J Pediatr Orthop* 1983;3:141–148.

59. Hjelmstedt A, Sahlstedt B: Talo-calcaneal osteotomy and soft-tissue procedures in the treatment of clubfeet: II. Results in 36 surgically treated feet. *Acta Orthop Scand* 1980;51:349–357.

60. Roberts JM, Drvaric DM: Comprehensive release for infantile idiopathic clubfeet: A review of 217 cases. *Orthop Trans* 1985;9:416–417.

CHAPTER 12

Gait Analysis and Intoeing

Frank M. Chang, MD

Identification of the Problem

In treating intoeing, the physician must frequently practice the art as well as the science of medicine. The history and the manner in which it is taken are important. The parents' perception of the problem and their level of concern must be determined. The concern of grandparents, the child, or the pediatrician must be gauged. The physician must determine whether or not the deformity is progressing. A progressive deformity may suggest a neurologic disorder instead of a mechanical or anatomic variation. The physician must also determine if the torsional abnormality has resulted in any functional impairment or disability, such as excessive tripping, fatigue, or pain.

Etiology

Determining the cause of intoeing is usually simple; a systematic examination is the key. Intoeing has three common causes: femoral anteversion, internal tibial torsion, and metatarsus adductus. The correct diagnosis is made by analyzing the data gathered from the torsional profile.[1] The torsional profile consists of five clinical measurements listed as follows: (1) FPA (foot progression angle); (2) TFA (thigh-foot angle); (3) HIR (hip internal rotation); (4) HER (hip external rotation); (5) HBL (heel bisector line).

The foot progression angle is the most difficult measurement to reproduce. The child should be observed while attempting to walk in a straight line. The angle between the longitudinal axis of the foot and the imaginary straight line the child is walking determines the foot progression angle. By convention, intoeing has been assigned a negative angular value and outtoeing a positive value. Each foot is recorded separately. Of course, toddlers never walk in a straight line, which makes this measurement more difficult to reproduce. The time of day may also influence the foot progression angle; with increasing fatigue, the child is less able to compensate actively for the torsional abnormality.

The remaining measurements are best done with the child prone on the examining table and the knees flexed 90 degrees. Distracting the child during this part of the examination is helpful. An inexpensive wind-up toy works well most of the time. The thigh-foot angle is determined by measuring the angle between the longitudinal axis of the foot and the long axis of the thigh.

Again, medial deviation of the foot, or intoeing, is assigned a negative value. A reproducible technique of measuring hip internal rotation is to use the leg to rotate the hip internally from the neutral or zero-degree position to maximum internal rotation. External rotation of the hip is also measured in this manner by maximally externally rotating the hips. Finally, the heel bisector line as described by Bleck,[2] is determined by constructing a line that bisects the hindfoot and then observing which toe or interspace is intersected. These data can be organized by listing the values obtained from these measurements for both the left and the right foot.

Femoral Anteversion

Femoral anteversion is defined as anterior deviation of the femoral head and neck with respect to the femoral shaft and condyles. The natural history of femoral anteversion has been well documented in the literature.[3,4] Neonates are born with 40 degrees of anteversion, which decreases during normal growth and development to the adult measurement of 15 degrees. Most cases are idiopathic, although a familial tendency has been noted in some. Only the most severe cases will not correct spontaneously. A useful indicator is whether or not there is any residual anteversion in other affected family members; if so, the child is less likely to correct completely. If progressive anteversion has been documented, neuromuscular imbalance should be suspected.

The diagnosis is easily confirmed by analyzing hip rotation. The history typically describes an otherwise healthy toddler who intoes during ambulation. The intoeing frequently is worse when the child is fatigued. The older child runs awkwardly as a result of circumducting the legs to avoid tripping. Parents often are concerned about the child's "W" sitting posture. Observation of gait reveals intoeing, with the "kissing patella sign" being diagnostic. Rather than pointing anteriorly, the patellae tend to face each other medially. Rotation of the hips will demonstrate an increase in hip internal rotation and a decrease in hip external rotation.

Usually, no treatment is necessary. Parents are reassured that the gait will improve until the child is 7 or 8 years old and that active compensation can be learned if remodeling is not complete. Disability or limitation of activities is seen only rarely. Conservative treatment does not seem to change the natural course.

Modifying shoes with wedges or changing the last has been shown to be ineffective in changing the gait or progression. In fact, because prescription shoes are usually heavier than standard footwear, the gait frequently looks worse. The hip external rotators, which are active in compensating for the femoral malrotation, will fatigue sooner with heavier shoes. I usually suggest that parents try a light-weight canvas shoe.

Rarely, a rotational femoral osteotomy is considered for a child who is 8 years old or older and has a functional disability such as excessive tripping, is upset with the appearance of the feet, and who has less than 15 degrees of passive external hip rotation. The preferred operation is a supracondylar rotational osteotomy made through a 1- to 2-cm medial, longitudinal incision with minimal periosteal stripping and no internal fixation. The periosteal sleeve will tighten with rotation of the femur, leaving the osteotomy relatively stable when held with a spica cast. This procedure is acceptable cosmetically, and a second procedure to remove hardware is avoided.

Internal Tibial Torsion

The etiology of internal tibial torsion is virtually the same as for femoral anteversion. Some internal tibial torsion is normally present at birth; the extent is determined by familial tendencies and intrauterine positioning. The tibial rotation then slowly "unwinds" with normal growth and development. Again, only the children with the most severe familial tendencies will not correct spontaneously. The remodeling potential is so great that some children will even overcorrect their tibial rotation to compensate for residual femoral anteversion. Internal tibial torsion is certainly not a functional problem, and in fact, offers some advantage in running sports. It is common for children who intoe to run faster than their peers, and there are many examples of athletes who intoe.

The diagnosis of tibial torsion is also made simply by analyzing the data gathered in the torsional profile. The thigh-foot angle measurement determines the exact nature of the tibial rotation. The normal adult measurement is 10 to 15 degrees. At birth, the thigh-foot angle typically measures about 5 degrees; children with significant internal tibial torsion will have a thigh-foot an-

gle greater than −30 degrees.[5] Hip rotation is symmetric in isolated tibial torsion; the patellae should not appear medially deviated, as with femoral anteversion. The intermalleolar angle can also be used to determine tibial rotation, but I have had more difficulty reproducing it consistently.

Treatment is controversial. Altering the shoes does not seem to improve the gait or change the natural course. A still-popular treatment is the Denis-Browne bar, despite the fact that there has never been any convincing scientific evidence to support its use. The most common program is to use the bar as a night splint, with the legs externally rotated approximately 30 degrees. The Denis-Browne bar is best used before the child is 2 years old, somewhat more agreeable, and still in a crib at night. The bar is relatively indicated for a child 15 to 18 months old with significant torsion, who has not demonstrated any spontaneous correction, especially if it is unilateral or combined with femoral anteversion, or who has family members who have not corrected.

A rotational osteotomy is a last resort; there are even fewer indications for tibial osteotomy than for femoral osteotomy in anteversion. For a child with severe internal tibial torsion who has not corrected spontaneously, a rotational supramalleolar osteotomy can be performed through a 1-cm anterior incision, with minimal periosteal stripping, no internal fixation, and with the leg held in a bent-knee, long leg cast. A fibular osteotomy is also necessary and is performed through a separate 1-cm lateral incision. An oblique cut through the fibula increases the surface area to facilitate healing.

References

1. Staheli LT: Torsional deformity. *Pediatr Clin North Am* 1977;24:799.
2. Bleck EE: Metatarsus adductus: Classification and relationship to outcomes of treatment. *J Pediatr Orthop* 1983;3:2.
3. Ryder CT, Crane L: Measuring femoral anteversion: The problem and a method. *J Bone Joint Surg* 1953;35A:321.
4. Shands AR Jr, Steele MK: Torsion of the femur: A follow-up report on the use of the Dunlap method for its determination. *J Bone Joint Surg* 1958;40A:803–816.
5. Staheli LT, Corbett M, Wyss C, et al: Lower-extremity rotational problems in children. *J Bone Joint Surg* 1985;67A:39–47.

The Flexible Flatfoot

Frank M. Chang, MD

Differential Diagnosis

Flatfeet are a common presenting complaint to orthopaedists who see children in their practice, not because the children complain about their feet, but because their parents think flatfeet are a significant medical problem. The flexible flatfoot is rarely of much clinical significance, but before parents are casually reassured, the correct diagnosis must be established. The differential diagnosis includes calcaneovalgus foot, congenital vertical talus, congenital oblique talus, peroneal spastic flatfoot, paralytic flatfoot, and flexible flatfoot. The key diagnostic factor is the flexibility of the foot. If the foot is rigid and the arch not passively correctable, then further diagnostic evaluation is necessary.

The calcaneovalgus foot is commonly seen in neonates; the dorsum of the foot touches or nearly touches the anterior surface of the leg, and ankle plantar flexion is markedly limited. These feet will correct easily with simple passive stretching exercises. The congenital vertical talus is easily recognized clinically by the physician experienced in treating children's foot disorders. These feet are the most rigid, have a convex arch, and limited ankle dorsiflexion. The oblique talus may be mistaken for a vertical talus, but it can be distinguished both clinically and radiographically. The foot is flexible, with the arch being passively correctable; however, the tight posterior structures cannot be passively corrected, limiting ankle dorsiflexion. Lateral plantarflexion radiographs confirm the diagnosis, demonstrating reduction of the subluxated talonavicular joint in the oblique talus, as opposed to incomplete reduction of the dislocated talonavicular joint in the vertical talus. The peroneal spastic flatfoot, which is usually caused by a tarsal coalition, is most commonly manifested when children reach their teens, with complaints of pain frequently associated with activity. Examination of the involved foot reveals limitation of subtalar motion, and a coalition can usually be documented radiographically. The paralytic flatfoot is caused by neuromuscular imbalance and is associated with a neuromuscular disorder such as cerebral palsy or spina bifida.

Flexible Pes Planus

All children have flatfeet at birth. Some of these feet will remain flat and asymptomatic; they are a normal physiologic variant. The normal foot may appear flat until the child is 2 to 3 years old. Reasons include ligament laxity, flexibility of cartilage, neuromuscular development, and the presence of subcutaneous fat that occupies space in the arch. The support ligaments gradually tighten to give the longitudinal arch increasing definition with normal growth. Therefore, the true flexible flatfoot is difficult to diagnose clinically before the child is 2 years old.

The cause is primarily laxity of the ligaments that normally support the bones forming the arch. The laxity is frequently familial and is sometimes associated with Down's, Marfan's, and Ehlers-Danlos syndromes, all of which include excessive ligament laxity.

Clinical Features

The normal arch is formed by the bony architecture and ligament support. Muscles do not support the arch, as documented by Basmajian and Bentzon[1] with electromyographic studies. The classic clinical finding is an arch that flattens with weightbearing. This finding is easily demonstrated by having the child stand on tiptoes, which will actively reform the arch. When the child stands flatfooted with full weightbearing, the midfoot pronates and the hindfoot rolls into excessive valgus; weightbearing occurs medially instead of through the lateral column.

The flatfoot can be classified either by severity or by location of the primary deformity. A mild flatfoot has a depressed arch; a moderate flatfoot has no arch with weightbearing; and a severe flatfoot appears convex through the medial aspect of the midfoot. The joint laxity can occur primarily through the talonavicular joint, the naviculocuneiform joint, or both. Severity is most easily demonstrated by a simple footprint, and location best demonstrated radiographically. Location can also be demonstrated clinically with the "toe raising test" of Jack,[2] which implicates the naviculocuneiform joint. As described by Jack, reconstitution of the arch with dorsiflexion of the great toe indicates the naviculocuneiform joint is involved. Assessment of heelcord tightness with the heel held in the neutral position should always be included. A tight heelcord suggests an oblique talus.

Symptoms are rare in children with true flexible flatfeet. Excessive wear on the shoes and breakdown of the medial counter of the shoe are often the only indications of the flexible flatfoot. As the severity of the flatfoot increases, symptoms also increase and include aching in the arch, increased fatigue, leg aches, and leg cramps that usually occur at night.

Radiographic evaluation aids in confirming the diagnosis, localizing the malaligned joints, and ruling out other possibilities in the differential diagnosis. Anteroposterior and lateral radiographs should be obtained with the patient standing so that the feet are in the weightbearing position. On the lateral view, the longitudinal arch is well visualized. Méary's angle is constructed with a line through the long axis of the talus intersecting the line bisecting the first metatarsal. This is a straight line in the normal foot. The flatfoot produces an angle convex in the plantar direction. The location of the break in the longitudinal arch can be localized to the talonavicular, naviculocuneiform joints, or both. The increased talocalcaneal angle on the anteroposterior view demonstrates the severity of hindfoot valgus.

Treatment

Once the correct diagnosis has been established, several facts should be ascertained before treatment is begun: the age of the patient, severity of the flatfoot, problems with shoe wear, and the nature of the symptoms.

The mild flatfoot is usually asymptomatic and no treatment is necessary. If the heelcord is tight, then stretching should be performed with exercises or serial casting. Casting is very effective, but accurate neutral positioning of the hindfoot and molding of the longitudinal arch are requisite.

As severity increases, symptoms justify considering treatment. Unfortunately, there are no established criteria to determine who should be treated or for how long.

If associated with genu valgus, a 3/16-inch medial heel and sole wedge may relieve leg aches or leg cramps. Heel cups or custom-molded inserts are effective in preventing excessive wear on the shoe.

Shoe modifications, heel cups,[3] and arch supports[4] have all been advocated by those who believe that the flatfoot can be corrected. The classic shoe prescription has been a laced, leather oxford shoe with a reinforced medial counter, medial heel wedge, Thomas heel, and some arch support. Various brands of heel cups are also popular and are definitely the most cost-effective. They support the hindfoot, preventing excessive valgus. Custom-molded orthotics are the most expensive and come in many varieties. The custom-molded insert, popular with many orthopaedic surgeons, provides excellent control of the hindfoot and can be molded to support the arch. All of these forms of treatment may alleviate symptoms, but will not alter the ultimate shape of the arch in the flexible flatfoot.

Wenger and associates[5] observed 179 feet in four groups. The four groups included a control group; a group wearing modified shoes; a group with Helfet heel cups in their shoes; and a group with custom-molded orthotics. The feet were analyzed clinically and roentgenographically both before and after the completion of treatment. The study concluded that there was no significant difference in the shape of the foot or arch in any of the groups.

Although surgery can alter the natural course and change the shape of the arch, it is rarely indicated because most flatfeet are asymptomatic.

References

1. Basmajian JR, Bentzon JW: An electromyographic study of certain muscles of the leg and foot in the standing position. *Surg Gynecol Obstet* 1954;98:662.
2. Jack EA: Naviculo-cuneiform fusion in the treatment of the flat foot. *J Bone Joint Surg* 1953;35B:75.
3. Bleck EE, Berzins UJ: Conservative management of pes valgus with plantar flexed talus, flexible. *Clin Orthop* 1977;122:85–94.
4. Helfet AJ: A new way of treating flat feet in children. *Lancet* 1956;1:262.
5. Wenger DR, Maulden D, Speck G, et al: The effect of corrective shoes and inserts on flexible flatfoot—A prospective randomized trial. *J Pediatr Orthop* 1986;6:732.

CHAPTER 14

Surgical Management of the Flatfoot

Gerard L. Glancy, MD

Introduction

The child with a flatfoot can be a source of confusion and anxiety to parents. "His ankles roll in" is a frequent observation of the worried parents. The lack of a longitudinal arch implies functional impairment. This concept was supported in the early orthopaedic literature by Whitman[1] who described the hypermobile flatfoot as a "weak foot." Today we know more about the natural course of untreated flatfoot. Therefore, we are able to advise our patients and their parents that in most cases the outcome is benign and without functional impairment. Occasionally, a symptomatic flatfoot occurs that demands diagnostic attention and surgical intervention. This chapter is concerned with the symptomatic flatfoot that requires surgical treatment.

Clinical Evaluation

The severity of the flatfoot deformity can be judged by the sag of the longitudinal arch during weight-bearing. The deformity is mild if there is some concavity to the arch. The deformity is moderate if the medial border of the sole is straight, and severe if there is convexity to the medial border. The convexity indicates that the navicular is falling into a weight-bearing position. It is important to determine if the deformity is supple or rigid initially. If the foot develops a normal longitudinal arch in an off-weighted position, or when the patient is standing on tiptoes, then it is classified as a supple flatfoot deformity. If the foot remains flat in an off-weighted position, intrinsic foot disease is likely (tarsal coalition, juvenile rheumatoid arthritis, or tumor). If a tight heelcord is present, it causes a secondary break in the midfoot resulting in a flatfoot attitude. Therefore, the amount of foot dorsiflexion should be measured with the hindfoot in a neutral and the knee in an extended position. Tight heelcord is not a consideration if at least 10 degrees of dorsiflexion is present.

Radiographic examination of any symptomatic flatfoot is mandatory. Radiographs should be taken in the weightbearing position. The normal bony alignment consists of a Kite angle of 20 to 35 degrees in the anteroposterior (AP) projection and 20 to 45 degrees in the lateral projection,[2] and a Méary's angle of 0 to +10 degrees (Fig. 14–1, *top left*) with a tarsal to first metatarsal angle of 0 to −10 degrees.[3] In contrast, the flatfoot is characterized by an increased talocalcaneal angle in both the AP and lateral projections, and a sag (negative Méary's line) at either the talonavicular or the naviculocuneiform, or both. A sag of 0 to −15 degrees is a mild deformity, −15 to −40 degrees is a moderate deformity, and over −40 degrees is a severe deformity (Fig. 14–1, *top right* and *bottom left*). Furthermore, an inclination of talus with respect to the calcaneus that exceeds 55 degrees should be regarded as an oblique talus. This is often associated with tight heelcord.

The Hypermobile Flatfoot

Bleck and Berzins[4] have proposed a comprehensive classification system of the symptomatic flatfoot. The hypermobile flatfoot is one that is a result of ligamentous laxity, not of bony deformity. In particular, the talonavicular (spring) ligament is responsible for support of the talar head. Generalized ligamentous laxity and laxity localized to the medial column of the midfoot will result in collapse of the longitudinal arch by eversion of the heel at the subtalar joint and disruption of the axial alignment of the talus, navicular, first cuneiform, and first metatarsal. The foot in an off-weighted position has a normal longitudinal arch.

Surgery for the Hypermobile Flatfoot

Surgery is indicated for the hypermobile flatfoot when plantar and medial foot pain with activity persists despite conscientious and prolonged use of orthotic devices. The patient is unable or unwilling to alter his activity in deference to symptoms. Because of the severe abductovalgus deformity, ordinary shoes are deformed and worn out at a frequency far in excess of their normal life span. With these criteria, children qualifying for surgery for hypermobile flatfoot are a very select group. Furthermore, since the majority of effective surgical procedures involve alteration of bony anatomy, it is best to delay any surgical procedure until the foot is at or near maturity. Maturity is generally considered to be age 10 in a girl and age 12 in a boy. The child at this age is better able to communicate the severity of symptoms.

The choice of surgical procedures are (1) soft tissue rebalance; (2) osteotomy; (3) arthroereisis; (4) fusion, or combinations of these procedures. The most com-

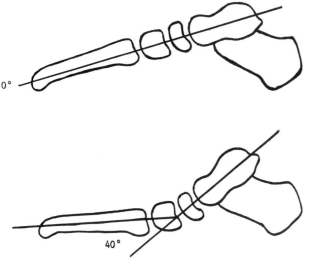

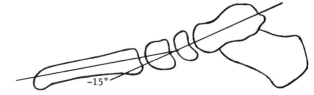

Fig. 14-1 **Top left:** Normal Méary angle is 0 to +10 degrees. **Top right:** In mild flatfoot the angle is 0 to −15 degrees. **Bottom left:** In severe flatfoot the angle is more than −40 degrees.

mon finding associated with the symptomatic, nonparalytic, flexible flatfoot is a tight heelcord. Initial treatment should consist of heelcord stretching exercises. If these exercises are not effective, then a heelcord lengthening can be accomplished with a series of short leg walking casts. Each cast is applied with the hindfoot in a neutral or slightly inverted position with the knee flexed to 90 degrees. Three casts are applied. Each cast is worn for two weeks. If this treatment is not effective, or if heelcord tightness recurs, a tendo Achillis lengthening is indicated.

A number of osteotomies have been described. Chambers[5] and Selakovich[6] have described procedures for the calcaneus. Evans[7] has described lengthening, and Dwyer[8] and Koutsogiannis[9] have described realignment procedures. All of these procedures are extra-articular; however, they are technically demanding. It is difficult to judge in the anesthetized patient the amount of osteotomy necessary for a satisfactory functional outcome.

Arthroereisis was initially described many years ago and consisted of placing a bony plug beneath the lateral process of the talus to prop open the subtalar articulation and thus reduce hindfoot valgus.[10] Recently, arthroereisis has been used by podiatrists with a Silastic plug devised to block the excessive hindfoot eversion. In contrast, orthopaedic surgeons have recognized that Silastic plugs can produce a synovitis, and often pain persists despite correction of the deformity by arthroereisis. Furthermore, the continued use of orthoses is recommended following arthroereisis.

Available hindfoot fusions include talonavicular, talonavicular and subtalar joints, triple arthrodesis, and the Grice[11] subtalar extra-articular fusion. In my opinion, hindfoot fusion for the hypermobile flatfoot in an otherwise neurologically normal and healthy child is surgery on a secondary component of the pathoanat-

omy. Furthermore, it results in the sacrifice of one or more major hindfoot articulations.

Surgical correction should be confined to the midfoot medial column.

Table 14–1 lists the major features of several correction procedures. The Scottish-Rite procedure[12] appears to provide satisfactory radiographic correction. Most importantly, this procedure provides reliable symptom relief, which is the primary goal of treatment. Internal fixation of the osteotomy site is recommended. Both the Scottish-Rite[12] and the Durham[13] procedures have stood the test of time and are recommended by this author. The Giannestras procedure[14] may involve excessive shifting of soft tissues in the surgical area.

Prehallux Syndrome

The prehallux syndrome results from the presence of an accessory navicular or an especially prominent navicular. The typical patient is female, preadolescent, and describes localized pain in the prominence of the navicular. If there is an associated tendonitis, there may also be pain along the posterior tibialis insertion. A hypermobile flatfoot sometimes occurs with the accessory navicular. The diagnosis is confirmed radiographically and initial treatment should consist of pressure relief, modification of the patient's shoes, and an arch support for flatfoot, if present. If symptoms persist with this conservative treatment, surgery can be performed.

The surgeon should exercise care regarding patient selection for surgery. All foot surgery is characterized by several weeks to months of disability in the postoperative period. The adolescent patient is not immune to reflex sympathetic dystrophy. Therefore, a specific diagnosis is mandatory, and patient expectations of postsurgical results should be discussed preoperatively.

Table 14-1
Surgical procedures for the hypermobile flatfoot

Investigators	Soft-Tissue Procedure	Joints Fused	Additional Features
Miller[25]	Osteal/periosteal flap, proximally based	Naviculocuneiform; first cuneiform; first metatarsal	Achilles tendon lengthening as indicated
Hoke[26]	Osteal/periosteal flap, proximally based	Naviculocuneiform; first cuneiform; second cuneiform	Achilles tendon lengthening as indicated
Duncan and Lovell[12]	Osteal/periosteal flap	Open dorsal wedge osteotomy of naviculocuneiform joint with wedge graft from navicular	Achilles tendon lengthening as indicated
Durham[13]	Distally based flap with rerouting of posterior tibialis	Closing wedge osteotomy, medially based; naviculocuneiform	—
Giannestras[14]	Rerouting of anterior and posterior tibialis to navicular	Naviculocuneiform	—

The patient with diffuse foot pain is a poor surgical candidate.

Kidner described a procedure to restore the longitudinal arch by rerouting the posterior tibialis to a more plantar location after excising the accessory navicular.[15] Recent surveys, however, have failed to confirm his results.[16] Therefore, I recommend simple excision of the accessory navicular and any prominent navicular remaining. Rerouting the posterior tibialis contributes little, if anything, to the functional outcome.

Spastic Flatfoot

Deformity of the foot secondary to cerebral palsy is common. Typically, the spastic flatfoot occurs in an ambulatory diplegic. Contracture of the tendo Achillis is a primary problem. Secondarily, the midfoot deforms into abductovalgus, enabling the foot to stay somewhat plantargrade at midstance (Fig. 14–2). With time, the foot becomes less responsive to the application of casts, orthoses, or both, and a decrease in ambulatory stamina and progressive deformity is observed. This foot should respond favorably to a surgical procedure. However, it is unusual that only a tendo Achillis lengthening is sufficient. It is also necessary to perform soft-tissue imbrication of the medial midfoot structures including the spring ligament and posterior tibialis. It is difficult to balance these feet with respect to extrinsic muscle forces. Therefore, in contrast to the hypermobile flatfoot, stabilization of the subtalar joint with a Grice procedure is appropriate.[11] Internal fixation should be used for a minimum of six weeks. A radiographic nonunion or disappearance of the bone graft, or both, is sometimes noted in the months following a Grice procedure. However, the foot is often maintained in a satisfactory neutral position because of secondary adaptive changes in the subtalar and transverse tarsal articulations. Therefore, nonunion of a Grice subtalar arthrodesis is not necessarily a surgical failure.

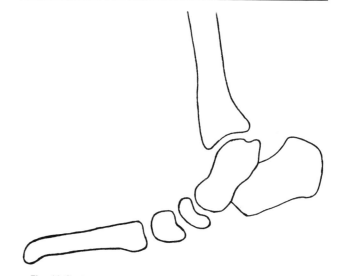

Fig. 14-2 Spastic flatfoot with tight heelcord. Note the equinus attitude of the calcaneus. This produces a secondary break in the midfoot.

Tarsal Coalition

Tarsal coalition is a rare disorder occurring in less than 1% of the general population.[17] In those affected, it is bilateral 5% to 50% of the time and is often inherited as an autosomal dominant trait.[18] Tarsal coalition is frequently asymptomatic and often not discovered until well into adulthood. Those who do become symptomatic in childhood, do so during early adolescence. The characteristic signs and symptoms include midfoot and instep pain, antalgic gait, and a foot progressively stiff and altered in shape. Occasionally, true peroneal tendon spasm can be observed. More commonly, we note a flatfoot that does not change shape in an off-weighted position and a marked decrease in subtalar joint motion. In general, symptoms increase with an increase in valgus.

Diagnosis of tarsal coalition is confirmed radiographically. The coalitions can occur between the calcaneonavicular (most common), talocalcaneal, or talonavicular bones. Multiple coalitions may exist in the same foot. The oblique projection of the foot shows a calcaneonavicular coalition best. The other coalitions may be more subtle radiographically, and diagnosis can be confirmed by secondary signs of abnormal foot mechanics. Secondary signs include beaking of the talar neck, elongation of the lateral process of the talus, and diminished joint space in the posterior facet of the subtalar joint (Fig. 14–3). Beaking of the talar neck is an adaptive change to compensate for the diminished mobility of the subtalar articulation secondary to abnormal mobility of the transverse tarsal joint. If standard radiographs fail to define the coalition, a ski-jump view, described by Harris and Beath,[19] may be helpful. For this view, the radiograph tube should be angled parallel to the posterior facet of the talus. Hypoplasia of the sustentaculum tali and obliteration of the middle facet are characteristic of a middle facet coalition. Tomograms will define middle and anterior facet coalitions but computed tomography (CT) is a more definitive study. A CT scan should be performed in both the coronal and axial planes of the foot to pick up multiple coalitions.

On rare occasions what appears to be a tarsal coalition clinically is not verified radiographically. Other forms of localized pathology should then be considered, such as juvenile rheumatoid arthritis, low-grade sepsis, or osteoid osteoma. An erythrocyte sedimentation rate, antinuclear antibody, rheumatoid factor, and a technetium bone scan are diagnostically useful.

Initial treatment of tarsal coalition should be nonsurgical, using either an orthosis or a short leg walking cast. The orthosis or cast should be kept in place for six weeks and then used on an as-needed basis. If intermittent immobilization fails to relieve symptoms, surgical intervention is justified. If the coalition is cartilaginous, resection can be considered. If the coalition is entirely bony, then arthrodesis is appropriate. The CT scan should be carefully evaluated preoperatively to determine on which side of the joint the coalition occurs. The bone contributing most to the coalition should be excised. In the case of middle and posterior facets, it is important to find the normal joint on either side to insure complete removal of the coalition. Fat, Silastic, or wax should be interposed into any excised coalition. For calcaneonavicular coalition, interposition of the origin of the extensor digitorum brevis works well.[20]

Immediately after coalition removal, range of motion should be assessed. Suspect multiple coalitions if there is not significant restoration of range of motion. If significant degenerative changes are seen either radiographically or intraoperatively, then a fusion should be done. However, beaking of the talus is an adaptive not a degenerative change.[21] Postoperative management consists of a short leg cast for three to six weeks. A postoperative CT scan should be obtained to confirm the extent of resection and any possible regrowth of the coalition.

Skewfoot

The skewfoot is also referred to as serpentine foot, S-foot, and zed foot. The skewfoot deformity is regarded as rare. Peterson,[22] in a thorough search of the literature, found only 50 reported cases. His own series at the Mayo Clinic consisted of four patients.[22] However, Berg[23] recently indicated that skewfoot may be more common than previously thought. The natural history of untreated skewfoot is unknown. Berg's series did not find the skewfoot resistant to manipulation and application of serial casts. He did note that children with skewfoot ended up with a flatfoot deformity.

The deformity itself consists of adduction and supination of the forefoot, abduction and lateral shift of the midfoot, and valgus of the hindfoot (Fig. 14–4). Despite the obvious deformity, the patient may be completely asymptomatic. Indications for surgery are disabling pain, clumsiness (especially during the swing phase with the forefoot striking the opposite leg), and inability to find comfort in ordinary shoes. While cosmesis is not a surgical indication, the skewfoot deformity is striking and is a source of embarrassment to the child.

A variety of surgical procedures have been described for the skewfoot. The most logical corrections of the forefoot deformity are either capsulotomies as described by Heyman and associates[24] or multiple metatarsal osteotomies. Multiple metatarsal osteotomies are

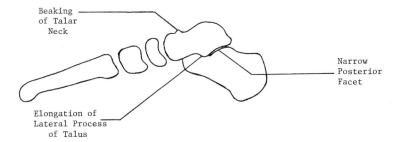

Beaking
of Talar
Neck

Narrow
Posterior
Facet

Elongation of
Lateral Process
of Talus

Fig. 14–3 Secondary signs of tarsal coalition.

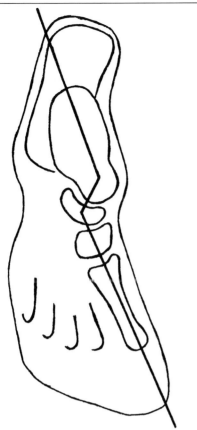

Fig. 14-4 Skewfoot. Note the lateral subluxation of the navicular.

preferred because the Heyman-Herndon procedure often produces joint stiffness. Injury to the physis at the base of the first metatarsal must be avoided. David Hahn has described correcting the midfoot with an opening wedge osteotomy of the cuboid and realignment of the navicular on the talus (personal communication). Other authors correct the hindfoot by either a Grice[11] or triple arthrodesis. In the Mayo Clinic series,[22] recurrence of the skewfoot deformity was frequent, although most patients eventually enjoyed a satisfactory outcome.

Summary

The flatfoot in a child with sufficient deformity and symptoms to warrant surgery occurs infrequently. A prolonged trial of nonsurgical measures is always indicated. With the exception of the spastic paralytic foot, surgery involving alteration of the bony anatomy should be postponed until the child's foot matures. Restoration of the longitudinal arch at the midfoot naviculo-cuneiform articulation is a reliable solution to the symptomatic hypermobile flatfoot. The spastic paralytic foot requires tendo Achillis lengthening, medial imbrication, and Grice subtalar stabilization. The symptomatic, cartilaginous tarsal coalition will respond to resection. Treatment of the skewfoot must be individualized de-

pending on the severity and location of symptoms, age of the patient, and joint mobility.

References

1. Whitman R: Observations of forty-five cases of flat foot with particular reference to aetiology and treatment. *Boston Med Surg J* 1888;118:598.
2. Simons GW: Analytical radiography of club feet. *J Bone Joint Surg* 1977;59B:485–489.
3. Méary R: Le pied creux essentiel. *Rev Chir Orthop* 1967;53:389.
4. Bleck EE, Berzins UJ: Conservative management of pes valgus with plantar flexed talus, flexible. *Clin Orthop* 1977;122:85–94.
5. Chambers EFS: An operation for correction of flexible flat-feet of adolescents. *West J Surg* 1946;54:77.
6. Selakovich WG: Medical arch support by operation: Sustentaculum tali procedure. *Orthop Clin North Am* 1973;4:117–144.
7. Evans D: Calcaneo-valgus deformity. *J Bone Joint Surg* 1975;57B:270–278.
8. Dwyer FC: Osteotomy of the calcaneum in the treatment of grossly everted feet with special reference to cerebral palsy, in *Huitième Congrès de la Société International de Chirurgie Orthopedique et de Traumatologie, New York, 4–9 September 1960.* Brussels, Imprimerie des Sciences, 1961, pp 892–897.
9. Koutsogiannis E: Treatment of mobile flat foot by displacement osteotomy of the calcaneus. *J Bone Joint Surg* 1971;53B:96–100.
10. DuCroquet C, Launay: Arthrodese du pied. *Presse Medicale,* June 30, 1909.
11. Grice DS: An extra-articular arthrodesis of the subastragular joint for correction of paralytic flat foot in children. *J Bone Joint Surg* 1952;34A:927.
12. Duncan JW, Lovell WW: Modified Hoke-Miller flatfoot procedure. *Clin Orthop* 1983;181:24–27.
13. Durham HA, cited by Caldwell GD: Surgical correction of relaxed flatfoot by the Durham flatfoot plasty. *Clin Orthop* 1953;2:221.
14. Giannestras NJ: Flexible valgus hindfoot resulting from naviculocuneiform and talonavicular sag: Surgical correction in the adolescent, in Bateman JE (ed): *Foot Science.* Philadelphia, WB Saunders, 1976, pp 67–105.
15. Kidner FC: The prehallux (accessory scaphoid) and its relation to flatfoot. *J Bone Joint Surg* 1929;11:831.
16. Macnicol MF, Voutsinas S: Surgical treatment of the symptomatic accessory navicular. *J Bone Joint Surg* 1984;66B:218.
17. Mosier KM, Asher M: Tarsal coalitions and peroneal spastic flat foot: A review. *J Bone Joint Surg* 1984;66A:976–984.
18. Cowell HR, Elener V: Rigid painful flatfoot secondary to tarsal coalition. *Clin Orthop* 1983;177:54–60.
19. Harris RI, Beath T: Etiology of peroneal spastic flat foot. *J Bone Joint Surg* 1948;30B:624.
20. Cowell HR: Extensor brevis arthroplasty. *J Bone Joint Surg* 1970;52A:820.
21. Swiontkowski MF, Scranton PE, Hansen S: Tarsal coalitions: Long-term results of surgical management. *J Pediatr Orthop* 1983;3:287.
22. Peterson HA: Skewfoot (forefoot adduction with heel valgus). *J Pediatr Orthop* 1986;6:24.
23. Berg EE: A reappraisal of metatarsus adductus and skewfoot. *J Bone Joint Surg* 1986;68A:1185–1196.
24. Heyman CH, Herndon CH, Strong JM: Mobilization of the tarsometatarsal and intermetatarsal joints for the correction of resistant adduction of the fore part of the foot in congenital clubfoot or congenital metatarsus varus. *J Bone Joint Surg* 1958;40A:299–310.
25. Miller OL: A plastic flat foot operation. *J Bone Joint Surg* 1927;9:84.
26. Hoke M: An operation for the correction of extremely relaxed flat feet. *J Bone Joint Surg* 1931;13:773.

Pelvic Ring Disruptions

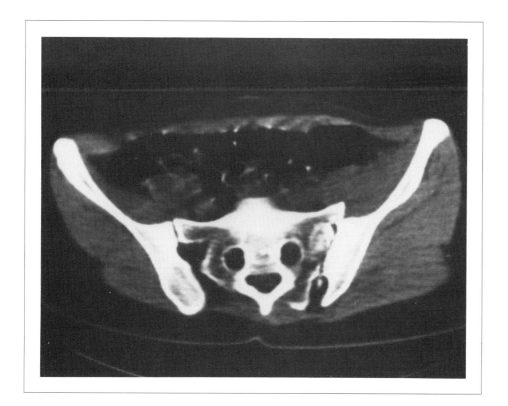

CHAPTER 15

Assessment of Pelvic Stability

Robert W. Bucholz, MD

Paul Peters, MD

Introduction

The term "pelvic disruption" has been applied to a spectrum of different injuries to the pelvic ring. The continuum stretches from simple, hairline fractures in elderly patients after minor falls to the severely displaced open pelvic fractures in young patients with polytrauma. The only common feature in this diverse group of injuries is disruption of the pelvic ring in two or more sites. All gradations of injuries between these two extremes may be encountered. Thus, the general term pelvic disruption should be avoided unless there are clear distinctions between major and minor pelvic ring injuries, stable and unstable lesions, and low-energy and high-energy injuries.

The potential for acute complications (including hemorrhage, neurologic deficits, and visceral injuries) and long-term disability (arising from leg-length discrepancy, pelvic obliquity, nonunion, and chronic sacroiliac arthritis) is significantly different in stable and unstable pelvic ring injuries. The initial orthopaedic evaluation of the patient with a pelvic injury includes two major tasks: assessing the effect of the injury on pelvic stability and deciding on the proper form of pelvic stabilization, thereby minimizing the acute and chronic complications of the injury. The first issue of assessment of pelvic stability constitutes our topic.

Normal Anatomy and Biomechanics

The transmission of load from the trunk to the lower limbs occurs through the posterior arch of the pelvis. This complex of the sacrum, sacroiliac joint, and adjacent ilium serves functionally as the weightbearing portion of the pelvis. The anterior pelvic ring provides a tie arch or strut that maintains the ring structure but is subjected to little physiologic loading during normal gait. As is evident in patients with exstrophy of the bladder and in patients who have undergone pubic symphyseal resection for urethral surgery, the normal load transmission from the trunk to the legs does not necessitate an intact anterior arch.

The sacrum and ilia form broad, strong cortical pillars between the spine and the hips. The sacroiliac joint, however, possesses little or no inherent osseous stability. Since the sacrum does not lock in a keystone configuration with the ilia, the only bony stability of the joint is provided by the concave-convex shape of the opposing joint surfaces and by a small anterior shelf of bone on each ilium.[1] The prime stabilizing structures of the joint are the supporting ligaments. The stout posterosuperior sacroiliac ligament complex confers the most stability while the anterior sacroiliac ligaments, sacrotuberous ligament, sacrospinous ligament, and iliolumbar ligament function as supplemental stabilizers. These posterior ligaments combine to form a strong posterior tension band to the joint.

When the posterior osseous elements are fractured and displaced or the sacroiliac joint has been rendered unstable, the hemipelvis tends to be displaced cephalad by muscle forces, posteriorly by supine positioning of the patient, and externally by the transmitted forces of the extended and externally rotated hips on the hemipelvis.

Pathoanatomy

The pathoanatomy of pelvic ring disruptions has been the subject of a number of different cadaver studies. In a study of 150 consecutive victims of fatal motor vehicle accidents, 47 (31%) cadavers had either detectable pelvic fractures or dislocations, or both.[2] The dissection of 26 hemipelves with double vertical breaks resulted in an anatomic classification scheme consisting of three distinct groups.

Group I (14 cadavers) showed radiographic evidence of an anterior ring injury only (Fig. 15–1, *top left*). Dissection of the anterior and posterior aspects of the pelvis after routine autopsy, however, revealed either a nondisplaced vertical fracture of the sacrum or a slight tearing of the anterior sacroiliac ligament in all 14 cases. Loading the hemipelvis resulted in no significant displacement of these injuries.

Group II (five cadavers) demonstrated partial disruption of the sacroiliac joint in addition to anterior ring injury on plain radiographs (Fig. 15–1, *top right*). Anatomic dissection disclosed complete tearing or avulsion of the anterior sacroiliac ligament from the sacrum, with sparing of the posterosuperior sacroiliac ligament complex. The hemipelvis tended to rotate externally, hinging open like a book on the intact posterior ligaments.

Group III (11 cadavers) included all grossly unstable injuries. Triplanar displacement of the hemipelvis on the sacrum was obvious both radiographically and anatomically. The posterior arch injury consisted of com-

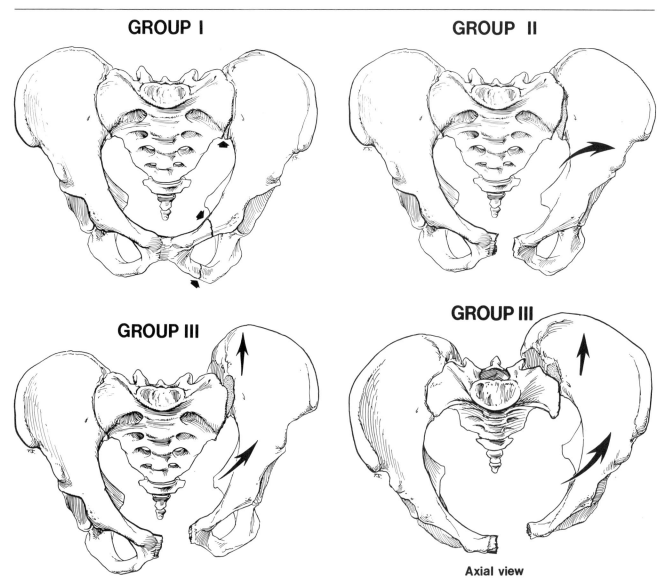

GROUP I

GROUP II

GROUP III

GROUP III

Axial view

Fig. 15-1 Classification of injuries. **Top left:** Radiographs show only anterior disruption of the pelvic ring but on dissection all have either a nondisplaced vertical fracture of the sacrum or a slight tearing of the anterior sacroiliac ligament. **Top right:** In addition to anterior injury to the pelvic ring, there is complete tearing or avulsion of the anterior sacroiliac ligament from the sacrum, with sparing of the posterosuperior sacroiliac ligament complex. **Bottom left:** Complete disruption of all sacroiliac ligaments allows triplanar displacement of the hemipelvis on the sacrum. An anteroposterior radiograph shows superior displacement. **Bottom right:** An axial radiograph shows posterior and external rotation displacement of the hemipelvis. (Reproduced with permission from Bucholz R: The pathological anatomy of Malgaigne fracture-dislocations of the pelvis. *J Bone Joint Surg* 1981;63A:400–404.)

plete sacroiliac ligament disruption or unimpacted, unstable fractures of the sacrum or ilium or both. The hemipelvis most frequently was displaced cephalad, posteriorly, and in external rotation (Fig. 15–1, *bottom left* and *bottom right*).

A number of interesting and clinically pertinent anatomic features were disclosed in the dissections. Ten of the 19 cadavers with sacroiliac disruptions had multiple avulsion fractures of the anterior surface of the sacrum. These fragments were firmly attached to the anterior sacroiliac ligament. Infolding of the ligament and attached fragments along with intra-articular de-

bris tended to block reduction attempts in both group II and group III. Group III injuries were so unstable that even anatomically reduced fractures/dislocations immediately redisplaced once the reduction force was released. The undulations of the opposing articular surfaces of the sacroiliac joint were not prominent enough to afford stability.

A similar anatomic study by Huittinen and Slatis[3] of 26 cadavers showed 12 injuries with wide separation and displacement of the detached hemipelvis. The majority were juxta-articular fractures of the ilium or sacrum extending into the sacroiliac joint. Bilateral hem-

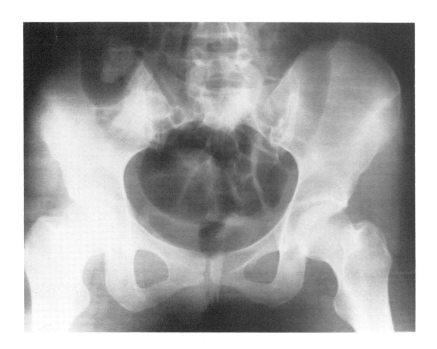

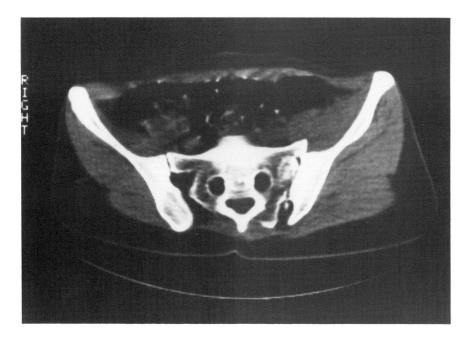

Fig. 15–2 A 25-year-old victim of a motor vehicle accident. **Top:** Anteroposterior radiograph shows a seemingly intact pelvic ring. **Bottom:** A computed tomographic scan, however, demonstrates a previously unsuspected locked sacroiliac joint and extensive comminution of the posterior part of the sacrum. (Reproduced with permission from Gill K, Bucholz R: The role of computerized tomographic scanning in the evaluation of major pelvic fractures. *J Bone Joint Surg* 1984;66A:34–39.)

ipelvic injuries were present in more than one half of the cases.

Radiographic Assessment

The standard radiographs used in evaluating pelvic ring disruptions include the anteroposterior, inlet, and tilt views. The latter two views are taken with the patient lying supine and the radiographic beam directed 40 degrees caudad and 40 degrees cephalad, respectively. These two views are directed at approximately right angles to each other and yield useful information on the amount of superior migration and anteroposterior translation of the hemipelvis. The inlet radiograph visualizes the anterior aspect of the sacral pars lateralis, the sacroiliac joint, and the adjacent part of the ilium, and can be used to detect anteroposterior displacement of the hemipelvis. The tilt radiograph discloses the extent of cephalad displacement.

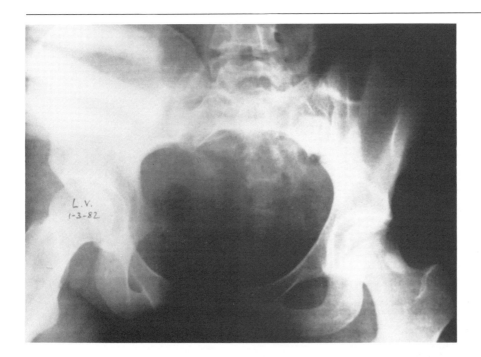

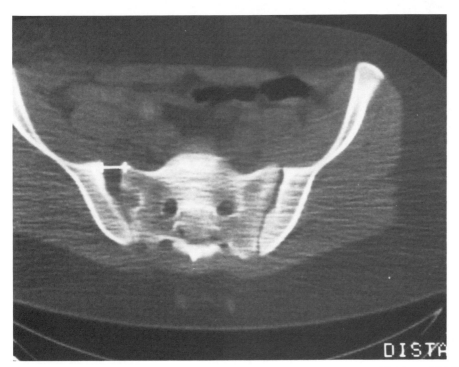

Fig. 15–3 Anteroposterior compression injury to the pelvic ring. **Top:** Anteroposterior radiograph shows the wide diastasis of the pubic symphysis without cephalad displacement of the hemipelvis. **Bottom:** Computed tomographic scan of the mid-portion of the sacroiliac joint demonstrates hinging of the hemipelvis on the intact posterior sacroiliac ligaments.

The plain radiographs are often misinterpreted. The clarity of the radiographs is frequently compromised by bowel gas, visceral shadows, and the posterior inclination of the sacrum. The true planes of displacement of the hemipelvis, as well as the status of the posterior aspect of the sacroiliac joint and the amount of comminution of sacral or sacroiliac fractures, may be difficult to assess. Bone scans using technetium polyphosphate aid in detecting hidden injuries in the pelvic ring distant from the site of obvious injury but are of primarily academic interest in the more unstable injuries.[4]

Computer-assisted tomographic scans significantly aid in the delineation of the pathologic anatomy of double vertical fractures of the pelvic ring. With a high-resolution whole-body scanner, 5-mm contiguous cross-sectional images suffice to demonstrate the pertinent anatomy. Only an average of eight to ten axial cuts is necessary to evaluate the posterior elements of the pelvic ring. Computed tomographic scanning of the an-

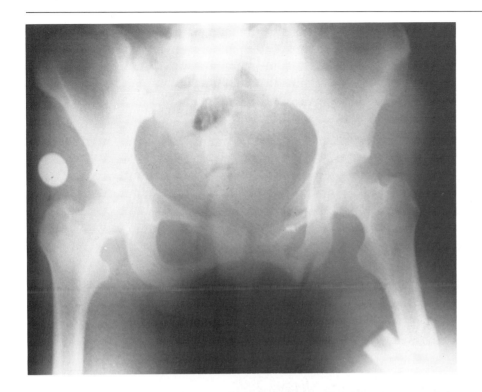

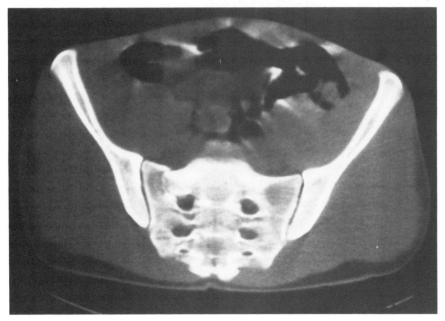

Fig. 15–4 Stable lateral compression injury. **Top:** Radiograph shows overriding of the pubic and ischial rami but no apparent posterior ring disruption. **Bottom:** Computed tomographic scan shows a vertical fracture through the sacral foramina with impaction of the sacral fragments. The ring has not been severely disrupted.

terior part of the pelvic ring is not routinely helpful and should be avoided to minimize the total radiation dose to the patient. Similarly, acetabular cuts provide no additional information unless there is a concomitant acetabular fracture. Sagittal reconstruction of the axial images has not been found helpful in assessing pelvic ring injuries.

In a recent comparative study of plain radiographs and computed tomographic scans in 25 pelvic disruptions, one third of the injury classifications were changed on the basis of the additional anatomic information provided by the computed tomographic scan.[5] Four injuries that originally had been classified as stable by plain radiographs were reclassified as unstable vertical shear injuries (Fig. 15–2). The authors concluded that computed tomographic scans offer several distinct advantages over routine radiographs. These include (1) an unobstructed cross-sectional image of the severity of the posterior pelvic arch injury, (2) a clear display of the planes of displacement of the hemipelvis, and

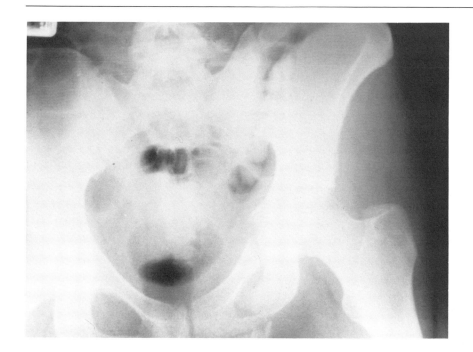

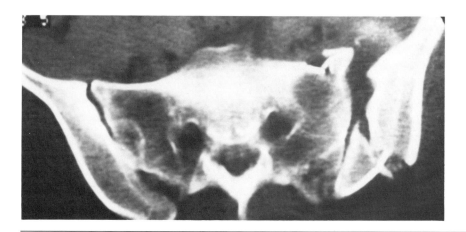

Fig. 15–5 Unstable lateral compression injury. **Top:** Radiograph shows cephalad displacement of the left hemipelvis. **Bottom:** Computed tomographic scan demonstrates a buckle fracture of the anterior cortex of the sacrum. Additionally, there is sacroiliac disruption and fracture of the posterior ilium, permitting posterior translation of the hemipelvis.

(3) in patients treated by internal fixation, an accurate method of evaluating the adequacy of fracture reduction, the position of implant, and the progress of osseous healing. Computed tomography is recommended in all cases in which plain radiographs are inadequate to judge pelvic stability, in fractures with extension into the adjacent acetabulum, and in major injuries to the hemipelvis that are to be treated by open reduction and internal fixation. Because of its increased cost and radiation exposure, routine computed tomographic scanning of all injuries to the pelvic ring is not justified.

Classification of Pelvic Ring Disruptions

A mechanistic classification scheme popularized by Tile is the most commonly used categorization system of pelvic disruptions in North America.[6,7] The three types of injuries are based on injurious force patterns. Anteroposterior compression injuries result from external rotation forces secondary to a direct posterior blow to the posterior ilium or direct pressure on the anterior iliac spines or femurs. The pelvis opens like a book, hinging on the intact posterosuperior sacroiliac ligaments (Fig. 15–3). This class of disruption corresponds to the group II anatomic pattern in the cadaver studies. Since the pelvis is not at risk for superior or anteroposterior displacement, these open-book injuries are relatively stable. A rarer cause of this anteroposterior compression pattern is a bucking horse injury when the rider is thrown onto the pommel of the saddle (P. Berg and W. Randall, personal communication, 1984). The resultant tensile forces on the pubic symphysis result in a similar anatomic lesion.

The second class of injuries consists of lateral compression fractures secondary to a direct blow on

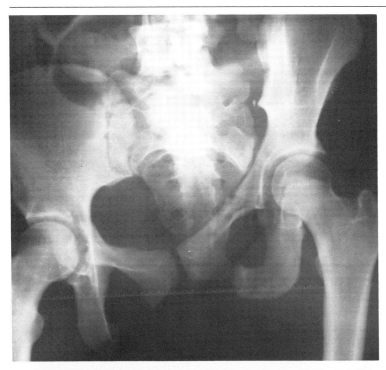

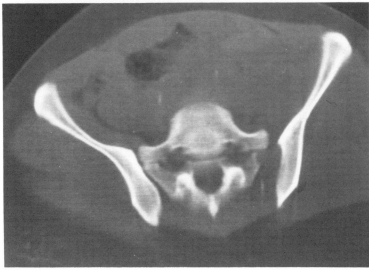

Fig. 15–6 Vertical shear injury. **Top:** Radiograph shows 3 to 4 cm of cephalad displacement. **Bottom:** Computed tomographic scan shows a completely disrupted sacroiliac joint with injury to the posterior sacroiliac ligament complex.

the iliac crests. This common mechanism of injury leads to either a stable or unstable lesion depending on the magnitude of the force. A stable lateral compression injury is characterized radiographically by overriding of pubic and/or ischial rami fractures and by an impacted posterior arch injury that is often missed on the plain radiographs. Computed tomographic scans usually demonstrate impaction of the cancellous bone of the sacral ala and a small buckle fracture of the anterior sacral cortex (Fig. 15–4). The remaining intact structures of the posterior ring are sufficient to provide stability to the ring.

Unstable lateral compression injuries occur by a similar mechanism but involve greater disruption of the posterior elements. In addition to the telltale buckle fracture of the anterior sacrum, the fracture line commonly extends into the sacroiliac joint and/or posterior sacrum and ilium. Subluxation of the posterior structures in the superior and anteroposterior planes is evident (Fig. 15–5). Vertical shear fractures constitute the third class of injuries. Forces perpendicular to the posterior ring bony trabeculae result in gross displacement of the hemipelvis. Wide diastasis of the sacroiliac joint and unimpacted sacral or ilial fractures are evident on computed tomography (Fig. 15–6). The pelvis is rendered unstable in all planes by these high-energy injuries.

Limitations of Classification Schemes

Both the anatomic and mechanistic classification schemes suffer from several inherent limitations. Ac-

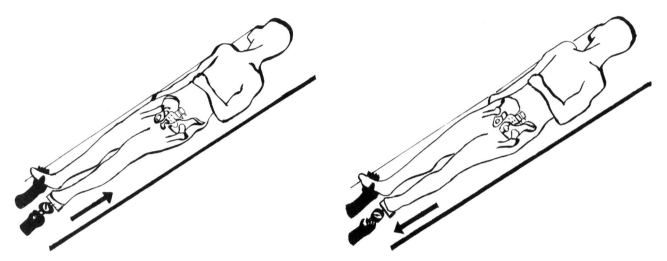

Fig. 15-7 Dynamic push-pull radiographs may be useful in distinguishing between stable and unstable ring injuries. A known longitudinal load is applied to the ipsilateral leg while the pelvis is stabilized through the opposite extremity. Plain radiographs are taken to detect cephalad translation of the hemipelvis during loading. This technique is experimental and should be used only in selected cases.

curate radiographic assessment is critical for both systems. Even with the advent of computed tomographic scanning, radiographic evaluation of a pelvic disruption provides only a static view of the injury. Unless there is gross displacement of the hemipelvis, the status of the primary and secondary stabilizing ligaments of the posterior arch cannot be deduced. An unstable hemipelvis may reduce spontaneously when the patient undergoes radiographic assessment, resulting in a false impression of a stable injury. Conversely, a slightly subluxated hemipelvis may be interpreted as grossly unstable even though there has been only partial disruption of the ligaments, with further displacement unlikely even after early mobilization of the patient.

Routine radiographic assessment of many pelvic injuries, therefore, yields only some inference of pelvic stability. Both the anatomic and mechanistic classification schemes are hampered by data from routine radiographs insufficient to categorize accurately many pelvic ring injuries. The use of push-pull or stress radiographs in the anesthetized patient assists in differentiating some of these borderline unstable injuries (Fig. 15–7). Anteroposterior radiographs of the pelvis during the application of strong longitudinal traction and then longitudinal load through the ipsilateral lower extremity can be obtained safely three to five days after injury. The degree of superior migration on the push film reflects the severity of the soft-tissue injury to the posterior arch. The pull film should reduce most of the cephalad displacement of acute injuries. A study is now in progress to determine the efficacy of such stress radiographs in supplementing routine radiographs and computed tomography in the assessment of pelvic stability.

Criteria for Pelvic Stability

Despite the limitations of currently available radiographic studies and classification schemes, an accurate statement on the effect of any given injury on pelvic stability can still be made in most cases. A qualitative definition of pelvic instability is straightforward. A pelvic disruption is unstable if there is sufficient osseous and/or ligamentous damage to the posterior arch so that normal physiologic forces displace the hemipelvis to such a degree that significant functional loss results. A similar objective or quantitative definition of pelvic stability is difficult and by the nature of the problem, necessarily arbitrary.

Tile[7] described specific signs of instability. Clinical signs of instability include (1) severe displacement of the hemipelvis that results in a leg-length discrepancy, (2) gross instability on manual palpation of the pelvic ring, (3) severe associated injuries to the viscera, blood vessels, or nerves, and (4) the presence of an open wound. The absence of all of these clinical signs, however, does not ensure that a particular pelvic injury is stable. Radiographic guidelines for instability recommended by Tile are (1) displacement of the posterior sacroiliac complex of more than 0.5 cm by fracture, dislocation, or a combination of these and (2) the presence of a gap rather than impaction posteriorly. Even with good-quality radiographic studies, the application of these criteria involves some degree of subjective evaluation. Additionally, the accuracy of these criteria has not been tested in large series of pelvic disruptions.

As a general rule, if a posterior ring injury is nondisplaced or impacted, the pelvis is probably stable. If there is superior or anteroposterior displacement of the hemipelvis of 1 cm or more, the pelvis is clearly unstable. All injuries between these two extremes may or may not be stable, and must be evaluated and treated individually. We hope that new classification schemes and diagnostic tests to identify the pathomechanics of any given pelvic disruption will be developed, thereby improving our ability to treat these challenging injuries.

References

1. Dommisse G: Diametric fractures of the pelvis. *J Bone Joint Surg* 1960;42B:432–443.

2. Bucholz RW: The pathological anatomy of Malgaigne fracture-dislocations of the pelvis. *J Bone Joint Surg* 1981;63A:400–404.

3. Huittinen V, Slatis P: Postmortem angiography and dissection of the hypogastric artery in pelvic fractures. *Surgery* 1973;73:454–461.

4. Gertzbein S, Chenoweth DR: Occult injuries of the pelvic ring. *Clin Orthop* 1977;128:202–207.

5. Gill K, Bucholz RW: The role of computerized tomographic scanning in the evaluation of major pelvic fractures. *J Bone Joint Surg* 1984;66A:34–39.

6. Tile M: Pelvic fractures: Operative versus nonoperative treatment. *Orthop Clin North Am* 1980;11:423–464.

7. Tile M: *Fractures of the Pelvis and Acetabulum.* Baltimore, Williams & Wilkins, 1984.

Initial Management of Pelvic Ring Disruptions

Bruce D. Browner, MD

J. Dean Cole, MD

Introduction

Pelvic fractures continue to be a primary source of morbidity and mortality in victims of severe blunt trauma despite advances in early identification of potential complications and their management. The incidence of pelvic fractures as the cause of death is reported to vary between 5% and 30%.[1-5] This variation can be explained by the difficulty in determining the significance of pelvic fractures that are associated with other major injuries[2,5,6] and by the difference in severity of trauma encountered at different institutions.

Fractures of the pelvic ring occur when the magnitude of injuring forces disrupts both the anterior and posterior arches.[7,8] The anterior defects consist of pubic symphysis diastases and vertical ramus fractures. Genitourinary tract and vascular injuries are often seen with these fractures. Posterior defects include vertical fractures of the sacrum, ilium, and sacroiliac joints. Displaced fractures such as these often are accompanied by soft-tissue injury to the pelvic vasculature, viscera, and nerves. First priority should be given to pelvic hemorrhage during the acute management of pelvic ring disruptions. A high incidence of late sequelae has been noted in several studies following displaced pelvic ring fractures.[9-12] The long-term morbidity is felt to be attributable to inadequate reduction and stabilization of the posterior arch defects. This long-term morbidity has led to the use of open reduction and internal fixation.

Field Management

Pelvic stability can be identified quickly by field personnel. They should hold iliac crests and compress and distract them to assess pelvic ring stability. Additionally, palpation of the pubis enables detection of pubic symphysis diastases and fractures of the vertical rami. Vital signs should be assessed and, if the patient is hemodynamically compromised with pelvic instability, Pneumatic Anti-Shock Garments (PASG) should be applied and inflated to a pressure of 40 to 50 mm Hg.[13,14] The PASG suit is similar to an air splint, acting to tamponade venous and small arterial bleeding; it may also decrease hemorrhage because of its stabilizing effect on mobile fracture lines (Fig. 16–1).

If femoral fractures or hip dislocations are present, traction splints may be applied over the PASG suit.

Additional stabilization should be obtained by using a long backboard or scoop before transporting the patient to a definitive care facility. Since other significant major injuries often accompany pelvic fractures caused by high-energy vehicular accidents, patients should be sent to level I or II trauma centers without delay. The mechanism of injury and other relative circumstances should be reported by the field personnel to the medical team in the hospital.

Emergency Management

Patients with pelvic fractures should be evaluated immediately to permit early and accurate intervention. Resuscitation priorities have been standardized and precedence should be given to the cardiopulmonary ABCs (airway, breathing, and circulation).[15] It is essential to determine immediately if the patient is in shock. If the PASG has been applied by field personnel it should be left in place. Severity of the shock state should be determined and subsequently used as a guideline for fluid resuscitation. Patients with severe pelvic fractures require several large-bore intravenous lines and the rapid infusion of large volumes of crystalloid. Constant monitoring of arterial and central venous pressure and urinary output will ensure adequate fluid management. Patients in moderate shock will respond to this fluid infusion, and there will be time to obtain properly cross-matched blood for transfusion. Patients in more profound shock will require type-specific, uncross-matched or O-negative blood. Exsanguination from pelvic hemorrhage is one of the major causes of death in patients with pelvic fractures, so they must be resuscitated aggressively.[14,16,17]

Hypothermia develops readily in patients with hemorrhagic shock who are undergoing massive fluid resuscitation. A variety of factors result in the lowering of the body's core temperature. A principal cause of hypothermia is the replacement of endogenous blood, which has been lost, with refrigerated blood products and room-temperature crystalloid. Additional radiant heat loss occurs through the skin, with the removal of the patient's clothing, and through the lungs with artificial ventilation. Once developed, hypothermia will cause coagulopathy that will substantially reduce the chances of controlling any hemorrhage associated with the pelvic fractures. Profound hypothermia can also lead to fatal cardiac arrhythmia. To avoid these prob-

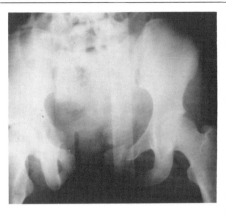
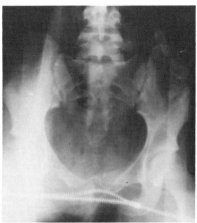
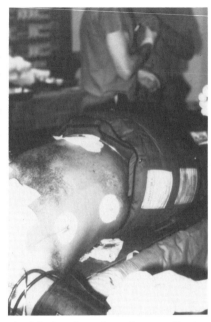

Fig. 16–1 Demonstration of effect of Pneumatic Anti-Shock Garment (PASG). **Left:** Displaced pelvic ring disruption prior to application of PASG. **Center:** Reduced pelvic ring disruption after application and inflation of PASG. **Right:** PASG maintained on patient in emergency room during resuscitation.

lems, it is important to remember that hypothermia occurs rapidly and to take early preventive measures. One such measure is to mix cold packed red blood cells with prewarmed crystalloid prior to infusion (R. Fischer, personal communication, 1986). New blood warmers have become available recently that incorporate large-diameter heat exchangers and large-bore tubing. These units overcome the restrictive low flow rate seen with the older machines. Radiant heat loss can be reduced by actively warming the patient with water-circulating heating blankets and covering the patient with reflective Mylar space blankets. Heat loss through the lungs can be decreased by warming the gases administered through the ventilator with a heated humidifier.

Significant coagulopathy can also result from depletion of clotting factors. This depletion occurs from the combination of lost clotting factors from massive hemorrhage and the infusion of large volumes of packed cells that are deficient in platelets and active clotting factors. The mortality from pelvic fractures increases dramatically with the development of this coagulopathy.[1] Early detection of this complication requires vigilance for diffuse bleeding and oozing from injured surfaces and routine measurement of clotting parameters. The hemostatic screen should include platelet count, prothrombin time, partial thromboplastin time, fibrinogen, and fibrin split products.[5] Clotting capacity can be improved by the administration of fresh-frozen plasma, calcium, platelets, and cryoprecipitate. One unit of fresh-frozen plasma generally is given after every four units of packed cells. When massive transfusion is

required to maintain hemodynamic stability, one unit of fresh-frozen plasma is given after every two units of packed cells administered. Definitions of massive transfusion vary widely, so no standard description can be given. The calcium citrate used in blood bags has an anticoagulant that combines blood calcium to make it less available for metabolic functions. For this reason, a gram of calcium generally is administered after every six to eight units of packed cells is transfused. The administration of platelets and cryoprecipitate is guided by the results of the coagulation tests. Platelets are given when there is generalized oozing and when the platelet count drops below 100,000 cells/mm³. Cryoprecipitate administration is reserved for evidence of frank disseminated intravascular coagulation.

Once the resuscitation is underway, efforts should be turned to investigation for major intrathoracic and intra-abdominal injuries. Initial radiographic studies should be performed according to a scheme of priorities with the PASG still inflated. A lateral view of the cervical spine that includes the C_7-T_1 junction should be obtained first to assess the alignment and stability of the cervical spine. Assuming that there is no evidence of injury to the spine, the second study should be an anteroposterior or posteroanterior radiograph of the chest taken with the patient sitting upright and inclining slightly forward. In this position, the abdominal contents and diaphragm descend to permit better visualization of the mediastinum, and signs of aortic injury can be detected more easily. Visualization of an enlarged aortic knob or widened mediastinum indicates the need for formal aortic arch angiography. Antero-posterior views of the abdomen and pelvis complete the radiographic survey. Significant hemorrhage is associated with superior displacement of the hemipelvis or posterior disruption of the pelvic ring.[1,2,18] When pelvic ring disruption is noted, the initial pelvic views should be supplemented with pelvic inlet and outlet views. The pelvic inlet view is taken with the tube tilted 45 degrees toward the head. Since the pelvic inlet view is taken perpendicular to the plane of the pelvic inlet, it gives an excellent view of both the anterior and posterior arches. The pelvic outlet view is taken with the tube tilted 45 degrees toward the feet. Since the pelvic outlet view is directed perpendicular to the sacrum, it provides a good anteroposterior view of this bone and permits identification of fracture patterns. The sites of pelvic ring disruption, direction, and magnitude of displacement can be determined from these radiographic studies. The surgeon should combine the information obtained from radiography with the findings from manual examination of the pelvic ring to determine the degree of pelvic instability. Since the lumbosacral nerves originate centrally in the spinal canal and arborize laterally, significant disruption of the posterior arch with displacement frequently causes neural injury.[8,19]

After adequate resuscitation and completion of the radiographic studies, the abdominal section of the PASG should be deflated cautiously to allow access to the abdomen and perineum. Gynecologic injury occasionally is associated with fractures of the pelvis. The labia and perineum should be inspected to determine the presence of hematomas or lacerations. A bimanual pelvic examination should be undertaken to identify blood in either the vaginal vault or rectal ampulla. If blood is found during these manual examinations, visual inspection of both the vaginal vault and rectal ampulla is indicated. Information can be gained with the use of an enema containing water-soluble contrast.[20,21] When the laceration communicates with the fracture site, this constitutes an open pelvic fracture and is associated with an increased risk of infection. Some of these wounds communicate with a significant defect in the muscular floor of the true pelvis. Since this floor represents an important restraint to pelvic hemorrhage, vaginal packing may be necessary in the emergency department to tamponade fracture bleeding that would otherwise flow unobstructed through the perineal wound.[22]

Great variation has been reported in the incidence of accompanying urinary tract injuries[20,23–25]; however, these injuries are associated most commonly with anterior arch pelvic fractures.[25] The cardinal signs of significant injury to the lower urinary tract are the presence of gross hematuria, blood at the urethral meatus, or inability to insert a Foley catheter. Inability to void should not be considered an accurate indicator of uri-nary tract injury. A complete tear of the membranous urethra in males can be detected on rectal examination by superior migration of the prostate gland. All patients with pelvic fractures should be suspected of having urinary tract injury, and appropriate screening examinations should be performed. In general, the greater the energy of injury and degree of pelvic fracture displacement, the greater the chance of associated urinary tract injury. The aid of a urologist should be enlisted in the management of these patients. Ideally, catheterization should be preceded by a retrograde urethrogram.[23] In practice, the retrograde urethrogram is usually performed when there is blood at the urethral meatus. After the integrity of the urethra is visualized by means of a contrast study, the urethral catheter is passed and cystography is performed to evaluate the bladder. Postvoiding views will help exclude posterior bladder rupture. The urologic contrast studies are completed by performing an intravenous pyelogram to evaluate the upper urinary tract. Urologic injuries are not as urgent as vascular injuries, and time-consuming diagnostic studies directed toward identifying urologic injuries should follow exclusion of major intraperitoneal hemorrhage.

History and physical examination are unreliable in evaluating intra-abdominal injury in patients with pelvic fractures who have associated head injuries, are under the influence of alcohol or drugs, or are chemically paralyzed early in their course to facilitate ventilation. Recognition of associated visceral injury and intraperitoneal hemorrhage can be enhanced through the use of diagnostic peritoneal lavage (DPL).[20,21,26] After filling the extraperitoneal space, blood from a pelvic fracture hemorrhage will often move up the anterior abdominal wall in the properitoneal layer. To avoid the possibility of a false-positive DPL, the portal for introducing the catheter should be established in the midline above the umbilicus.[27] The DPL has very high sensitivity, and negative findings are an extremely reliable indication that there is no intraperitoneal bleeding.[28] A positive DPL, on the other hand, must be interpreted cautiously. Blood from the retroperitoneal hematoma produced by a pelvic fracture hemorrhage can produce a false-positive DPL by spilling into the peritoneal cavity through rents or as a result of diapedesis of red cells through the peritoneum.[21,27,29] Clinical experience is required to make an accurate judgment concerning the necessity of laparotomy.

When the emergency diagnostic and therapeutic examinations and procedures requiring access to the abdomen and perineum are completed, it is important to obtain provisional reduction and stabilization of the displaced pelvic fracture to reduce bleeding from ruptured veins and fracture surfaces. This can be accomplished by reassembling and inflating the PASG or by early application of anterior external fixation.[18,26,30,31]

External fixation yields excellent immobilization and pain relief.[32,33] Fixation is obtained readily by the percutaneous insertion of two pins into the superior aspect of each iliac crest just posterior to the anterior superior spine (Fig. 16–2). After insertion of a spinal needle or Kirschner wire parallel to the internal iliac fossa, the pins can be guided safely into the dense column of bone immediately above the acetabulum. Five-millimeter pins, which are twice as stiff as the 4-mm pins originally used, enhance the fixation. A shallow drill hole is made through the cortical cap of the iliac crest, and then the pin is allowed to find its way down between the two tables of the pelvis. A simple anterior frame such as the Slätis trapezoidal design is then erected. The couplings are left loose, and the patient is rolled onto the unaffected side. After the displaced hemipelvis is reduced by gravity in this position, the couplings on the frame can be tightened. If laparotomy is anticipated, the frame is tilted caudally to allow the surgeons adequate access to the abdomen (Fig. 16–3). While anterior external fixation cannot maintain ideal reduction of vertical shear injuries in which the posterior arch is completely disrupted, it still should be used under these circumstances to aid in the resuscitation and control of the hemorrhage.[31,32] Reduction of the displaced pelvis will reduce the intrapelvic volume significantly. The reduced intrapelvic volume, in turn, diminishes the potential space for hematoma formation. Stabilization also may prevent dislodgement of newly formed hemostatic clots by decreasing the movement of fracture fragments. In comparison with such older therapies as traction and pelvic slings, the use of anterior external fixation permits greater patient mobility and decreases the likelihood that patients will develop post-traumatic respiratory distress syndrome and multiple organ system failure.[34]

Open pelvic fractures are a particularly serious problem, with mortality rates reported to be between 5% and 50%.[35,36] The difference in mechanism of injury explains this wide variation, as pedestrians and motorcyclists are more likely to sustain life-threatening open pelvic fractures.[36] Hemorrhage associated with open pelvic fractures is sometimes uncontrollable because of the loss of the tamponade afforded by the parietal peritoneum and the muscular floor of the pelvis. Sepsis also has been a major cause of death in these cases. Early stabilization with PASG or external fixation aids in control of the bleeding and helps reduce the likelihood of infection. While packing may be necessary in the emergency department, perineal wounds ultimately must undergo formal debridement and irrigation in the operating room. Antibiotic prophylaxis aimed at gram-positive and gram-negative organisms as well as anaerobes is recommended. Diverting colostomy and distal loop washout is essential to prevent fecal contamination of the large perineal wounds.[1,14,36,37] The combination of all of these measures will reduce substantially the risk of death from an open pelvic fracture.

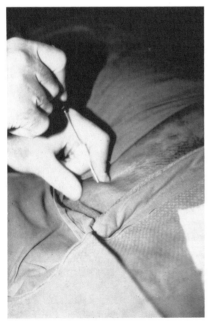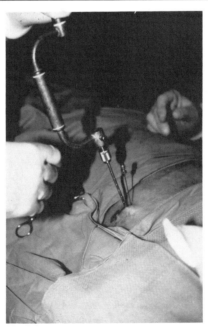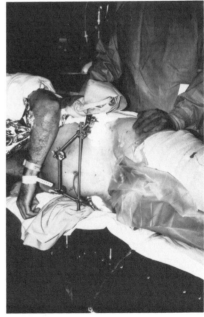

Fig. 16–2 Technique for early application of anterior pelvic external fixation. **Left:** Spinal needle inserted along the internal iliac fossa against the bone defines the inclination of the ilium. **Center:** Safe percutaneous insertion of a 5-mm pin is guided by the previously inserted spinal needle. **Right:** After two pins are inserted in each iliac crest, the frame is assembled and the patient is rolled onto the unaffected side to perform a gravity reduction. The frame components are tightened with the patient in this position.

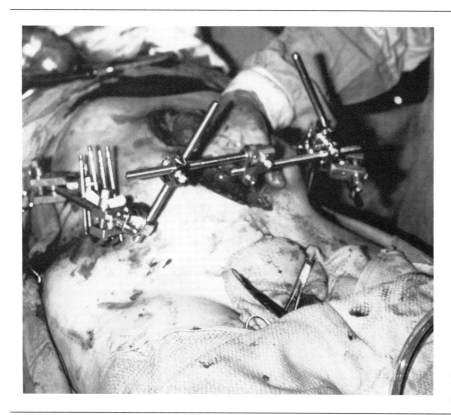

Fig. 16-3 Laparotomy being performed after previous early application of anterior external fixation. Note that the frame is tilted inferiorly to allow adequate access to the abdomen.

Radiographic Management

At this stage in the management, information obtained from the history, physical examination, radiographic survey, and special diagnostic procedures should permit the confirmation or exclusion of significant injuries in the cranial, thoracic, or abdominal cavities. Initial identification of musculoskeletal injuries should also have been possible. The pace of activity, which moves so rapidly during the initial resuscitation, often tends to slow at this stage. When indicated, computed tomographic (CT) scans and angiography should be completed expeditiously to avoid delays in essential definitive surgical management. One physician, usually the general surgeon in charge, must serve as the team leader to coordinate the efforts of the various surgical and medical services caring for the patient. Setting priorities and strategic planning are critical to patient survival and avoiding significant complications.

Careful interpretation of plain radiographic studies of the pelvis, including the anteroposterior and pelvic inlet views, reveals much information about the injury but fails to characterize the exact pathoanatomy of posterior arch disruptions. Better definition of the structures at the back of the pelvis can be obtained through the use of computed axial tomography. Studies have shown that this information can change management plans.[9,38] The value of this information, how-ever, must be balanced against the risk introduced by keeping the patient in the radiology department for a greater period of time. If posterior fixation is not planned immediately, a CT study should be deferred. If, however, the patient with an associated head injury is already on the scanner for a cranial study, little additional time is required to obtain views of the pelvis. It is important to maintain the same level of hemodynamic and respiratory monitoring in the radiology suite as in the emergency department and the operating room.

Angiography represents a powerful tool for both diagnosis and treatment of arterial bleeding associated with pelvic fractures (Fig. 16-4). However, the timing of and indications for angiography in pelvic fracture management have been controversial. Although certain fractures have a higher incidence of specific vascular trauma,[39] it is difficult to determine initially whether a patient has an arterial injury, or if hemodynamic instability also results from the more frequent sources of disrupted veins and fracture surfaces. Identification of patients with arterial injuries is critical since the higher rate of blood loss represents a greater risk of mortality. Selective catheterization of the pelvic vasculature permits accurate diagnosis of the site and magnitude of arterial bleeding. Control of these arterial bleeding points has been achieved successfully by embolization with a variety of agents, including

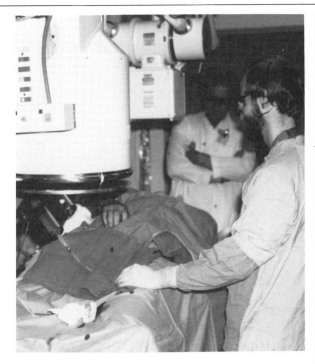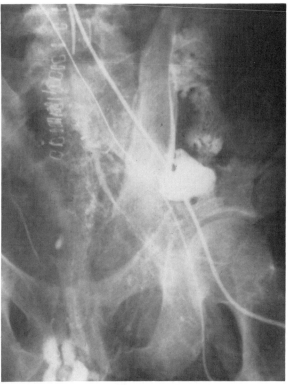

Fig. 16-4 Demonstration of diagnostic pelvic angiography. **Left:** With catheters inserted through an incision in the groin, selective catheterization is performed under fluoroscopic control. **Right:** A displaced pelvic fracture with associated arterial bleeding identified by selective catheterization.

autologous blood clot, detachable balloons, Gelfoam, and metal coils.[17,28,39,40] It is questionable whether all hemodynamically unstable patients with pelvic fractures should undergo angiography, as this procedure requires a variable amount of time, and since major arterial bleeding accounts for only approximately 10% of pelvic hemorrhage.[4,16,39] The presence of arterial injury is indicated by a continued need for transfusion to maintain hemodynamic stability following resuscitation and application of PASG or anterior external fixation. Unfortunately, waiting for arterial injuries to declare themselves in this way can result in death from arterial bleeding that could have been diagnosed and controlled by angiography. Resolution of the dilemma of whether or not to use angiography awaits the development of new techniques for diagnosing arterial injury.

Surgical Management

After the completion of resuscitation and diagnostic evaluation, some patients will require emergency surgery. The evacuation of intracranial masses and the treatment of aortic injuries should be the first priority in surgical repair. Patients with closed head injuries should have intracranial pressure monitoring using a Richman screw or intraventricular catheter. Intracranial pressure monitoring will permit the accurate measurement and control of intracranial pressure during the subsequent hours of emergency surgery. Vascular repair of major arterial injuries and laparotomy for control of intraperitoneal hemorrhage should be the next priorities.[16] At the time of laparotomy, it is important not to disturb a stable, nonpulsatile, nonexpansile retroperitoneal hematoma.[17,26] Opening the hematoma results in loss of the tamponade effect and can result in profuse hemorrhage with exsanguination.[2,14] The management of an expanding hematoma remains controversial. Direct exploration is difficult at best and attempted ligation of bleeding vessels has not proven to be an effective means of controlling pelvic hemorrhage.[4,7,13,39] Pelvic hemorrhage is difficult to control because of the extensive venous and arterial collateral network of the hypogastric vascular system. In addition, opening the posterior parietal peritoneum seriously increases the risk of infection in this area. In cases in which the anterior component of the pelvic ring disruption is a diastasis of the symphysis pubis, the laparotomy incision can be extended inferiorly to permit reduction and plate osteosynthesis of the displaced symphysis.

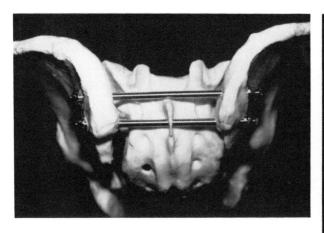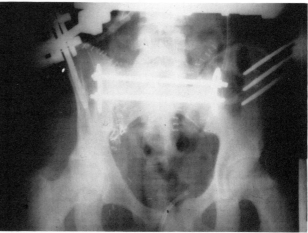

Fig. 16-5 Combination of anterior exterior fixation and posterior internal fixation with transiliac rods. **Left:** Posterior view of pelvic model shows the transiliac rods with associated plates and nuts. **Right:** Post-fixation radiograph of an unstable vertical shear injury fixed with a combination of anterior external fixation and transiliac rods.

Postoperative Management

Continued stabilization of the reduced pelvic ring is important postoperatively to maintain hemostasis and allow mobilization of the patient. Reinflated PASG can be used successfully for this purpose. To avoid pressure necrosis of the soft tissue, the garment should not be left inflated longer than 48 hours. Spica casts have been used by Hansen and associates (personal communication, 1986) as an adjunct for postoperative pelvic stabilization. In addition to providing compression of the iliac wings, these casts immobilize the hips and reduce the movement of ischial fragments. Anterior external fixation applied earlier in the management is maintained to provide continued stabilization and to permit patient and joint mobility. While succeeding with some of these goals, many centers have noted an inability to maintain reduction of posterior arch disruptions using anterior external fixation alone. This has been of concern since a number of studies have noted a high incidence of late sequelae following persistent displacement of the pelvic ring.[9-12] The addition of skeletal traction has not overcome this difficulty.

Posterior Internal Fixation

In most studies, almost half the patients with persistent posterior displacement following severe pelvic fracture complain of moderate-to-severe low back pain. While some pain can be attributed to associated lumbosacral nerve injuries and undetected lumbar spine fractures, most pain probably is related to malunion or nonunion of the posterior arch disruption. With this thought in mind, surgeons have begun to treat these fractures and dislocations by internal fixation. Many surgical approaches and fixation techniques have been attempted. The choice of specific technique is related to the exact pathoanatomy of the pelvic ring disruption. Anterior external fixation can be used to immobilize the anterior disruption in combination with internal fixation of the posterior defect (Fig. 16-5). Initial fixation of a diastasis of the symphysis pubis can restore anatomic relationships and facilitate subsequent reduction and fixation of a sacroiliac disruption or sacral fracture (Fig. 16-6).

Since the ilium projects over the sacrum posteriorly, reduction through posterior approaches is difficult. Incisions in this area, made through skin contused at the time of injury, are complicated by a high incidence of infection. Insertion of screws from the external iliac surface into the ala and body of the first and second sacral vertebrae provides excellent fixation, but there is a great risk of neurovascular injury. The proximity of the sacral nerve roots, cauda equina, and iliac vessels restricts the space through which these implants must be inserted to avoid neurovascular injury. Transiliac rods (Fig. 16-5) provide less ideal biomechanical fixation, but can be inserted with greater safety using a knee ligament drill guide. Thus, reduction and fixation of posterior iliac fractures is accomplished with greater ease and less danger of neurovascular injury.

Anterior access can be gained to the sacroiliac joint through the Aville approach to the internal iliac fossa. Definite landmarks on both the anterior ilium and sacral ala can be used to guide accurate reduction of the sacroiliac joint. Fixation can be achieved by the application of plates to the superior surface of the ala and corresponding ilium. While this approach avoids dissection of the potentially contused posterior skin, it

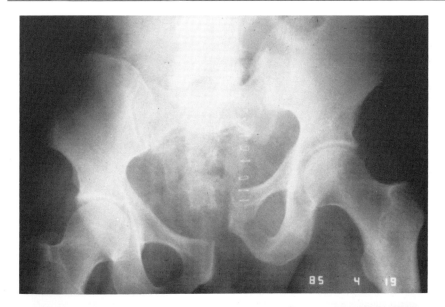

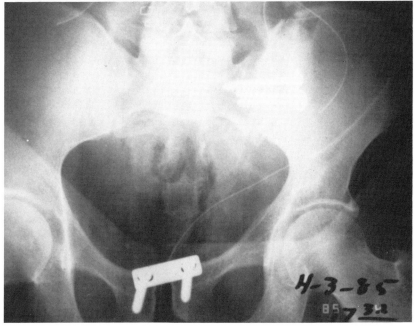

Fig. 16–6 Internal fixation of unstable vertical shear injury with a two-hole plate anteriorly and sacroiliac screws posteriorly. **Top:** Displaced fracture prior to fixation. **Bottom:** Reduced fracture after fixation.

enters the retroperitoneal space and increases the risk of decompressing the tamponaded hemorrhage. Many surgeons utilize preoperative pelvic angiography with embolization to identify and control arterial bleeding prior to an anterior approach to the sacroiliac joint. The fifth lumbar nerve passes over the top of the ala tip to form the lumbosacral plexus and is injured easily during this procedure.

More experience will be necessary to determine if reduction and internal fixation of unstable posterior pelvic ring disruption will decrease the incidence of low back pain and other problems reported following these injuries. It must be remembered that an orthopaedic surgeon's first priority in the care of a serious pelvic

fracture is the recognition and treatment of associated hemorrhage. The early use of anterior external fixation is a valuable adjunct to the control of bleeding. Although external fixation cannot maintain the reduction of certain unstable injuries, it should be used to reduce the pelvic volume and obtain provisional stabilization.

References

1. Gilliland MD, Ward RE, Barton RM, et al: Factors affecting mortality in pelvic fractures. *J Trauma* 1982;22:691–693.
2. Looser KG, Crombie HD Jr: Pelvic fractures: An anatomic guide to severity of injury. *Am J Surg* 1976;132:638–642.

3. Mucha P Jr, Farnell M: Analysis of pelvic fracture management. *J Trauma* 1984;24:379–386.

4. Rothenberger D, Fischer R, Perry J, et al: The mortality associated with pelvic fractures. *Surgery* 1978;84:356–360.

5. Trunkey DD, Chapman MW, Lim RC Jr, et al: Management of pelvic fractures in blunt trauma injury. *J Trauma* 1974;14:912–923.

6. Bucholz RW: The pathological anatomy of Malgaigne fracture-dislocations of the pelvis. *J Bone Joint Surg* 1981;63A:400–404.

7. Patterson FP, Morton KS: The cause of death in fractures of the pelvis: With a note on treatment by ligation of the hypogastric (internal iliac) artery. *J Trauma* 1973;13:849.

8. Tile M, Pennal GF: Pelvic disruption: Principles of management. *Clin Orthop* 1980;151:56–64.

9. Gill K, Bucholz RW: The role of computerized tomographic scanning in the evaluation of major pelvic fractures. *J Bone Joint Surg* 1984;66A:34–39.

10. Handley JM: Ununited unstable fractures of the pelvis, abstract. *J Bone Joint Surg* 1966;48A:1025.

11. Semba RT, Yasukawa K, Gustilo RB: Critical analysis of results of 53 Malgaigne fractures of the pelvis. *J Trauma* 1983;23:535–537.

12. Slatis P, Huittinson VM: Double vertical fractures of the pelvis: A report of 103 patients. *Acta Chir Scand* 1972;138:799–807.

13. Brown JJ, Greene FL, McMillin RD: Vascular injuries associated with pelvic fractures. *Am Surg* 1984;50:150–154.

14. Flint LM Jr, Brown A, Richardson JD, et al: Definitive control of bleeding from severe pelvic fractures. *Ann Surg* 1979;189:709–716.

15. Tile M: Pelvic fractures: Operative versus nonoperative treatment. *Orthop Clin North Am* 1980;11:423–464.

16. Rothenberger D, Fischer R, Perry J: Major vascular injuries secondary to pelvic fractures: An unsolved clinical problem. *Am J Surg* 1978;136:660–662.

17. Yellin AE, Lundell CJ, Finck EJ: Diagnosis and control of post-traumatic pelvic hemorrhage. *Arch Surg* 1983;118:1378–1383.

18. Slatis P, Karaharju EO: External fixation of the pelvic girdle with a trapezoid compression frame. *Injury* 1975;7:53–55.

19. Jackson H, Kam J, Harris JH Jr, et al: The sacral arcuate lines in upper sacral fractures. *Radiology* 1982;145:35–39.

20. Kane WJ: Fractures of the pelvis, in Rockwood CA, Green DP (eds): *Fractures in Adults*. Philadelphia, JB Lippincott Co, 1984, pp 1093–1209.

21. Ward RE, Clark DG: Management of pelvic fractures. *Radiol Clin North Am* 1981;19:167–170.

22. Levine JI, Crampton RS: Major abdominal injuries associated with pelvic fractures. *Surg Gynecol Obstet* 1963;116:223–226.

23. Colapinto V: Trauma to the pelvis: Urethral injury. *Clin Orthop* 1980;151:46–55.

24. Fallon B, Wendt JC, Hawtrey CE: Urological injury and assessment in patients with fractured pelvis. *J Urol* 1984;131:712.

25. Palmar J, Benson G, Corriere J: Diagnosis in initial management of urological injuries associated with 200 consecutive pelvic fractures. *J Urol* 1983;130:712–714.

26. Murr PC, Moore EE, Lipscomb R, et al: Abdominal trauma associated with pelvic fracture. *J Trauma* 1980;20:919–923.

27. Hubbard SG, Bivins BA, Sachatello CR, et al: Diagnostic errors with peritoneal lavage in patients with pelvic fractures. *Arch Surg* 1979;114:844–846.

28. Gilliland MG, Ward RE, Flynn TC, et al: Peritoneal lavage and angiography in the management of patients with pelvic fractures. *Am J Surg* 1982;144:744–747.

29. de Vries JE, van der Slikke W: False positive peritoneal lavage due to retroperitoneal haematoma. *Injury* 1980;12:191–193.

30. Slätis P, Karaharju EO: External fixation of unstable pelvic fractures: Experiences in 22 patients treated with a trapezoid compression frame. *Clin Orthop* 1980;151:73–80.

31. Slätis P, Karaharju EO, Kaukonen JP, et al: External fixation of pelvic fractures: Principles of the trapezoid compression frame, in Uhthoff HD (ed): *Current Concepts of External Fixation of Fractures*. Berlin, Springer-Verlag, 1980, pp 273–280.

32. Lansinger O, Karlsson J, Berg U, et al: Unstable fractures of the pelvis treated with a trapezoid compression frame. *Acta Orthop Scand* 1984;55:325–329.

33. Slätis P: External fixation of pelvic fractures, in Johnson RM (ed): *Advances in External Fixation*. Chicago, Year Book Medical Publishers, 1980, pp 77–92.

34. Gylling SF, Ward RE, Holcroft JW, et al: Immediate external fixation of unstable pelvic fractures. *Am J Surg* 1985;150:721–724.

35. Richardson JD, Harty J, Amin M, et al: Open pelvic fractures. *J Trauma* 1982;22:533–538.

36. Rothenberger D, Velasco R, Strate R, et al: Open pelvic fracture: A lethal injury. *J Trauma* 1978;18:184–187.

37. Maull KI, Sachatello CR, Ernst CB: The deep perineal laceration—An injury frequently associated with open pelvic fractures: A need for aggressive surgical management. *J Trauma* 1977;17:685–696.

38. Pennal GF, Tile M, Waddell JP, et al: Pelvic disruption: Assessment and classification. *Clin Orthop* 1980;151:12–21.

39. Kam J, Jackson H, Ben-Menachem Y: Vascular injuries in blunt pelvic trauma. *Radiol Clin North Am* 1981;19:171–186.

40. Ben-Menachem Y, Handel SF, Ray R, et al: Embolization procedures in trauma: The pelvis. *Semin Interv Radiol* 1985;2:158–181.

Pelvic Fractures: Diagnostic and Therapeutic Angiography

Yoram Ben-Menachem, MD

Introduction

The fractured pelvis, a minority of the total admissions for trauma, continues to contribute significantly to trauma's overall death rate[1] because of delays in diagnosis and control of hemorrhage.[2-7] This chapter reviews some of the challenges and pitfalls in diagnosing hemorrhage in patients with pelvic ring disruption, and proposes early and aggressive angiographic diagnosis and hemostasis, in tandem with orthopaedic management, as the primary mode of assessment and control of hemorrhage immediately following trauma.

Rationale for Angiography in Pelvic Fractures

Pelvic ring disruption is usually part of a complex, multisystem wounding pattern[1,8-11] caused by extremely violent, wide-impact, blunt trauma.[1,4,12]

The Causes of Death in Pelvic Fractures

Several factors add to the risk of death in patients with pelvic fractures; among these are (1) the degree of violence of the impact, (2) the type of pelvic ring disruption, (3) a high injury severity score, (4) hemorrhagic shock on admission, (5) requirements for great quantities of blood, (6) perineal lacerations, (7) associated injuries, and (8) advancing age.[1,8,9,12-15] In the absence of injury to the central nervous system, hemorrhage is the common denominator in all these causes of death, with most deaths occurring either directly from hemorrhage (exsanguination) or from its complications.[1,8,13,15] Therefore, diagnosis and treatment of hemorrhage are matters of great urgency that must take precedence over diagnosis and treatment of other injuries.

Sites and Sources of Hemorrhage

In a patient with borderline or unstable hemodynamics from pelvic fractures, any or all of six primary sources contribute to the hemorrhage: arterial, venous, and osseous/capillary sources within the pelvis, and sources in the abdomen, thigh, and chest. The two most common sources are the internal iliac arteries and, in the abdomen, the spleen and liver.[12] A normal chest radiograph on admission is usually sufficient to rule out intrathoracic bleeding, but still leaves five unidentified sources of hemorrhage. The actual contribution to the hemorrhage from any source cannot be estimated with certainty either by clinical criteria or by plain radiographic findings.[16]

The Case Against Laparotomy

Exploratory laparotomy, a relatively benign procedure in penetrating injuries and in isolated blunt abdominal trauma, is often lethal when performed on an unstable patient with pelvic fractures, because it accelerates the extraperitoneal hemorrhage and thus further exacerbates the patient's shock state.[1,17-20] Laparotomy also expands the volume of the extraperitoneal hematoma to the extent that it may occupy the entire abdominal cavity. Evacuation of the hematoma, either to allow closure of the abdomen or to find and ligate the internal iliac arteries, accelerates the hemorrhage even more and may culminate in exsanguination.

Surgical ligation of the internal iliac arteries is not recommended for control of pelvic hemorrhage. The proximal position of the ligature of the internal iliacs leaves all their first-generation branches open to collateral flow from large regional arteries, as well as from the internal iliacs themselves. Thus, the operation not only fails to stop the hemorrhage but may greatly accelerate it.[1,17]

The Case Against Diagnostic Peritoneal Lavage

Peritoneal lavage, although extremely sensitive in detecting intraperitoneal blood, is not designed to determine the source of that blood. Even though a positive lavage is traditionally an indication for exploratory laparotomy, in the presence of pelvic fractures, laparotomy is contraindicated. In pelvic ring disruptions there is always some tearing of the peritoneum and leakage of extraperitoneal blood into the abdominal cavity. This leakage causes a high rate of false-positive lavage in these patients.[1,8,10,20] The danger of laparotomy in the presence of pelvic fractures is serious enough for this author and others[1,4] to conclude that the peritoneal lavage tray does not belong on the resuscitation cart of patients with pelvic fractures.

Radiologic Diagnosis of Hemorrhage: Need for Direct Evidence

Reliable radiographic information can be obtained only by direct evidence of injury or normalcy. Therefore, the radiographic modality capable of giving such direct evidence is the examination of choice. In soft-tissue wounds, there is concern with vascular and/or parenchymal injuries, and with hemorrhage and/or hematomas. The diagnostic procedure should be selected accordingly. Angiography provides direct evidence of vascular injury and hemorrhage, and computed tomography (CT) shows parenchymal injury and hematoma. Plain-film radiography, with or without added contrast media, provides no direct evidence of soft-tissue injury and must be discarded. Thus, for the patient with borderline or unstable hemodynamics from pelvic fractures, angiography is the examination of choice.[4,17]

The Case for Angiographic Hemostasis

Control of arterial hemorrhage by angiographic techniques is well established as the method of choice in an ever-increasing number and variety of injuries.[3,4,12] In the fractured pelvis the angiographic approach to hemostasis is simpler, faster, and far safer than attempting to approach hemostasis through "the swamp of the extraperitoneal hematoma."[17] Angiographic hemostasis is applicable not only in the management of hemorrhage from the internal iliac arteries but also in arterial and severe parenchymal bleeding elsewhere in the body.[3,4,12]

Exploratory Angiography in Patients With Pelvic Fractures

Timing and Priorities for Angiography

The initial assessment of patients with pelvic ring disruptions must adhere to the rules that apply to the investigation of all multitrauma victims. The most important rule states that all critical injuries should be treated before any injury that does not pose an immediate risk to life.[2,5] Death can be avoided by obeying the law of inverse proportionality with regard to the number of radiographs allowed in the emergency room. The severely injured patient requires only three radiographs: chest, pelvis, and lateral cervical spine.[2]

Angiography must be performed as soon as possible after the patient's arrival at the emergency room and, except for the three basic admission radiographs mentioned above, it must precede all other radiologic investigations. It is especially important to avoid all urologic investigation prior to angiography.[2,4] Except for a massive renal hemorrhage—which will be found and treated by the angiographer—no injury to the urinary tract is of concern in the first hours after admission. Intravenous pyelogram (IVP) and cystourethrography must not be done: they are unnecessary to save life, and, if positive, their extravasated contrast medium will prevent diagnosis of an arterial hemorrhage.[2,4] All the information that an IVP can offer will be obtained by angiography, or by CT if the patient does not need an angiogram. The cystourethrogram should be done in the angiographic suite after completion of angiography and embolization.

Which First: Reduction-Fixation or Angiography? The answer

to this question depends on the condition of the patient, the availability of specialists, supportive personnel, and proper equipment, and on the degree of coordination and cooperation between the various specialists. Ideally, the patient should undergo angiography and embolization first, then open reduction and internal fixation.[21] However, the attending surgeon must make that decision after considering the patient's needs in light of available support to manage the hemorrhage.

Should Unstable Patients Be Transported to Angiography? Unequivocally, yes. An unremitting hemorrhage must be controlled by surgical or angiographic intervention. Despite shock, patients must be transported for treatment in the operating suite or angiographic suite to avoid exsanguination in the emergency room.[3]

Planning and Performance of the Angiogram

The angiographic exploration should be designed to diagnose all active and potential arterial bleeding points beginning with the pelvis and continuing into the abdomen and other suspected areas, if necessary.[4] The diagnostic study is stopped temporarily whenever significant arterial hemorrhage is encountered and is continued after the bleeding artery has been embolized. A complete diagnostic investigation of the torso, including midstream pelvic arteriography, midstream thoracic and abdominal aortography, and selective splenic arteriography need not take more than 20 minutes.[12] Except for the inability of angiography to diagnose or rule out bowel wall injury, there is great reliability in negative findings of vascular or parenchymal wounding.

Angiographic Control of Hemorrhage in Pelvic Ring Disruption

The angiographer contributes to patient stabilization by controlling arterial hemorrhage and managing extrapelvic parenchymal hemorrhage, primarily from the spleen.[4,12] Reduction and fixation of the fractures reduces or stops osseous and capillary bleeding and the great majority of venous hemorrhages.

Angiographic Embolic Agents

The angiographic embolic agent I prefer is Gelfoam,[4,12,16] because its life in the artery is limited to two to 12 weeks. Gelfoam is the preferred agent when temporary long-term occlusion is needed. Steel coils are best when Gelfoam cannot be used, either because of the target's caliber or its nearness to the central nervous system, and when permanent occlusion of the artery is acceptable.[4] Fixed occlusion balloon catheters are useful as a means of short-term (a few hours) occlusion of a major artery until it can be surgically repaired.[3] Fixed occlusion balloon catheters can also be used to aid in identifying the site of injury at the time of exploration.[12] Other occluding agents are available and, with the exception of powders and of destructive agents such as ethanol or phenol, can be employed by an experienced angiographer.

Techniques of Embolization

Ideally, only the target artery should be embolized. However, in many patients, more than one branch of the internal iliac artery may be bleeding. Attempts to embolize each one will waste time. Arteries bleeding in more than one branch should be embolized with a suspension of 2-mm cubes of Gelfoam in diluted contrast medium ("Gelfoam pudding").[4] An injection of 3 to 4 cc of this "pudding" into the internal iliac artery creates an almost simultaneous embolization of all its first- and second-generation branches and leaves the smaller arteries patent. Thus, slow collateral perfusion of the tissues can continue without negating the hemostatic effect of the embolization.

Steel coils are not good substitutes for Gelfoam pudding, because, like a surgical ligation, the coil occludes only the main artery and may provide only partial and temporary control of hemorrhage.

Patient Management After Embolization

Embolization is one step in patient stabilization. Total patient care must continue in earnest at the conclusion of embolotherapy. In many instances, patients suffer from coagulopathy and hypothermia at the time of angiography. If these are not reversed, the beneficial effect of the embolization will be short-lived, because hemorrhage will quickly resume via the collateral blood vessels. The severely injured patient must undergo reduction and fixation of the fractured pelvis, if these were not done prior to angiography, and then be treated supportively to allow restoration of normal body temperature and clotting activity. All surgery should be postponed until the patient is stabilized to this degree.[4]

Summary

Pelvic ring disruption is part of a complex wounding pattern that challenges our ability to diagnose and manage hemorrhage.

The conventional methods of diagnosis and control of abdominopelvic bleeding—peritoneal lavage and exploratory laparotomy—should be replaced by exploratory abdominopelvic angiography and transcatheter embolization.

Angiography should be performed as soon as possible after the patient is admitted to the emergency room, and shock should not delay transfer of the patient to the angiography suite.

References

1. Mucha P Jr, Farnell MB: Analysis of pelvic fracture management. *J Trauma* 1984;24:379–386.
2. Ben-Menachem Y: Logic and logistics of radiography, angiography, and angiographic intervention in massive blunt trauma. *Radiol Clin North Am* 1981;19:9–15.
3. Ben-Menachem Y, Handel SF, Ray RD, et al: Embolization procedures in trauma: A matter of urgency. *Semin Interv Radiol* 1985;2:107–117.
4. Ben-Menachem Y, Handel SF, Ray RD, et al: Embolization procedures in trauma: The pelvis. *Semin Interv Radiol* 1985;2:158–181.
5. Foley RW, Harris LS, Pilcher DB: Abdominal injuries in automobile accidents: Review of care of fatally injured patients. *J Trauma* 1977;17:611–615.
6. Certo TF, Rogers FB, Pilcher DB: Review of care of fatally injured patients in a rural state: 5-year follow-up. *J Trauma* 1983;23:559–565.
7. Dove DB, Stahl WM, DelGuerico LRM: A five-year review of deaths following urban trauma. *J Trauma* 1980;20:760–766.
8. Gilliland MD, Ward RE, Barton RM, et al: Factors affecting mortality in pelvic fractures. *J Trauma* 1982;22:691–693.
9. Faist E, Baue AE, Dittmer H, et al: Multiple organ failure in polytrauma patients. *J Trauma* 1983;23:775–787.
10. Ward RE, Clark DG: Management of pelvic fractures. *Radiol Clin North Am* 1981;19:167–170.
11. Kane WJ: Fractures of the pelvis, in Rockwood CA, Green DP (eds): *Fractures*. Philadelphia, JB Lippincott, 1975, pp 923–973.
12. Ben-Menachem Y: *Angiography in Trauma: A Work Atlas*. Philadelphia, WB Saunders Co, 1981.
13. Grieco JG, Perry JF Jr: Retroperitoneal hematoma following trauma: Its clinical importance. *J Trauma* 1980;20:733–736.
14. Richardson JD, Harty J, Amin M, et al: Open pelvic fractures. *J Trauma* 1982;22:533–538.
15. Rothenberger D, Velasco R, Strate R, et al: Open pelvic fracture: A lethal injury. *J Trauma* 1978;18:184–187.
16. Kam J, Jackson H, Ben-Menachem Y: Vascular injuries in blunt pelvic trauma. *Radiol Clin North Am* 1981;19:171–186.
17. Peltier LF: Comments to the 43rd annual session of the AAST. *J Trauma* 1984;24:385.
18. Shah R, Max MH, Flint LM Jr: Negative laparotomy: Mortality and morbidity among 100 patients. *Am Surg* 1978;44:150–154.
19. Yellin AE, Lundell CJ, Finck EJ: Diagnosis and control of posttraumatic pelvic hemorrhage. *Arch Surg* 1983;118:1378–1383.
20. Hubbard SG, Bivins BA, Sachatello CR, et al: Diagnostic errors with peritoneal lavage in patients with pelvic fractures. *Arch Surg* 1979;114:844–846.
21. Goldstein A, Phillips T, Sclafani SJA, et al: Early open reduction and internal fixation of the disrupted pelvic ring. *J Trauma* 1986;26:325–333.

Posterior Pelvic Disruptions Managed by the Use of the Double Cobra Plate

Dana C. Mears, MD, PhD

Charles P. Capito, MD

Henry Deleeuw, MD

Introduction

Reconstruction of a displaced unstable sacral fracture or of bilateral sacroiliac dislocations has presented a formidable or unsolvable fracture problem.[1,2] With nonsurgical management, a late painful nonunion or malunion of the posterior pelvic injury is inevitable. The application of external fixation generally gives an equally poor prognosis, even if an initial closed reduction results in a reapproximation of the disruption or disruptions. Usually, with limitation of activity to bed rest or bed-to-chair transfers, the reduction is lost when the patient moves in bed.

Previous attempts to employ internal fixation for sacral stabilization have used lag screws or sacral bars.[2,3] In a simple sacral fracture through the alar portion of the bone, the use of two or three lengthy, cancellous lag screws can provide effective stability.[1] The screws are inserted through the posterior wing of the ilium and across the ipsilateral sacroiliac joint. Biplane image intensification has been used to insert the screws because of the numerous neurovascular hazards and the proximity of the rectum. The application of image intensification is thwarted by the limited field of view and the poor resolution that is typically achieved on patients who weigh more than 180 lb.

If the sacral fracture is a midline variant or is complicated by comminution, then the use of lag screws is inadequate and can be very hazardous. As an alternative, one or two Harrington compression rods have been used to span the back of the pelvis to anchor in the posterior iliac crests.[2] Either sacral hooks or nuts are used to achieve anchorage in the ilia. The proponents of this method advocate it as a minimally invasive surgical exposure in which a closed reduction is accompanied by internal fixation. Since the bars are inserted superficial to the paraspinous muscles, a relatively limited dissection is needed.

This method of using Harrington compression rods has substantial shortcomings. Since the bars span from one posterior ilium to the other, the sacrum itself, which is the site of the injury, is not anchored. Isolated use of sacral bars is inadequate with a highly comminuted double vertical sacral fracture, bilateral sacroiliac dislocations, or combinations of these injuries. In an attempt to extend its applications, special washer-plates have been devised that are situated near the ends of the bars on the superficial surfaces of the ilia. The washer-plates have holes so that cancellous lag screws

can be inserted that cross either sacroiliac joint. With or without the use of the washer-plates, the rotational stability of this fixation is marginal. Unless the method of fixation is accompanied by an anatomic reduction of the fracture, the inadequacy of the fixation is likely to result in a persistent malunion. Complications of pelvic malalignment that are likely to ensue include apparent limb-length discrepancy, sitting imbalance, pelvic obliquity, uncomfortable bony prominences, and cosmetically significant asymmetry of the pelvis.

About eight years ago at the Orthopaedic Research Laboratories of the University of Pittsburgh, an anatomic and biomechanical study on various pelvic stabilization techniques was initiated.[1,4] A novel technique called the Double Cobra plate was developed in an attempt to provide effective stabilization for unstable sacral fractures or bilateral sacroiliac disruptions. The results of the biomechanical studies have been presented by Rubash and associates.[5] These results indicated that the application of a Double Cobra plate with supplementary simple internal or external fixation of an anterior pelvic lesion provided rigid fixation to bilateral sacroiliac dislocations. This was accompanied by a diastasis of the symphysis pubis that rivaled the stability of the intact pelvic ring. Subsequently, a clinical evaluation of this fixation technique was initiated. The results are presented in this chapter.

Surgical Technique

After induction of general anesthesia, the patient is turned to a prone position on a standard operating table. For a reduction of a comminuted displaced sacral fracture accompanied by an anterior injury, the sacral fracture is anatomically reduced and stabilized before approaching the anterior injury. In bilateral sacroiliac dislocations accompanied by a diastasis of the symphysis pubis, the symphysis is anatomically reduced first, which helps to realign the posterior injuries. Generally, an accurate reduction of the pelvis, particularly with regard to rotation, is more easily achieved by initial anterior exposure prior to surgical approach of the sacroiliac joints.

To expose the sacrum or both sacroiliac joints, a straight or curvilinear transverse incision is made across the mid portion of the sacrum about 1 cm inferior to the posterior superior spines of the ilium (Fig. 18–1, *top left*). Typically, a straight transverse incision is made.

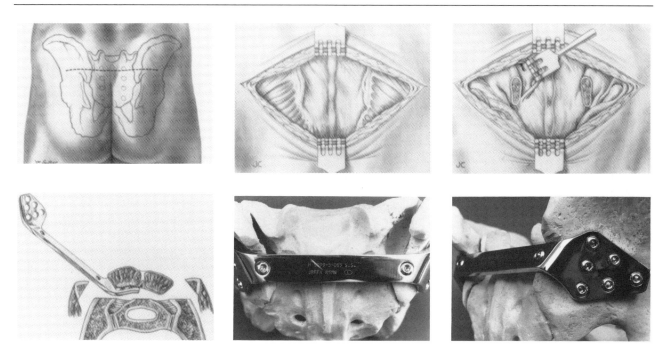

Fig. 18–1   Insertion techniques for the Double Cobra plate. **Top left:** Cutaneous incision. **Top center:** Exposed posterior iliac crests, gluteus maximus, and paraspinous muscles. **Top right:** Preparation of subperiosteal tunnel deep to paraspinous muscles. The gluteus maximus muscles have been reflected and an osteotomy performed on the posterior superior spines. **Bottom left:** Insertion of the Double Cobra plate into the tunnel deep to the paraspinous muscles. **Bottom center:** Posterior view of the Double Cobra plate across the sacrum with its recessed position in the posterior superior spines. **Bottom right:** A posterolateral view of one end of the Double Cobra plate.

If exploration of one or both sciatic nerves from the sacral foramina to the greater sciatic notch is indicated, then the ends of the incision are curved distally to facilitate such an exposure. If one or both iliac crests are to be visualized for concomitant stabilization of an iliac fracture, then the appropriate side of the incision is curved in a superior direction. The incision is sharply extended through the deep fascia. The superior portions of the origins of the gluteus maximus from the posterior superior spines are visualized. The oblique origin of the gluteus maximus from the posterior superior spine to the midline of the sacrum is sharply incised (Fig. 18–1, *top center*). Subperiosteal elevation is undertaken on the adjacent parts of either iliac wing until the roof of either greater sciatic notch can be palpated. The paraspinous muscles are elevated from the sacrum (Fig. 18–1, *top right*). The elevation is begun along the midline of the sacrum with continuation in either lateral direction. Also, the muscles are elevated from the lateral borders of the sacrum adjacent to the posterior superior spines. Ultimately, a tunnel deep to either paraspinous muscle is created that extends from approximately the superior border of the sacrum to the fourth sacral body. Retraction of the appropriate paraspinous muscle permits direct visualization of the sacral fracture. The fracture is gently debrided of hematoma to facilitate the subsequent reduction. Alternatively, in the presence of bilateral sacroiliac dislocations, the sa-

croiliac joints are debrided to the level of subchondral bone. The debridement is needed to encourage an ultimate fusion of the sacroiliac joints.

Typically, the sacral fracture or the disrupted sacroiliac joints are reduced by using tenaculum bone-holding forceps applied to 3.2-mm unicortical drill holes. For a vertical sacral fracture that propagates along the foramina, the forceps are applied from the contralateral side of the sacral spinous processes to the iliac wing. Multiple forceps are needed to correct a vertical malalignment as well as to approximate the fracture. In a rotational malalignment of a hemipelvis, a 5- or 6-mm Steinmann pin or half-pin is inserted between the inner and outer tables of the pelvis at the level of the posterior superior spine. Manipulation of the pin facilitates the reduction. When an anatomic reduction is accomplished, an osseous bed for the Double Cobra plate is prepared. At the level of the posterior superior spines, the posterior ilia are trimmed to create a notch that is flush with the posterior surface of the sacrum. Also, the adjacent posterior superior spines of the sacrum are removed.

To determine the optimal size of the Double Cobra plate, both clinical and radiologic measurements can be employed. The seven sizes of the plate differ in width to fit across the sacrum. These sizes were selected from the appropriate anthropometric documentation with 10-mm increments between the adjacent models. By a computed tomographic (CT) scan taken through the posterior superior spines, the width of the appropriate plate can be estimated. Alternatively, at this stage of the surgical procedure, the corresponding width of the pelvis can be measured. Where the measurement is between two sizes of available plate, the smaller size is selected. If the measurement is less than 75 mm, the size of the smallest available plate, a 4.5-mm reconstruction plate of an appropriate length is selected. This plate should have three holes for application to either lateral ilium as well as an appropriate length to bridge the back of the pelvis. The reconstruction plate is contoured to rival the shape of the Double Cobra plate.

The plate is inserted into the tunnel deep to the paraspinous muscles and inverted into its final position (Fig. 18–1, *bottom left*). Two lengthy, 6.5-mm threaded cancellous screws are inserted into the posterior surfaces of the osteotomized posterior superior spines (Fig. 18–1, *bottom center*). During the insertion of the screws, as the plate impinges upon the pelvis, it forces the ilia together to obliterate the fracture gap of the sacral fracture. While the mechanical advantage for approximation of the fracture surfaces is a major asset of the technique, overenthusiastic compression of a sacral fracture that violates the foramina jeopardizes the adjacent sacral roots. Next, the three screw holes in the broadest parts of the plates are filled with 6.5-mm cancellous screws that are 45 to 55 mm long (Fig. 18–1,

bottom right). These lag screws are inserted through the ilia into the sacral ala. In the presence of bilateral sacroiliac dislocations, they provide effective lag screw fixation of the injuries. Finally, two or three 4.5-mm cortical screws are inserted in both ends of the plate. These screws anchor the plate to the ilia to augment the rotational stability of the pelvis.

Before the wound is closed, the bone fragments that were harvested from the posterior superior spines and the spinous processes of the sacrum are morsellized to provide autologous bone graft for the posterior fracture site or sites.

Postoperative Regimen

In the typical case of both the posterior and the anterior pelvic lesions stabilized with internal fixation, the patient is encouraged to undertake bed-to-chair transfers and a touchdown gait within a few days after surgery. Six weeks later, with a successful clinical and radiographic evaluation, the patient is advanced to substantial partial weightbearing, with the restoration of full weightbearing at ten to 12 weeks.

In an acute sacral fracture complicated by a four-part ramus disruption, only posterior fixation with a Double Cobra plate has been undertaken. In these cases, bed-to-chair transfers were undertaken for four weeks

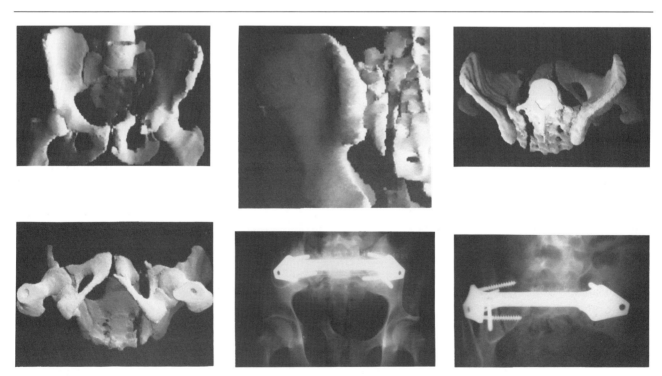

Fig. 18–2 Use of the Double Cobra plate for a simple vertical sacral fracture. Three-dimensional CT views, anterior (**top left**), posterior (**top center**), superior (**top right**), inferior (**bottom left**). Postoperative radiographic views with the Double Cobra plate: Anteroposterior (AP) view (**bottom center**), obturator oblique view (**bottom right**).

before starting a touchdown gait. Subsequently, weight-bearing progresses to full, independent ambulation within ten to 12 weeks.

Clinical Results

During the past five years, 30 patients have been managed for various posterior pelvic disruptions using a Double Cobra plate or a comparable technique with a 4.5-mm reconstruction plate. The 14 male and 16 female patients ranged in age from 16 to 63 years, with an average age of 28 years. There were 23 injuries resulting from motor vehicle accidents, four from industrial incidents, and five falls from heights including one equestrian injury. Fourteen of the cases were seen at the time of injury and five individuals were seen between six and 20 weeks after the time of injury. There were 11 cases of nonunion or malunion, including one nonunion in a 35-year-old woman who was seen three years after a chondrosarcoma of the sacral ala had been removed. The other injury patterns included 12 sacral fractures, three bilateral sacroiliac disruptions, and 14 complex posterior injuries with sacral fractures accompanied by unilateral or bilateral sacroiliac disruptions. In 26 cases, a Double Cobra plate was employed, and in four others, a 4.5-mm reconstruction plate was used. Three of the last cases were undertaken prior to the availability of the 75-mm Double Cobra plate.

Supplementary anterior internal fixation was employed in 25 of the cases. Two of the remaining five cases were managed with an anterior external pelvic frame although one of these was removed one week after the surgery because of pin-track drainage. The remaining three cases of sacral fracture complicated by a four-part ramus fracture were managed solely with posterior internal fixation.

All of the acute traumatic disruptions and the delayed presentations progressed to an uneventful union that was documented clinically and radiographically within three months of the pelvic reconstruction. Two other patients who were managed for a malunion of the pelvis also progressed to an uneventful union within three months after posterior osteotomies of the pelvis were undertaken to correct marked rotational deformities accompanied by superior migration of the hemipelvis. Of the nonunion group, two patients complained of persistent posterior pelvic pain. In one of these, a surgical exploration was undertaken and a Double Cobra plate was removed. At that time, a bony union of the sacrum and adjacent sacroiliac joint was documented. The remaining patient shows radiographic features that are consistent with a union; however, there is still the possibility of a persistent nonunion.

There were no deaths immediately after the surgical reconstructions. One patient, who underwent a surgical correction for a malunion about three years after his

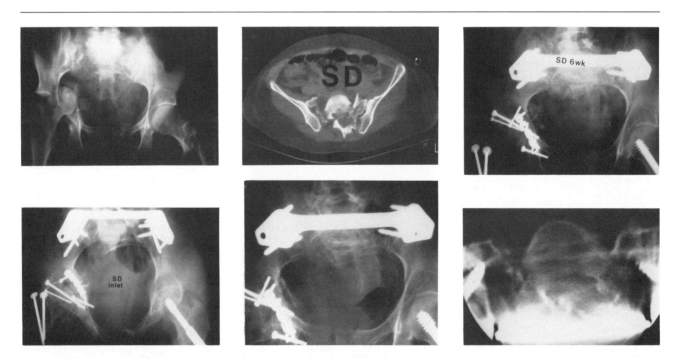

Fig. 18–3 Use of the Double Cobra plate for a comminuted sacral fracture complicated by a T-type acetabular fracture and a left intertrochanteric femoral neck fracture. **Top left:** Preoperative AP radiograph. **Top center:** Preoperative CT scan of sacral fracture. **Top right:** Postoperative AP view. **Bottom left:** Postoperative inlet view. **Bottom center:** One year postoperative AP view. **Bottom right:** One year postoperative CT scan of sacral repair.

initial pelvic injury, ultimately developed and died of acquired immune deficiency syndrome apparently related to the multiple blood transfusions he received after his initial injury. Three patients complained of hypesthesia or dysesthesia in their buttocks or genitalia. Three other patients had postoperative features of partial foot drop or weakness of the extensor hallucis longus. In the latter case, there was spontaneous resolution during the six-month period after the surgery. There were no postoperative wound infections or clinically documented thromboembolic problems.

Clinical Case Reports

Case 1

Case 1 was a 19-year-old man involved in a motor vehicle accident that resulted in a simple vertical fracture of the sacrum through the left foramina (Fig. 18–2). The sacral fracture was accompanied by a disruption of the left rami. An open reduction was performed without difficulty with the application of a Double Cobra plate. After the surgery, he undertook bed-to-chair transfers for one month followed by a partial weightbearing gait for one month. Within four months of surgery, he had resumed full activities. The surgical procedure provided an anatomic reduction of the sacrum (Fig. 18–2, *bottom center* and *bottom right*), although no attempt was undertaken to reconstruct the rami.

Case 2

Case 2 was a 29-year-old woman involved in a motor vehicle accident that caused multiple traumatic insults, including a comminuted sacral fracture with an ipsilateral T-type acetabular fracture and a contralateral intertrochanteric femoral neck fracture (Fig. 18–3, *top left* and *top center*). For the surgical reconstruction, the acetabular and femoral neck fractures were repaired prior to the surgical reconstruction of the sacrum by a Double Cobra plate (Fig. 18–3, *top right* and *bottom left*). For eight weeks she was limited to a bed-to-chair transfer regimen, after which time a four-point gait was started. One year later she was fully ambulatory, although she complained of localized discomfort at the site of the posterior pelvis. Because of her lean body habitus, the ends of the plate could be palpated deep to the skin. Assessment by conventional radiographs and a CT scan (Fig. 18–3, *bottom center* and *bottom right*) was consistent with a solid union of the sacrum. The plate was removed when complete healing of the sacral fracture was documented. Plate removal alleviated the patient's discomfort.

Case 3

Case 3 was a 16-year-old youth involved in an unusual motor vehicle accident. He was a passenger in the back seat of a car and his legs were spread over the top of the front seat. When the vehicle struck a tree, he was catapulted into the windshield, which caused dislocations of both sacroiliac joints (Fig. 18–4). Because of

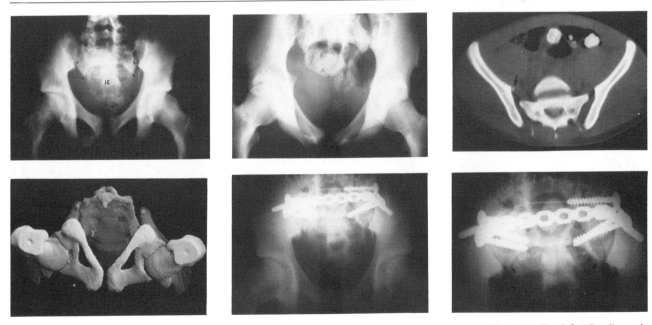

Fig. 18–4   Use of the Double Cobra technique with a 4.5-mm reconstruction plate for bilateral sacroiliac dislocations. **Top left:** AP radiograph. **Top center:** Inlet radiograph. **Top right:** CT scan of sacroiliac joints. **Bottom left:** Three-dimensional CT scan, inferior view. **Bottom center:** Postoperative AP view with 4.5-mm reconstruction plate and a supplementary cancellous lag screw. **Bottom right:** Postoperative close-up inlet view highlights the accuracy of the reduction.

his small stature, the open reduction and internal fixation of the sacroiliac joints was done with a 4.5-mm
reconstruction plate and a supplementary cancellous
lag screw across the left sacroiliac joint (Fig. 18–4,
bottom center and *bottom right*). Following an eight-week
period of four-point gait, he rapidly resumed full
activities.

Case 4

Case 4 was a 34-year-old male pedestrian struck by
a tractor trailer traveling at high speed. He sustained
multiple traumatic insults including a comminuted sacral fracture with a fracture-dislocation of the left sacroiliac joint, a diastasis, and a transverse, posterior-
wall acetabular fracture (Fig. 18–5). Other injuries included a hemopneumothorax, a ruptured spleen, and
multiple lacerations. Six weeks after his initial management of laparotomy, splenectomy, and the insertion of
chest tubes, he was transferred to our care for pelvic
reconstruction. Following open reduction and internal
fixation of the acetabulum, the patient was repositioned
for posterior pelvic repair using a Double Cobra plate.
He was managed with bed-to-chair transfers for eight
weeks followed by a four-point gait for a period of six
weeks. Four months later he was able to walk without
limitations. Radiographs are consistent with oblitera-

tion of the fracture lines (Fig. 18–5, *bottom center* and
bottom right), although Brooker Grade II ectopic bone
is an incidental finding without clinical significance evident at the involved hip joint.

Case 5

Case 5 was a 44-year-old woman who sustained
injuries when the school bus that she was driving
plunged from a height of more than 50 ft. She sustained a right-sided sacral fracture with an associated fracture-dislocation of the sacroiliac joint complicated by contralateral ramus fractures. Initially, she
was managed with bedrest for eight weeks. Subsequently, she developed a mobile painful nonunion of
the right hemipelvis including the left rami. Three
years later she had a symptomatic nonunion and an
open reduction and internal fixation of the posterior injury was performed using a Double Cobra
plate (Fig. 18–6). She continued to complain of a
painful grating at the site of the left ramus disruptions. One year later, internal fixation of the superior pubic ramus was performed. Subsequently, she
was managed with a six-week period of bed-to-chair
transfers followed by six weeks of a partial weightbearing gait. Six months after the second procedure,
she was able to return to work.

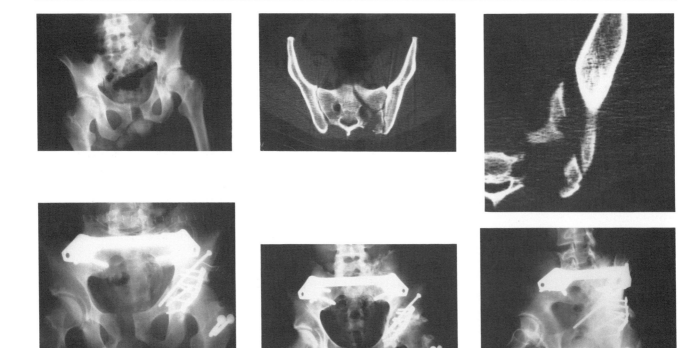

Fig. 18–5 Use of the Double Cobra Plate for a complex pelvic injury following a delayed presentation. The injury includes a comminuted sacral fracture with a fracture-dislocation of the left sacroiliac joint, a diastasis, and a transverse, posterior-wall acetabular fracture. **Top left:** AP radiograph. **Top center:** CT scan of the sacrum. **Top right:** CT scan of the left sacroiliac joint. **Bottom left:** Postoperative AP view. **Bottom center:** Four months later, postoperative AP view. **Bottom right:** Four months later, left obturator oblique view.

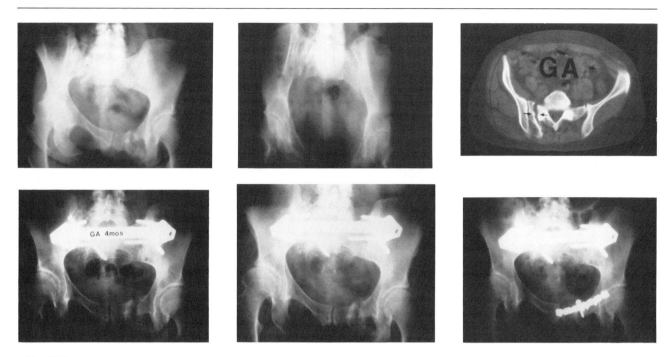

Fig. 18-6 Use of the Double Cobra Plate for a nonunion of a sacral fracture with a fracture-dislocation of the right sacroiliac joint, and fractures of the left rami. **Top left:** Preoperative AP radiograph. **Top center:** Preoperative inlet view. **Top right:** Preoperative CT scan of the sacrum and right sacroiliac joints. **Bottom left:** Initial postoperative AP view after posterior fixation. **Bottom center:** Initial postoperative inlet view, supplementary anterior fixation. **Bottom right:** AP view one year after supplementary anterior fixation.

Discussion

In the presence of a displaced sacral fracture or bilateral sacroiliac disruption, especially when the injury is accompanied by an acetabular fracture, an accurate radiologic evaluation of the pelvis is crucial to appropriate preoperative planning.[3] The use of anteroposterior inlet and outlet radiographs accompanied by the five standard CT views of the pelvis is strongly recommended. Three-dimensional CT scans provide the optimal method for the recognition of crucial rotational deformities.[1] With the substantial magnitude of posterior pelvic reconstruction and its potential for profuse intraoperative hemorrhage, the surgical reconstruction is deferred until hemodynamic stability has been achieved. The use of a "cell saver" during the surgery is advised. In the presence of a concomitant acetabular fracture, the acetabulum is reconstructed prior to the posterior reduction, since the former requires a more accurate reduction. Within the scope of these constraints, the use of the Double Cobra plate, or in smaller patients, a posterior reconstruction plate, appears to provide effective stable fixation with an acceptable incidence of morbidity. The principal complication appears to be the risk of injury to posterior sensory nerves, although this problem is not of great functional significance. The risk of intraoperative hemorrhage is minimized by a careful dissection of the principal muscles from bone, especially the gluteus maximus and paraspinous muscles. The tunnel of paraspinous muscles is optimally prepared by dissection from the midline working in the lateral direction, as well as elevation of the muscles from the posterior superior spinous processes working in a medial direction. During the subperiosteal elevation on the lateral ilia, the roof of either greater sciatic notch is carefully visualized to minimize a risk of injury to the sciatic nerves.

A cautious debridement of a sacral fracture that includes the neural foramina is crucial to avoid injury to the sacral nerve roots. Large pelvic bone-holding forceps are needed to facilitate the reduction. Rotational realignment of a displaced hemipelvis may require the use of a supplementary Steinmann pin inserted between the inner and outer tables of the displaced ilium. When bilateral sacroiliac dislocations are encountered, a posterior confirmation of an accurate reduction can be difficult to achieve. In the presence of a concomitant diastasis of the symphysis pubis, an initial realignment of the symphysis is preferred to facilitate a rotational realignment of the posterior injuries. The rotational realignment is much more readily confirmed by a scrutiny of the symphysis than by a visualization of the sacroiliac joints. For documentation of the accuracy of the posterior realignment, the flat, opposing undersurfaces of the sacroiliac joint at the roof of the greater sciatic notch can be palpated and the superior interface of the sacroiliac joint above the posterior superior spine examined. The anatomic reapproximation of the posterior superior spine and the adjacent ilium is then documented. In a sacroiliac dislocation, the joint is thoroughly debrided to encourage the formation of a solid fusion so that the incidence of later posterior pelvic pain is minimized.[1]

When the Double Cobra plate is positioned across the back of the sacrum, the insertion of two lengthy, 6.5-mm cancellous lag screws between the inner and outer tables of the ilia provides a highly effective mechanical tool for reapproximation of the sacral fracture or sacroiliac joints. During the tightening of these screws, the Double Cobra plate serves as a wedge to approximate the bony disruption. When the injury is a sacral fracture through the neural foramina, however, cautious reapproximation is necessary so that the adjacent nerve roots are not compressed. When the initial cancellous lag screws are inserted across the sacroiliac joints, the drill bit is limited to a maximum insertion of 55 mm. Also, the drill bit is not advanced for more than three cortices, representing the superficial ilium, the deep iliac table, and the alar cortex. These recommendations greatly lessen the likelihood of injury to the sacral nerve roots or the neurovascular structures anterior to the sacrum and the rectum.

In the presence of an acute sacral fracture or bilateral sacroiliac disruptions, isolated use of the Double Cobra plate for posterior reconstruction appears to stabilize the pelvis adequately. In persons weighing more than 200 lb, or in persons with osteoporosis who present late, the reduction can be anticipated to be less accurate. In these cases, a supplementary anterior fixation is strongly recommended to maintain posterior fixation until union of the pelvis is documented.

Summary

From five years of experience with 30 patients on whom the Double Cobra plate technique was employed for reconstruction of a variety of acute and late posterior pelvic injuries, this method appears to be highly suitable for effective stabilization of both sacral fractures and bilateral sacroiliac dislocations. With late presentations and larger individuals, associated anterior reconstruction of the pelvic ring is strongly recommended. The surgical complications have been sufficiently uncommon to recommend more widespread application of the protocol. Nevertheless, the potential for major complications, including life-threatening problems associated with pelvic reconstruction, should not be underestimated. These surgical techniques of internal fixation are potentially formidable undertakings that should be limited to those surgeons who possess appropriate training, instrumentation, and experience.

References

1. Mears DC, Rubash HE: *Pelvic and Acetabular Fractures.* Thorofare, NJ, Slack Inc, 1986, p 218.
2. Tile M, Pennal GF: Pelvic disruption: Principles of management. *Clin Orthop* 1980;151:56–64.
3. Tile M: *Fractures of the Pelvis and Acetabulum.* Baltimore, Williams & Wilkins, 1984, p 24.
4. Mears DC, Rubash HE: External and internal fixation of the pelvic ring, in Murray JA (ed): American Academy of Orthopaedic Surgeons *Instructional Course Lectures, XXXIII.* St. Louis, CV Mosby Co, 1984, p 144.
5. Rubash HE, Brown TD, Nelson DD, et al: Comparative mechanical performances of some new devices for fixation of unstable pelvic ring fractures. *Med Biol Eng Comput* 1983;21:657–663.

Nonunion of Long Bones

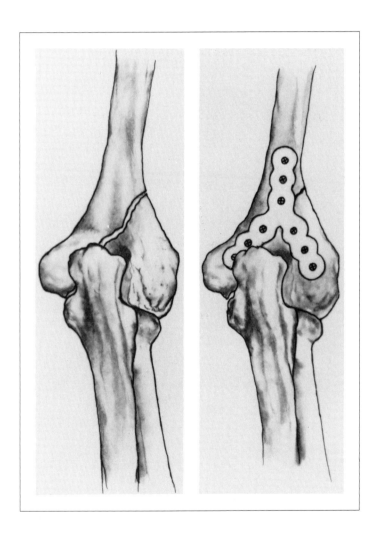

Historical Overview of Treatment of Nonunion

Sir Dennis Paterson, MD, FRCS, FRACS

Introduction

Few subjects have commanded a greater share of surgical literature than the growth and repair of bone. In 1948, Edgar Bick[1] reported that an estimated 5000 papers concerning bone growth and repair had been published in established journals. Certainly, there have been many papers published on this topic in the *Journal of Bone and Joint Surgery* since its first volume in 1918.

It can safely be assumed that nonunion of fractures has always been a problem. One of the early descriptions of the "false joint" that occurs at the site of nonunion appeared in an article by Edward Hartshorne published in 1841.[2] It is interesting to note the low incidence of nonunion reported by Hartshorne in the Pennsylvania Hospital at that time.

The treatment of delayed union and nonunion has always been controversial. Some advocate compression plating without bone grafts, others recommend the use of intramedullary nails, and others advocate cancellous bone grafting. Despite many theories, the mechanism of converting nonunion to union is not clear. However, three important factors are necessary for successful union: firm fixation, good apposition of the fragments, and an environment that will promote osteogenesis.

The History of Bone Grafting

Over 200 years ago, John Hunter demonstrated that separated fragments of bone could survive and grow. "Adhesion of detached splinters takes place . . . not only in those which are attached to the soft parts but in those which are entirely loose." In concluding that "these pieces must retain the living principle," Hunter made the first accurate though quite unconscious forecast of the possibility of bone transplantation.[3] The first successful bone transplantation was reported in 1878 by Macewen in Glasgow.[4]

Bone grafts may be used in the treatment of delayed union or nonunion. The objectives in grafting are to stimulate bony union, to replace lost tissues, and to assist in the revascularization of avascular segments of bone. In general there are three types of bone grafts: autologous (autograft), homogenous (allograft), and heterogenous (xenograft).

Onlay and Inlay Grafting

The pioneering work of Lane,[5,6] first published before 1900, and of Groves,[7,8] published some years later, had limited success mainly because they advocated massive onlay grafts and these were slow to revascularize. However, these methods incorporated two important treatment principles, namely, fixation and osteogenesis in the management of nonunion.

Various methods of grafting cortical bone have been developed over the years. Cortical bone is selected when there is bone loss or when stability is required. It is important to remember that cortical bone must first be resorbed by osteoclasts before significant osteoblastic activity can take place. Thus, cortical bone goes through a porous phase and will be less strong structurally for several weeks or months after implantation. Massive cortical grafts may never be resorbed.

Homogenous and Heterogenous Grafts

Orell[9,10] first advocated the use of cadaveric human or animal bone, and the modern counterpart of this concept is Kiel bone. These bone grafts are not as good as autogenous grafts.

Bone banks have gained more acceptance in recent years but should only be used when autogenous bone is not suitable to use.

Cancellous Bone Grafting

It has only been within the past 50 years that the special advantage of grafting with cancellous bone has been recognized. Cancellous bone grafts revascularize much more quickly and have greater osteogenic properties than other bone grafts. As a result, massive cortical grafting is used less often in surgical practice today.

The use of thin osteoperiosteal strip grafts to repair defects of bone was described in the early part of this century. However, in the 1940s, Phemister[11] described a method of onlay strip grafting without disturbing the pseudarthrosis. Phemister established that the callus associated with a nonunion would ossify spontaneously when an adequate surgical strip graft was performed, and that disturbance of the fibrous tissue was both unnecessary and undesirable. Wilson[12] and Charnley[13] modified the technique and used cancellous strip grafts from the iliac crest. A review of the use of cancellous bone grafting in nonunion of tibial fractures reveals a 92% success rate.[14]

Free Vascularized Fibular Grafts

Free vascularized grafts have been taken either from the iliac crest or the fibula. These grafts require time-consuming microsurgical techniques that have allowed many severely injured limbs to be salvaged. One disorder for which free vascularized grafts have become increasingly used is congenital pseudarthrosis of the tibia.

Electrical Stimulation

Electrical stimulation was first used to heal fractures almost 150 years ago, but only in the last two decades has this form of treatment gained acceptance. The clinical use of electrical stimulation has followed a period of intense and detailed scientific research to show that electrical stimulation is safe and that it significantly augments bone healing.

There are three basic techniques of electrical stimulation: a noninvasive,[15,16] a semi-invasive,[17,18] and a totally invasive technique of implanting a bone growth stimulator.[14,19,20] These methods of electrical stimulation are as effective as cancellous bone grafts in achieving success with nonunions.

Union is helped by bone that is actively osteogenic, has good fixation and bone contact, and is compressed. There are factors that impede union either relative to the injury itself, where the surgeon has no control, or relative to the treatment performed, where the surgeon has a significant role.

References

1. Bick EM: *Source Book of Orthopaedics.* Baltimore, Williams and Wilkins Co, 1948, p 102.

2. Hartshorne E: On the causes and treatment of pseudarthrosis and especially of that form of it sometimes called supernumerary joint. *Am J Med Sci* 1841;1(new series):143.

3. Watson-Jones R: Fractures and joint injuries, in Wilson JN (ed): *Ununited Fractures and the Transplantation of Bone.* Edinburgh, Churchill Livingstone Inc, 1982, pp 436–483.

4. Macewen W: *The Growth of Bone: Observations on Osteogenesis: An Experimental Inquiry Into the Development and Reproduction of Diaphyseal Bone.* Glasgow, James Maclehose and Sons, 1912.

5. Lane WA: *Cleft Palate and Hare Lip.* London, The Medical Publishing Co Ltd, 1908.

6. Lane WA: *The Operative Treatment of Fractures.* London, The Medical Publishing Co Ltd, 1914.

7. Groves EWH: Ununited fractures with special reference to gunshot injuries and the use of bone grafting. *Br J Surg* 1918;6:203.

8. Groves EWH: *On Modern Methods of Treating Fractures,* ed 2. Bristol, John Wright, 1921.

9. Orell S: Interposition of os purum in osteosynthesis after osteotomy: Resection of bones and joints (interposition osteosynthesis). *Surg Gynecol Obstet* 1934;59:638.

10. Orell S: Surgical bone grafting with 'os purum,' 'os novum,' and 'boiled bone.' *J Bone Joint Surg* 1937;19:873.

11. Phemister DB: Treatment of ununited fractures by onlay bone grafts without screw or tie fixation and without breaking down the fibrous union. *J Bone Joint Surg* 1947;29:946–960.

12. Wilson JN: Cancellous strip bone grafting. *J Bone Joint Surg* 1957;39B:585.

13. Charnley J: *Closed Treatment of Common Fractures.* Edinburgh, Churchill Livingstone Inc, 1961, p 245.

14. Paterson DC, Lewis GN, Cass CA: Treatment of delayed union and nonunion with an implanted direct current stimulator. *Clin Orthop* 1980;148:117–128.

15. Bassett CAL, Pawluk RJ, Pilla AA: Acceleration of fracture repair by electromagnetic fields: A surgically non-invasive method. *Ann NY Acad Sci* 1974;238:242.

16. Bassett CA, Pilla AA, Pawluk RJ: A non-operative salvage of surgically-resistant pseudarthroses and non-unions by pulsing electromagnetic fields: A preliminary report. *Clin Orthop* 1977;124:128–143.

17. Brighton CT, Friedenberg ZB: Treatment of non-union with electric current, abstract. *J Bone Joint Surg* 1974;56A:1542.

18. Brighton CT, Friedenberg ZB, Zemsky LM, et al: Direct-current stimulation of non-union and congenital pseudarthrosis. *J Bone Joint Surg* 1975;57A:368–377.

19. Paterson DC, Lewis GN, Cass CA: Treatment of congenital pseudarthrosis of the tibia with direct current stimulation. *Clin Orthop* 1980;148:129–135.

20. Paterson DC: Clinical use of the osteostim: An implanted bone growth stimulator for impaired bone healing, in American Academy of Orthopaedic Surgeons *Instructional Course Lectures, XXXI.* St. Louis, CV Mosby Co, 1982, pp 103–113.

The Use of Electricity in the Treatment of Nonunion

Sir Dennis Paterson, MD, FRCS, FRACS

Introduction

Since the early 1970s, electrical stimulation has been used increasingly in clinical practice for the treatment of nonunion of bone.

Basically, there are three methods of electrical stimulation used: noninvasive,[1,2] semi-invasive,[3-8] and totally invasive.[9-14] In treating nonunion of long bones, the results of all these methods of electrical stimulation are similar. The results of electrical stimulation are also similar to the results of cancellous bone grafting reported by Boyd and associates[15,16] and Paterson and associates.[11]

The Noninvasive Technique

The noninvasive method of treating nonunion by electrical stimulation developed by Bassett and his coworkers[1] requires the accurate placement of two coils around the fracture site. Nonweightbearing is important for successful union. The limb is immobilized in plaster, coil-placement blocks are fixed in exact locations on the plaster, and coils are placed according to standard intercoil distances supplied by the manufacturer. This accuracy is necessary to ensure the induction of a therapeutic voltage across the fracture site. The passage of current into the coils results in a pulsed electromagnetic field between the two coils. Initially, the daily treatment required is for a minimum of ten hours. The success of this treatment is not affected by the age or sex of the patient, the number of failed operations, the presence of hypertrophic or atrophic nonunion, the presence of a chronic discharge, skin or nerve loss, or the presence of nonmagnetic metal.

The Semi-Invasive Technique

The semi-invasive technique of electrical stimulation was first reported in 1971[17] and was used to achieve union for a fracture of the medial malleolus. The semi-invasive method consists of (1) a power pack that supplies a current of 20 μA, (2) an anode consisting of a stainless steel grid that is applied to the skin, and (3) one or more cathodes made of a stainless steel Kirschner wire that is insulated with Teflon except for the 1-cm tip. The tip of the cathode is inserted through the skin and into the site of nonunion using an image in-

tensifier. Nonweightbearing is an essential requirement of this method of treatment. Brighton and associates[4-6] reported their success rate and the complications of this method of treatment, and have pointed out three important factors that impair bone healing no matter what method of electrical stimulation is used. These three factors are the presence of a synovial pseudarthrosis, a gap in the bone fragments of more than half the diameter of the bone, and significant osteoporosis.

The Invasive Technique

The totally invasive technique I developed[11,13] involves a small operation to insert a generator that supplies a constant direct current of 20 μA. A platinized anode together with a titanium cathode is made into the form of a helix and placed across the site of the nonunion. Strict adherence to basic details of the operation is required for a successful result. It is essential that the slot in the bone be centered over the site of nonunion, that the medullary cavity be curetted of fibrous tissue, and that the generator be placed 8 to 10 cm from the cathode and beneath the deep fascia. In addition to delayed union and nonunion of long bones, this invasive technique can be used in small bones, such as the scaphoid, and for nonunion following osteotomies, arthrodesis, and failed posterior spinal fusion. The lithium iodine power source has a shelf life of three years and an implant life of nine months. A small operation is required to remove the generator, leaving the titanium cathode in the bone itself. The electrical implant can be used in the presence of metal implants, as long as there is no direct contact between the cathode and the metal implant itself, and the implant can also be used in the presence of chronic infection. Many of the original cases using this invasive technique had long standing nonunions with chronic discharge and were often cases where amputation had been advised.

Bassett and associates,[18] using the noninvasive technique, and Paterson and Simonis,[19] using the totally invasive technique, have reported encouraging results in the treatment of congenital pseudarthrosis of the tibia, perhaps one of the most difficult conditions to treat in orthopaedic surgery.

There is clearly a significant place in the treatment of nonunion for a totally invasive technique; however, a noninvasive method of electrical stimulation is preferable in certain situations. New forms of noninvasive electrical stimulation have been developed, such as the iron-cord electromagnet,[20] and Brighton and Pollack's[8] capacitive coupling technique. The results by these methods have also been very encouraging. The iron-cord electromagnet requires precise localization of the electromagnetic and treatment coils, but weightbearing must be avoided. Precise localization of the capacitive plates is not required and full weightbearing is allowed with the capacitive coupling technique. Capacitive coupling produces a time-varying electrical field.

The Future of Electrical Stimulation in the Treatment of Nonunions

It is now clear that the successful treatment of nonunions with electrical stimulation is as good as treatment with an autogenous cancellous bone graft. There are advantages to both the totally invasive and noninvasive techniques. Perhaps the most significant advantage of the totally invasive method is that, although a small operation is required, the need for patient compliance is avoided. Electrical stimulation should be an accepted form of management in the treatment of nonunion of long bones, and may be indicated when delayed union first becomes apparent.

References

1. Bassett CAL, Pawluk RJ, Pilla AA: Acceleration of fracture repair by electromagnetic fields: A surgically non-invasive method. *Ann NY Acad Sci* 1974;238:242.
2. Bassett CAL, Mitchell SN, Gaston SR: Treatment of ununited tibial diaphyseal fractures with pulsing electromagnetic fields. *J Bone Joint Surg* 1981;63A:511–523.
3. Brighton CT, Friedenberg ZB: Treatment of non-union with electric current, abstract. *J Bone Joint Surg* 1974;56A:1542.
4. Brighton CT, Friedenberg ZB, Zemsky LM, et al: Direct-current stimulation of non-union and congenital pseudarthrosis. *J Bone Joint Surg* 1975;57A:368–377.
5. Brighton CT, Friedenberg ZB, Mitchell EI, et al: Treatment of non-union with constant direct current. *Clin Orthop* 1977;124:106–123.
6. Brighton CT, Black J, Friedenberg ZB, et al: A multicenter study of the treatment of non-union with constant direct current. *J Bone Joint Surg* 1981;63A:2–13.
7. Brighton CT: The treatment of non-unions with electricity. *J Bone Joint Surg* 1981;63A:847–851.
8. Brighton CT, Pollack SR: Treatment of recalcitrant non-union with a capacitively coupled electrical field. *J Bone Joint Surg* 1985;67A:577–585.
9. Dwyer AF, Wickham GG: Direct current stimulation in spinal fusion. *Med J Aust* 1974;1:73–75.
10. Dwyer AF: The use of electrical current stimulation in spinal fusion. *Orthop Clin North Am* 1975;6:265.
11. Paterson DC, Lewis GN, Cass CA: Treatment of delayed union and nonunion with an implanted direct current stimulator. *Clin Orthop* 1980;148:117–128.
12. Paterson DC, Lewis GN, Cass CA: Treatment of congenital pseudarthrosis of the tibia with direct current stimulation. *Clin Orthop* 1980;148:129–135.
13. Paterson D: Clinical use of the osteostim: An implanted bone growth stimulator for impaired bone healing, in American Academy of Orthopaedic Surgeons *Instructional Course Lectures, XXXI.* St. Louis, CV Mosby Co, 1982, p 103–113.
14. Paterson D: Treatment of nonunion with a constant direct current: A totally implantable system. *Orthop Clin North Am* 1984;15:47–59.
15. Boyd HB, Lipinski SW: Causes and treatment of non-union of the shafts of long bones with a review of 741 patients, in American Academy of Orthopaedic Surgeons *Instructional Course Lectures, XVII.* St. Louis, CV Mosby Co, 1960, p 165.
16. Boyd HB, Lipinski SW, Wiley JH: Observations on non-union of the shafts of the long bones, with a statistical analysis of 842 patients. *J Bone Joint Surg* 1961;43A:159–168.
17. Friedenberg ZB, Harlow MC, Brighton CT: Healing of nonunion of the medial malleolus by means of direct current: A case report. *J Trauma* 1971;11:883–885.
18. Bassett CAL, Mitchell SN, et al: Electromagnetic repairs of non-unions, in Brighton CT, Black J, Pollack SR (eds): *Electrical Properties of Bone and Cartilage: Experimental Effects and Clinical Applications.* New York, Grune and Stratton, 1979, pp 605–630.
19. Paterson DC, Simonis RB: Electrical stimulation in the treatment of congenital pseudarthrosis of the tibia. *J Bone Joint Surg* 1985;67B:454–462.
20. Downes EM, Watson J: Development of the iron-cored electromagnet for the treatment of non-union and delayed union. *J Bone Joint Surg* 1984;66B:754–759.

Nonunion of the Diaphysis of the Radius and Ulna

Lewis D. Anderson, MD

Frederick N. Meyer, MD

As recently as the 1950s, fractures of the shaft of the radius and ulna in adults presented major treatment problems. In 1949, Knight and Purvis[1] found that nonunion developed in 46% of their patients treated by open reduction. This was primarily the result of the inadequate fixation devices then available. In this same study, Knight and Purvis found that 12% of fractures of the forearm bones treated by closed reduction developed nonunion; many of those that did unite had malunions with poor function. Smith and Sage[2] found that nonunion developed in 14% of their patients treated with the intramedullary nails available in 1957. When even less adequate Kirschner wires or Steinmann pins were used for medullary fixation of forearm fractures, the nonunion rate was 38%.[2]

Modern internal fixation for forearm fractures developed in the late 1950s. In 1960, Jinkins and associates[3] reported that the Eggers plate produced nonunions in only 4% of patients. Sage[4] introduced his prebent triangular nails in 1959 and reported a 6% nonunion rate. The Arbeitsgemeinschaft für Osteosynthesefragen group introduced the compression plate and a number of articles were subsequently published showing a low nonunion rate in the range of 2% to 3%.[5,6] Anderson and associates,[6] reviewing acute forearm fractures at the Campbell Clinic treated from 1960 through the following decade, found an overall nonunion rate of 2.7% in a large series of 330 patients. In 1984, Anderson and Bacastow[5] reviewed their experiences with dynamic compression plates at the University of South Alabama and found a nonunion rate of 1.4%. Thus, the nonunion rate has markedly decreased since the introduction of good internal fixation devices.

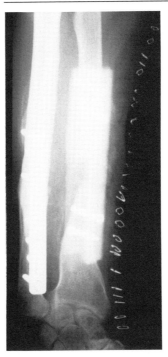

Fig. 21-1 Anteroposterior view of the left forearm of a 22-year-old man whose forearm had been caught in machinery at a sawmill three years previously. The open fracture of the radius and ulna with extensive loss of soft tissue and bone had been treated elsewhere. He had undergone 19 separate surgical procedures by the time this radiograph was made. The ulna had healed but there was a nonunion of the radius with a gap of 7 cm between good viable host bone.

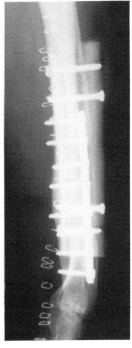

Fig. 21-2 Anteroposterior (**left**) and lateral (**right**) radiographs made one week after a dual onlay bone-grafting procedure. The cortical bone was from the right tibia. Cancellous bone from the proximal tibial metaphysis was packed into the defect.

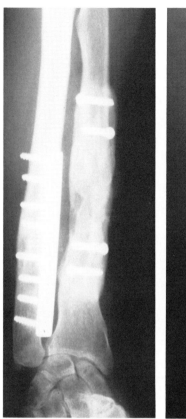
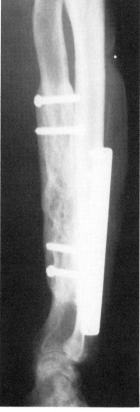

Fig. 21-3 Anteroposterior (**left**) and lateral (**right**) radiographs made three years after surgery. Union was evident at 12 weeks but the forearm was kept in a cast for six months to protect the grafts. The patient achieved surprisingly good function and when last seen was working as a bulldozer operator.

However, those nonunions that do develop tend to be difficult to treat because there is often a loss of bone and infection may also be present.

Predisposition

In the large series of 842 nonunions of all long bones reported by Boyd and associates[7] in 1961, 222 of the nonunions involved forearm bones (26.3%). Boyd and associates[8] later reported 55 nonunions of the radius and ulna treated with compression plates. Their success rate was 93%. There are no recent large series of nonunions for comparison, but forearm nonunions certainly constitute a much lower percentage of all nonunions. Boyd and associates[8] noted four factors predisposing a fresh fracture to nonunion: (1) compounding; (2) comminution; (3) disturbance of blood supply; and (4) infection. They also noted that four treatment factors predispose a fracture to nonunion: (1) ill-advised open reduction; (2) infection; (3) distraction; and (4) inadequate immobilization.

We now have better antibiotics to help prevent and control infection and better methods of internal fixa-

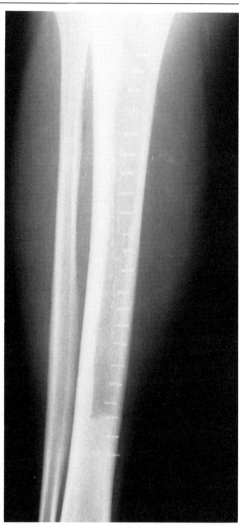

Fig. 21-4 Radiograph of the donor tibia one week after the extensive (32 cm long) cortical bone graft was taken. The extremity was protected in a long leg walking cast for four months.

tion that aid union and require less external immobilization.

Recognition

Recognition is usually not a problem in forearm nonunions. Polytomography and computed tomographic scans can sometimes be helpful if there is any doubt. Also, a bone scan frequently identifies a synovial pseudarthrosis that might preclude attempted treatment with electrical stimulation.

Treatment

Factors promoting union include osteogenesis, contact, fixation, and compression. Each forearm nonunion is different and each requires different treatment techniques. If good function, including pronation and

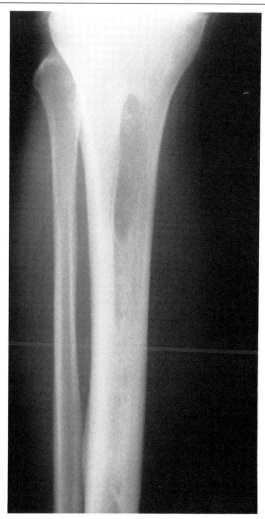

Fig. 21-5 Radiograph of the donor tibia three years after surgery demonstrates how slowly the defect filled in.

supination, is to be restored, the appropriate length of the radius and ulna must be maintained or restored. This can be a problem, especially when there is a gap with loss of bone at the nonunion site. For nonunions with no significant loss of bone, the appropriate treatment may be a compression plate with an outrigger compression device. The dynamic compression plate should not be used in nonunions because the bone is soft and adequate excursion for good compression may not be obtained. Once the compression plate is applied, barrel-stave grafts of cortical-cancellous iliac bone approximately 1.25 inches long are cut to the size of matchsticks and placed circumferentially around the nonunion. They are held in place with sutures to promote good contact and help prevent synostosis.

A gap of up to 1 cm may be bridged by a tricortical iliac graft. Fixation is achieved with a long compression plate and screws.[9] The tricortical graft should be drilled to provide several small holes for better vascularization. This method should not be used for defects much

greater than 1 cm because revascularization is slow and the procedure may fail. In defects longer than 1 cm, a step-cut fibular graft may be used. At times it is appropriate to use a vascularized fibular graft, especially if infection is present.[10-12] Another alternative is a dual onlay bone graft with bone taken from the anteromedial aspect of the tibia and applied so that the two grafts are opposite each other. The screws can then obtain good purchase and hold the radius or ulna as if it were in a vise[7] (Figs. 21-l to 21-3). Cancellous bone from the proximal tibia or from the ilium can then be packed between the cortical tibial grafts into the defect. Whenever a tibial cortical graft is taken, the leg must be carefully protected to prevent fracture of the tibia. Rounding off the ends of the defect so that they are oval helps prevent this from happening. A long leg walking cast should be worn for two to three months (Figs. 21-4 and 21-5). Also, whenever tibial or fibular cortical grafts are used on the forearm bones, revascularization of the graft is slow, and the graft may fracture if it is not protected for as much as six months.[7]

Finally, autogenous bone is preferable to homogenous bone. In Boyd and associates'[7] series, the success rate with autogenous bone was 88% in the overall series and only 70% for homogenous bone.

References

1. Knight RA, Purvis GD: Fractures of both bones of the forearm in adults. *J Bone Joint Surg* 1949;31A:755–764.
2. Smith H, Sage FP: Medullary fixation of forearm fractures. *J Bone Joint Surg* 1957;39A:91–98.
3. Jinkins WJ Jr, Lockhart LD, Eggers GWN: Fractures of the forearm in adults. *South Med J* 1960;53:669–679.
4. Sage FP: Medullary fixation of fractures of the forearm: A study of the medullary canal of the radius and a report of fifty fractures of the radius treated with a prebent triangular nail. *J Bone Joint Surg* 1959;41A:1489–1516.
5. Anderson LD, Bacastow DW: Treatment of forearm shaft fractures with compression plates. *Contemp Orthop* 1984;8:17–25.
6. Anderson LD, Sisk TD, Tooms RE, et al: Compression-plate fixation in acute diaphyseal fractures of the radius and ulna. *J Bone Joint Surg* 1975;57A:287–297.
7. Boyd HB, Lipinski SW, Wiley JH: Observations on non-union of the shafts of the long bones, with a statistical analysis of 842 patients. *J Bone Joint Surg* 1961;43A:159–168.
8. Boyd HB, Anderson LD, Johnston DS: Changing concepts in the treatment of nonunion. *Clin Orthop* 1965;43:37–54.
9. Shelton WR, Sage FP: Modified Nicoll-graft treatment of gap non-unions in the upper extremity. *J Bone Joint Surg* 1981;63A:226–231.
10. Dell PC, Sheppard JE: Vascularized bone grafts in the treatment of infected forearm nonunions. *J Hand Surg* 1984;9A:653–658.
11. Hurst LC, Mirza MA, Spellman W: Vascularized fibular graft for infected loss of the ulna: Case report. *J Hand Surg* 1982;7:498–501.
12. Osterman AL, Bora FW: Free vascularized bone grafting for large-gap nonunion of long bones. *Orthop Clin North Am* 1984;15:131–142.

CHAPTER 22

Nonunion of the Humerus

Charles H. Epps, Jr., MD

Although fractures of the humerus generally heal satisfactorily, in certain circumstances union may be delayed or may fail to occur. In these cases, the impairment caused by the nonunion may be disabling. In previous years, many investigators documented the difficulties of treating nonunions of the humerus.[1-10] The presence of a pseudocapsule, rounded sclerotic ends, and the complete absence of osteogenic potential remain the generally accepted criteria for nonunion. In delayed union, by contrast, repair is not complete, the spaces between fracture fragments are filled with granulation tissue, and there is still clinical and roentgenographic evidence that healing is taking place.

The hanging cast and the coaptation splint, which are widely accepted and easy to use, have made closed treatment of humeral fractures highly successful and preferred by most surgeons. However, some fractures of the humerus require open reduction and internal fixation. The generally accepted indications for surgical intervention are marked displacement, soft-tissue interposition, malposition, segmentation, and neurovascular compromise. The victim of polytrauma who has more than one extremity fracture or injury to a major organ may also require fixation of a humeral fracture. The patient's cooperation is also necessary.

Those fractures that go on to nonunion are associated with open fracture, failed open reduction, infection, metabolic bone disease, hematologic disorders, and tumors. Displacement and distraction of the fracture fragments also tend to predispose to nonunion. Soft-tissue interposition can prevent the requisite bony contact and result in nonunion. In a classic study by the Pennsylvania Orthopaedic Society, union rates were found to be 95% with closed treatment and 88% with open treatment of humeral fractures.[11] Moreover, it has been observed that nonunion is increased in fractures near joints. There is general agreement that stable fixation is essential to the successful treatment of nonunion of the humerus. The type of fixation varies with the local conditions of the fracture site and the location of the fracture.

Historically, orthopaedic surgeons in several countries contributed to the foundations that led to the concepts, techniques, and instruments used today. In 1947, Phemister[12] elaborated the concept of treating nonunions with onlay bone grafts without resecting the pseudarthrosis. The concept of compression was developed by Key[13] (1932) for treatment of knee tuberculosis and by Charnley[14] for arthrodesis (1953). In 1948, Eggers[15] introduced a sliding plate that produced compressive forces. However, it was the Arbeitsgemeinschaft für Osteosynthesefragen in 1959 that put compression plate fixation of fractures on a firm scientific basis, leading to this technique's wide acceptance.[16] Küntscher[17,18] used the intramedullary nail in the treatment of nonunion without resection of the pseudoarthrosis and without a bone graft.

The decision to apply a graft is generally based on the status of the bone ends. If the bone ends are inert, sclerotic, rounded, and avascular, local grafting is indicated. Conversely, if the bone ends are sclerotic but vascular and not completely inactive, firm fixation results in osseous union without bony augmentation. When the bone ends are separated or if there is comminution or insufficient blood supply to the area, bone grafting is also indicated. Today, bone scans can be used to determine the type of nonunion more accurately. This is necessary because the status of the bone ends cannot always be determined with complete accuracy. Fractures in the proximal and distal thirds of the humerus appear to be more susceptible to nonunion.

Nonunion in the Proximal Third

Epidemiologic studies suggest that fractures of the proximal third of the humerus are associated with a higher incidence of fractures of the upper end of the femur and the distal radius. These data indicate a relationship to osteoporosis and a specific and rapid increase with age. The incidence in women is twice that in men.[19]

Fractures complicated by nonunion in this region present difficult management problems because the proximal fragment is short and usually osteoporotic. The preferred methods of treatment are combined onlay and intraosseous graft, parallel cortical grafts extending into the humeral head, or a blade plate. All three methods are augmented by cancellous bone graft about the nonunion.[20]

Parallel or "forceps" grafts are applied so that they extend into the humeral head just below the articular cartilage and are transfixed to the shaft with screws. There seems to be some risk of delayed fracture of the graft in this technique. Cortical grafts are best obtained from the proximal tibia, a site that can also supply cancellous bone. However, the iliac crest is an excellent source of cancellous bone grafts. Various types of nail plates have been used (Fig. 22–1). Epps and Cotler[21] reported the successful use of a pediatric Jewett nail. In cases in which the articular cartilage of the humeral head proves to be inadequate, a Neer-type endoprosthesis may be considered.[22] The prosthetic stem traverses the fracture site and the cancellous bone graft is added. Less generally accepted is the use of a Rush nail in proximal-third nonunions.[23,24] The nail, which passes through the rotator cuff and the nonunion into the distal shaft, may back out and impinge against the acromion. This complication may limit shoulder motion enough to produce a frozen shoulder. The Rush nail in the osteoporotic proximal fragment may provide less-than-desirable fixation, and the overall effect on healing of the nonunion may be adverse.

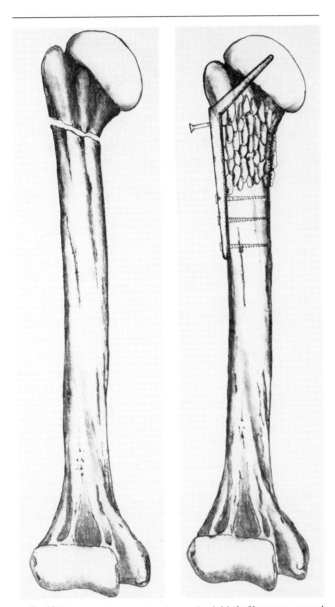

Fig. 22–1 Avascular nonunion in proximal third of humerus treated by reduction using angled plate and autogenous bone graft. Proximal screw may require insertion at an angle to engage the proximal fragment.

Nonunion in the Middle Third

The tubular anatomy of the middle third or shaft of the humerus lends itself well to two rather reliable methods of correcting nonunion.

The requisite stability can be achieved either by compression plate[20,25–29] or by intramedullary fixation.[20,29–31] Augmentation with a corticocancellous isograft, usually from the iliac crest, plays a vital role in most cases.

Compression Plate Fixation

In the middle third of the humerus, the anterolateral surgical approach, lateral to the biceps, offers ideal exposure for plating.

This approach allows identification and protection of the radial nerve, an important consideration at this level. The brachialis muscle is split and the fracture site is exposed by subperiosteal dissection. Before the development of modern compression techniques, Eggers[15] preferred a sliding plate with a single onlay graft. Today, most surgeons recommend six- or eight-hole compression plates with autogenous bone grafts as the treatment of choice.[25–29] A minimum of three screws should transfix both cortices of the main proximal and distal fracture fragments (Fig. 22–2). The length of the plate should be at least five times the bone diameter for optimum fixation. When the humerus is osteoporotic, nut or bolt fixation may offer additional protection against mechanical failure. Murray and associates[32] advocated the use of dual compression plates combined with bone grafts. This technique has not enjoyed wide use because of the risk of bone resorption and fracture at the plate sites.

The compression plate is usually placed laterally. In a combined technique, tibial onlay bone graft is utilized. The anteromedial aspect of the tibia is the preferred donor site, which should be 1 to 1.5 cm wide. The tibial graft is secured to the humerus anteriorly with cortical screws. Additional cancellous bone is placed around the nonunion site.

The rigidity provided by compression plating offers the best possible biologic and mechanical environment for satisfactory healing when augmented by autogenous bone graft. Rosen[25] achieved a healing rate of 92.6% with one compression in his series of humeral nonunions.

Intramedullary Fixation

The intramedullary nail can provide firm stable fixation for the nonunion. Küntscher,[17] Christensen,[30] and others have reported favorable experience with intramedullary nails combined with cancellous bone grafts. It may be necessary to ream the medullary canal to obtain a long enough segment on each side of the fracture site. Firm stability should result if approximately

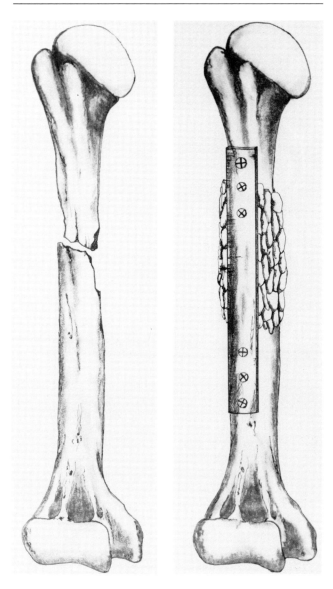

Fig. 22–2 Avascular nonunion in middle third of shaft of humerus treated by compression-plate fixation and autogenous bone graft.

25% of the length of the humerus both proximal and distal to the fracture site can be engaged (Fig. 22–3).

External Fixation

Coventry and Laurnen[5] reported favorable results with the application of external fixation devices to humeral nonunions associated with sepsis. The device provides both bony and soft-tissue stability and is excellent when a vascularized bone graft has been used. It is important that three or four half-pins be placed proximal and distal to the nonunion site in two planes at a 90-degree angle to each other. This technique allows wound observation and access for local wound care. Moreover, in complex injuries, elbow and glenohumeral joint motion may be permitted early when de-

sired. Caution must be exercised to avoid inserting pins through infected areas and neurovascular structures.

Nonunion in the Distal Third

Nonunion of the distal third of the humerus may occur in both surgically treated and nonsurgically treated fractures. Intramedullary fixation is usually not appropriate. Special plates, such as the "Y" plate, can be used to obtain firm fixation in some cases (Fig. 22–4). The nonunion of the medial humeral epicondyle may be excised, the ulnar nerve transposed, and the common origin of the flexor muscles attached to the medial condyle. The surgeon must be cautious in this region to protect the radial nerve and the ulnar nerve. Special care is necessary to mobilize the elbow joint when deal-

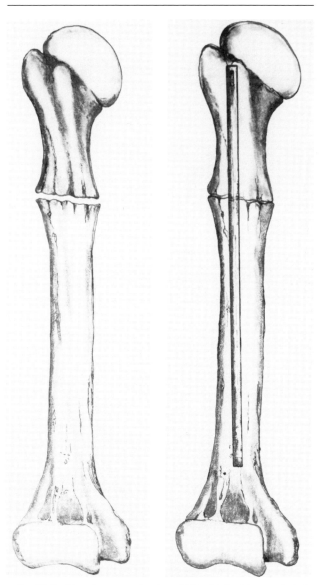

Fig. 22–3 Vascular nonunion in middle third of humeral shaft treated by intramedullary nail without bone graft.

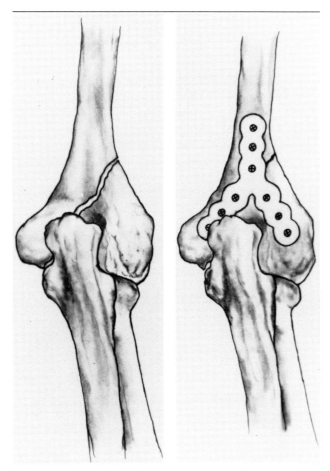

Fig. 22-4 Firm fixation of nonunion in distal third can be obtained with "Y" plate.

ing with a nonunion in this region. A cast brace may be useful in these cases.

Comminuted Fractures of the Distal End

In many cases, comminuted fractures (intercondylar) of the distal end of the humerus can only be reduced anatomically by open reduction and maintained by internal fixation. Fractures treated by surgery are at great risk for infection, nerve damage, and limited motion. Treatment requires exacting technique and is best accomplished through the transolecranon approach. Jupiter and associates[33] reported 13 excellent and 14 good results in 34 patients. Conversely, Riseborough and Radin[34] reviewed a series of 52 patients and concluded that gentle manipulation in traction was preferable to open reduction. Brown and Morgan[35] treated ten patients in collar-and-cuff slings with early active movement and obtained results they considered equal to the results of open reduction.

Nonunion With Infection

The infected nonunion offers a serious challenge. Many of these cases involve retained fixation devices

and active infection. All hardware, sequestra, methacrylate, and other foreign material must be removed. The septic process must be controlled locally and systemically. The wound is usually left open and delayed closure effected only after quantitative wound cultures and the clinical appearance indicate a healthy wound. Skin grafts or pedicle skin grafts may be necessary to obtain adequate skin coverage. Cancellous bone grafts can be applied. An alternate method is the technique of open wound treatment using cancellous bone grafting (Papineau technique) combined with skin grafting of the granulating base, local muscle flap, or free tissue myocutaneous flap for coverage.

In Rosen's[25] review of 24 infected nonunions (all in long bones), 20 (83%) healed primarily. Most were treated by plating and two required a second plating. The basic treatment was meticulous excision of sequestra and sinus tracts, the addition of cancellous bone grafts, suction antibiotic irrigation, and parenteral administration of antibiotics.

Nonunion With Loss of Substance

When there is a loss of intervening humerus with intact segments distally and proximally, a critical situation exists. In considering the feasibility of reconstruction, one must take into account basic local conditions that may justify the risk. Of prime importance is the presence of neuromuscular, osseous, and vascular components adequate for reasonable function. The patient must also have a cooperative attitude and willingness to accept the restraints of the long convalescence and its associated risks, including infection and even loss of the extremity.

In one report, a free vascularized fibular bone graft was used successfully in a nonunion of the humerus that had persisted for 14 months. Union was achieved in 3½ months.[36]

Radial Nerve Injury

The radial nerve is the nerve most commonly associated with injury in humeral fractures and surgical treatment for these fractures. Pollock and associates[37] reported radial nerve palsy in about 12% of displaced and comminuted fractures. The palsy is usually caused by compression or stretch and most palsies in closed fractures recover spontaneously. Exposure of the radial nerve is recommended in all operations or re-operations for nonunion of the humerus, especially for fractures in the middle or distal thirds.

Electrical Stimulation

Direct-current stimulation techniques have been developed by Paterson and associates[38] and Brighton and associates.[39] The use of pulsed electromagnetic fields has been advocated by Bassett and associates.[40] Although success rates in nonunion with both methods are reported to be better than 80%, the precise role of electrical stimulation remains controversial. However, there is accumulating evidence that electrical stimulation is useful in some cases of nonunion.

Humeral Sleeve

In some cases of humeral nonunion, the patient's general health contraindicates surgical intervention or the patient refuses surgical treatment. The application of a polyethylene orthosis can provide sufficient stability and comfort to allow a significant degree of function. The humeral sleeve was originally developed for use in acute fractures by Sarmiento and associates,[41] who reported nonunion in one pathologic fracture among 50 in the series.

Summary

Under certain circumstances, fractures of the humerus may not heal. Some fractures experience delayed union and some develop nonunion despite improved methods of treatment. This chapter discussed nonunion and fracture fixation methods in the proximal, middle, and distal thirds of the humerus. Special circumstances were discussed, such as infection, nerve palsy, comminution, and electrical stimulation.

References

1. Bennett G: Fractures of the humerus with particular reference to nonunion and its treatment. *Ann Surg* 1936;103:994–1006.
2. Campbell WC: Ununited fractures of the shaft of the humerus. *Ann Surg* 1937;105:135–149.
3. Dameron TB Jr, Grubb SA: Humeral shaft fractures in adults. *South Med J* 1981;74:1461–1467.
4. Stewart MJ, Hundley JM: Fractures of the humerus: A comparative study in methods of treatment. *J Bone Joint Surg* 1955;37A:681–692.
5. Coventry MB, Laurnen EL: Ununited fractures of the middle and upper humerus: Special problems in treatment. *Clin Orthop* 1970;69:192–198.
6. Christensen S: Humeral shaft fractures, operative and conservative treatment. *Acta Chir Scand* 1967;133:455–460.
7. Boyd HB, Lipinski SW, Wiley JH: Observations on non-union of the shafts of the long bones, with a statistical analysis of 842 patients. *J Bone Joint Surg* 1961;43A:159–168.
8. Mast JW, Spiegel PH, Harvey JP Jr, et al: Fractures of the humeral shaft: A retrospective study of 240 adult fractures. *Clin Orthop* 1975;112:254–262.
9. Fenyö G: On fractures of the shaft of the humerus: A review covering a 12-year period with special consideration of the surgically treated cases. *Acta Chir Scand* 1971;137:221–226.
10. Svend-Hansen H: Displaced proximal humeral fractures: A review of 49 patients. *Acta Orthop Scand* 1974;45:359–364.
11. Pennsylvania Orthopaedic Society, Scientific Research Committee: Fresh midshaft fractures of the humerus in adults: Evaluation of treatment in Pennsylvania during 1952–1956. *Pa Med J* 1959;62:848–850.
12. Phemister DB: Treatment of ununited fractures by onlay bone grafts without screw or tie fixation and without breaking down of the fibrous union. *J Bone Joint Surg* 1947;29:946–960.
13. Key J: Positive pressure in arthrodesis for tuberculosis of the knee joint. *South Med J* 1932;25:909.
14. Charnley J: *Compression Arthrodesis.* London, E and S Livingstone, 1953, pp 34–60.
15. Eggers GWN: Internal contact splint. *J Bone Joint Surg* 1948;30A:40.
16. Müller ME, Allgöwer M, Willenegger H: *Technique of Internal Fixation of Fractures.* New York, Springer-Verlag, 1965, pp 172–181.
17. Küntscher BG: Die Nagelung der malleolar Pseudarthrose. *Monatsschr Unfallheilkd* 1953;56:107.
18. Küntscher BG: The Küntscher method of intramedullary fixation. *J Bone Joint Surg* 1958;40A:17–26.
19. Horak J, Nilsoon BE: Epidemiology of fracture of the upper end of the humerus. *Clin Orthop* 1975;112:250–253.
20. Crenshaw AH: Delayed union and nonunion of fractures, in Edmonson AS, Crenshaw AH (eds): *Campbell's Operative Orthopaedics,* ed 6. St. Louis, CV Mosby Co, 1980, vol 1, pp 761–820.
21. Epps CH Jr, Cotler JM: Complications of treatment of fractures of the humeral shaft, in Epps CH Jr (ed): *Complications in Orthopaedic Surgery,* ed 2. Philadelphia, JB Lippincott, 1985, pp 231–243.
22. Neer CS II: Displaced proximal humeral fractures: I. Classification and evaluation. *J Bone Joint Surg* 1970;52A:1077–1089.
23. Weseley MS, Barenfeld PA, Eisenstein AL: Rush pin intramedullary fixation for fractures of the proximal humerus. *J Trauma* 1977;17:29–37.
24. Rush LV, Rush HL: Intramedullary fixation of fractures of the humerus by the longitudinal pin. *Surgery* 1950;27:268–275.
25. Rosen H: Compression treatment of long bone pseudarthroses. *Clin Orthop* 1979;138:154–166.
26. Müller ME: Treatment of nonunions by compression. *Clin Orthop* 1965;43:83–92.
27. Anderson LD, Boyd HB, Johnston DS: Changing concepts in the treatment of nonunion. *Clin Orthop* 1955;43:37.
28. Cooney WP III: Humeral fractures: Complications and reconstructive surgery, in Evarts CM (ed): *Surgery of the Musculoskeletal System.* New York, Churchill Livingstone, pp 185–209.
29. Stern PJ, Mattingly DA, Pomeroy DL, et al: Intramedullary fixation of humeral shaft fractures. *J Bone Joint Surg* 1984;66A:639–646.
30. Christensen NO: Küntscher intramedullary reaming and nail fixation for nonunion of the humerus. *Clin Orthop* 1976;116:222–225.
31. Nummi P: Intramedullary fixation with compression for the treatment of fracture in the shaft of the humerus: Fixation with supramid pin and two vitallium screws. *Acta Chir Scand* 1971;137:71–73.
32. Murray WR, Lucas DB, Inman VT: Treatment of non-union of fractures of the long bones by the two-plate method. *J Bone Joint Surg* 1964;46A:1027–1048.
33. Jupiter JB, Neff U, Holzach P, et al: Intercondylar fractures of the humerus: An operative approach. *J Bone Joint Surg* 1985;67A:226–239.
34. Riseborough EJ, Radin EL: Intercondylar T fractures of the humerus in the adult: A comparison of operative and non-operative treatment in twenty-nine cases. *J Bone Joint Surg* 1969;51A:130–141.
35. Brown RF, Morgan RG: Intercondylar T-shaped fractures of the humerus: Results in ten cases treated by early mobilisation. *J Bone Joint Surg* 1971;53B:425–428.

36. Solonen KA: Free vascularized bone graft in the treatment of pseudarthrosis. *Int Orthop* 1982;6:9–13.

37. Pollock FH, Drake D, Bovill EG, et al: Treatment of radial neuropathy associated with fractures of the humerus. *J Bone Joint Surg* 1981;63A:239–243.

38. Paterson DC, Lewis GN, Cass CA: Treatment of delayed union and nonunion with an implanted direct current stimulator. *Clin Orthop* 1980;148:117–128.

39. Brighton CT, Black J, Friedenberg ZB, et al: A multicenter study of the treatment of non-union with constant direct current. *J Bone Joint Surg* 1981;63A:2–13.

40. Bassett CA, Mitchell SN, Gaston SR: Pulsing electromagnetic field treatment in ununited fractures and failed arthrodeses. *JAMA* 1982;247:623–628.

41. Sarmiento A, Kinman PB, Galvin EG, et al: Functional bracing of fractures of the shaft of the humerus. *J Bone Joint Surg* 1977;59A:596–601.

Nonunion of the Tibia: Experience With Modified Phemister Bone Graft and With Compression Plates and Cancellous Bone Graft

Peter G. Carnesale, MD

Nonunion of the tibia has been of special interest to the physicians at the Campbell Clinic since Campbell's[1,2] introduction of the onlay tibial graft. Boyd and associates[3] published an extensive review of their experience (295 nonunions) in 1961. They concluded that operations for nonunion are in essence rewounding events and that none of the methods studied (medullary nailing and graft, onlay graft, Phemister graft, dual graft, plate and graft) was clearly superior to the others. Although methods changed with the availability of newer implants, these conclusions were unchanged five years later.[4]

Present Study

The records and roentgenograms of 80 patients with nonunion of the tibia treated at the Campbell Clinic by either Phemister grafting or compression plating and cancellous iliac bone grafting were reviewed.

Almost all of these patients were treated in the 20-year period from 1966 to 1985.

A modified Phemister graft technique was used in 49 patients (Fig. 23–1). In Phemister's[5] original description in 1947, the bone grafts were placed subperiosteally, bridging the site of nonunion. The site itself was minimally dissected. A modification of this technique involves partly decorticating the tibia near the site of nonunion, using only a cancellous iliac graft placed beneath the decorticated shavings. This technique should be used only in patients with a stable fibrous union (only 10 to 15 degrees of motion) with acceptable alignment. In addition, the soft tissues through which the incision is made should be healthy. When anterior drainage or extensive scarring is pres-

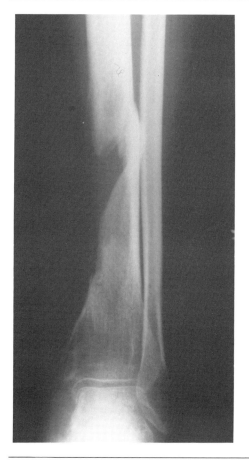
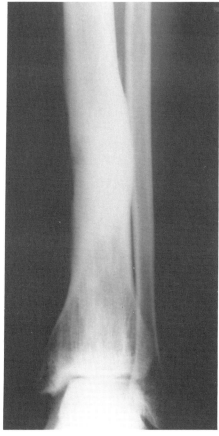

Fig. 23-1 A 16-year-old youth sustained a type III open fracture in a motor vehicle accident. The fracture was initially treated with wound debridement, closed reduction, and a long-leg cast. **Left:** "Spot-weld" union after five months. **Right:** Solid union was obtained after Phemister grafting.

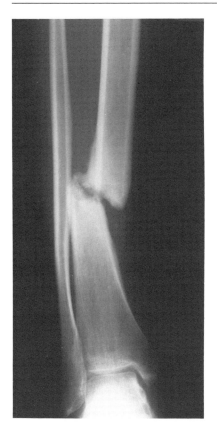

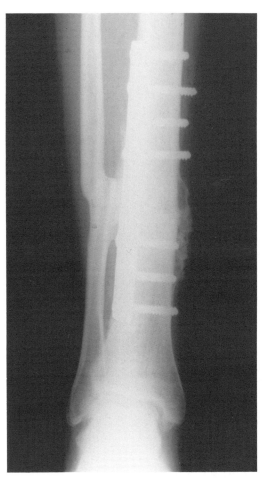

Fig. 23–2 An 18-year-old woman sustained multiple injuries, including an open tibial fracture that was initially treated with wound debridement, closed reduction, and cast immobilization. **Left:** Nonunion. **Right:** Eight months after injury, open reduction, compression plating, and iliac bone grafting were done. Solid union was obtained after 3.5 months of cast immobilization.

ent, the posterolateral approach of Harmon has been used.

The Arbeitsgemeinschaft für Osteosynthesefragen (AO) compression plate combined with iliac bone grafting was used in 31 patients (Fig. 23–2). Until recently this has been the Campbell Clinic's preferred method of treating tibial nonunions when Phemister's method could not be used.

When the pulsed electromagnetic field (PEMF) technique of electrical stimulation became available, a number of tibial nonunions were treated with this method. Ingram and Haynes[6] reported PEMF treatment of 26 tibial nonunions, of which 16 (61.5%) united. In several patients PEMF was combined with bone grafting (Fig. 23–3). This technique is especially useful in the presence of active infection.

Results

Phemister Grafts

The 49 patients in whom Phemister grafts were used ranged in age from 11 to 66 years (average, 40 years). Forty-two were male and seven were female. The right tibia was injured in 22 patients and the left in 27.

Twenty-three of the patients were involved in either car-truck or motorcycle accidents. The fracture was open in 33 patients and closed in 16. Eighteen patients had associated injuries. Four had fractures of the ipsilateral femur. Four patients had significant other health problems. The time from injury to Phemister grafting ranged from four to 61 months (average, 16 months). Fibular osteotomy was used in 16 patients and PEMF in 14. In two patients allografts were used and in all others cancellous iliac autogenous bone was employed. After Phemister grafting, immobilization ranged from two to 44 months (average, eight months). Union was obtained in 45 of 49 patients (92%) (Fig. 23–4). There was one known failure and three patients had inadequate follow-up and were classified as failures. Six patients had angulation greater than 10 degrees and three others had angulation greater than 5 degrees. Nine patients healed with more than 2 cm of shortening.

Compression Plates and Graft

Compression plating was used in 31 patients whose ages ranged from 17 to 88 years (average, 38 years). Twenty were male and 11 were female.

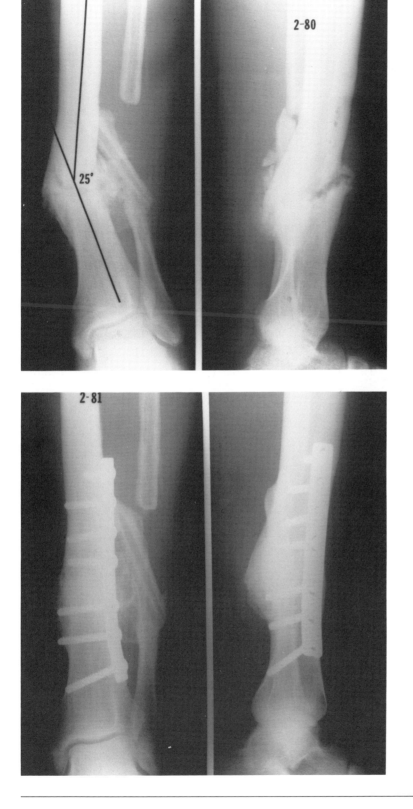

Fig. 23-3 An 18-year-old man had undergone several previous operations. **Top:** Infected nonunion. **Bottom:** Union was obtained after compression plating, autogenous iliac grafting, and the use of pulsed electromagnetic field stimulation.

Sixteen were injured by car-truck or motorcycle accidents. Nineteen patients had injuries to the left side and 12 to the right. There were 20 open fractures and 11 closed fractures. Fourteen patients had associated injuries. Three had fractures of the ipsilateral femur. Eleven patients had significant other health problems.

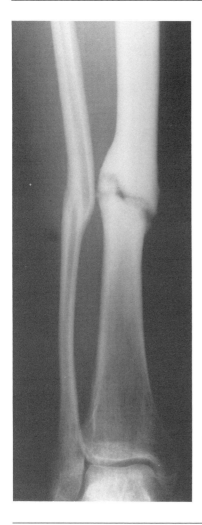 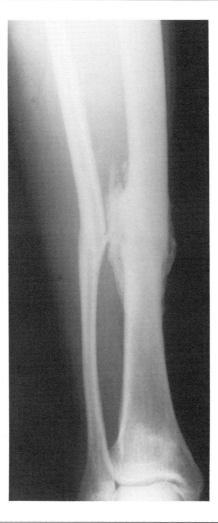

Fig. 23-4 A 15-year-old boy sustained a closed fracture that was initially treated with open reduction and screw fixation. **Left:** Nonunion of the middle third of the tibia. **Right:** After internal fixation was removed, Phemister grafting resulted in solid union 15 months after the injury.

The time from injury to compression plating and grafting ranged from three to 48 months (average, ten months). Fibular osteotomy was used in 18 patients and PEMF in six. In four patients the bone bank (allografts) was used; the other 27 had autogenous iliac grafts. After compression plating, patients were immobilized from three weeks to 27 months (average five months). Six patients (19%) had postoperative infections and seven patients (23%) had wound sloughs. Twenty-six patients had union after one operation (84%). Two patients had more than 10 degrees of angulation and another two had more than 5 degrees of angulation. One patient healed with more than 2 cm of shortening.

Discussion

The tibia is a common site of delayed union or nonunion. This occurs most often in young males subjected to high-velocity injury. In this series, two thirds of the patients had open fractures and many had delayed wound healing. If progressive fracture healing cannot be documented six to eight months after injury, it is reasonable to operate for delayed union or nonunion. The appropriate operative procedure, however, is not as easily determined. European authors[7] have suggested that nonunions are either viable (vascular) or nonviable (avascular) and that viable nonunions require only stabilization (no bone graft) for cure. Campbell and Boyd,[8] using tibial onlay grafts, reported a rate of union above 90%. The major disadvantage is obvious: violation of the uninjured extremity. The favorable biomechanics of intramedullary devices make their use in tibial nonunions attractive; however, their harmful effect on bone circulation must be considered carefully. A number of studies[6,9-12] have demonstrated the effectiveness of electrical stimulation in treating nonunion, especially when it is combined with grafting and stabilization.

When the criteria for modified Phemister grafting are met (acceptable alignment and less than 10 to 15 degrees of motion at the fracture), union rates above 90% can be achieved with one operation and little risk of complications. The fracture does require protection until union occurs; in the present series this averaged eight months. Electrical stimulation and functional bracing probably would shorten this period. Functional results in most patients were satisfactory, although ranges of motion of the knee and ankle were not recorded for all patients.

When free motion is present at the site of the nonunion or if alignment is not acceptable, then Phemister's method is not applicable. This series used compression plating and bone grafting in this situation. Twenty-six of 31 patients (84%) achieved union after one operation and almost all had good function. However, the complication rate was high: infection in 19% and wound slough in 23%. Although immobilization time was shorter than after Phemister grafting (average, five months), rough activities should be limited until plate removal because of the stresses concentrated at the ends of the plate. In addition, since the plates are load-sharing, the underlying bone is weakened and must be protected after plate removal; the risk of refracture is well documented.

In their classic studies of nonunion, Boyd and associates concluded that no one method of treatment was clearly superior to others. More recent data do not lead me to differ. When applicable, the modified Phemister graft is probably the method of choice for tibial nonunion; union was obtained in 92% of patients treated with Phemister grafting in this series. When criteria for Phemister grafting were not met, 84% of patients achieved union with compression plating and grafting procedures, but more than one fifth had complications such as infection or wound slough. Electrical stimulation may be a valuable adjunctive treatment when combined with bone grafting and stabilization.

References

1. Campbell WC: The treatment of ununited fractures. *Am J Surg* 1923;37:1–3.
2. Campbell WC: Onlay bone graft for ununited fractures. *Arch Surg* 1939;38:313–327.
3. Boyd HB, Lipinski SW, Wiley JH: Observations on non-unions of the shafts of the long bones, with a statistical analysis of 842 patients. *J Bone Joint Surg* 1961;43A:159–168.
4. Boyd HB, Anderson LD, Johnston DS: Changing concepts in the treatment of nonunion. *Clin Orthop* 1966;43:37–54.
5. Phemister DB: Treatment of ununited fractures by onlay bone grafts without screw or tie fixation and without breaking down of the fibrous union. *J Bone Joint Surg* 1947;29:946–960.
6. Ingram AJ, Haynes DB: *The Use of Pulsed Electromagnetic Fields in the Treatment of Nonunions: Campbell Clinic Experience*, videotape. Park Ridge, American Academy of Orthopaedic Surgeons, 1981.
7. Weber BG, Cech Ŏ: *Pseudarthrosis.* New York, Grune and Stratton, 1976, pp 45–46.
8. Campbell WC, Boyd HB: Fixation of onlay bone grafts by means of vitallium screws in the treatment of ununited fractures. *Am J Surg* 1941;51:748–756.
9. Bassett CAL, Mitchell SN, Gaston SR: Treatment of ununited tibial diaphyseal fractures with pulsing electromagnetic fields. *J Bone Joint Surg* 1981;63A:511–523.
10. Brighton CT: Treatment of nonunion of the tibia with constant direct current. *J Trauma* 1981;21:189–195.
11. De Haas WG, Watson J, Morrison DM: Non-invasive treatment of ununited fractures of the tibia using electrical stimulation. *J Bone Joint Surg* 1980;62B:465–470.
12. Heckman JD, Ingram AJ, Loyd RD, et al: Nonunion treatment with pulsed electromagnetic fields. *Clin Orthop* 1981;161:58–66.

Nonunions of Fractures of the Proximal and Distal Thirds of the Shaft of the Femur

Robert E. Zickel, MD

Nonunions of fractures of the subtrochanteric and supracondylar areas of the femur are more common than is generally appreciated. There are relatively few published reports on these complications and fewer still on methods of salvaging failures. Understanding the specific anatomic and biomechanical features of each area is essential to avoid pseudarthrosis, which should be the primary goal. When a nonunion does occur, apposition of fragments, adequate immobilization, healing of soft tissue, and stimulation of osteogenesis still remain the tenets of successful salvage.

Anatomy and Biomechanics

Proximal Femur

The pitfalls of both internal fixation and closed management of fractures of the proximal femur are well known. The subtrochanteric area has the highest stresses

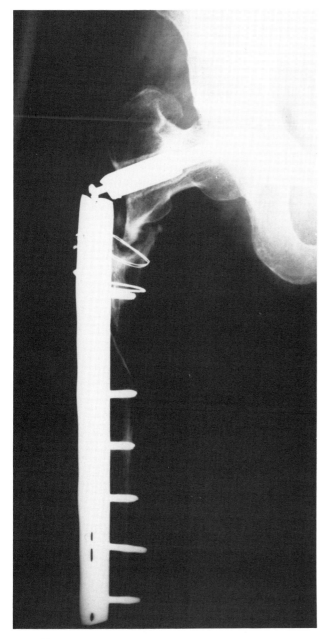

Fig. 24-1 Appliance breakage of strong screw-plate device after nonunion.

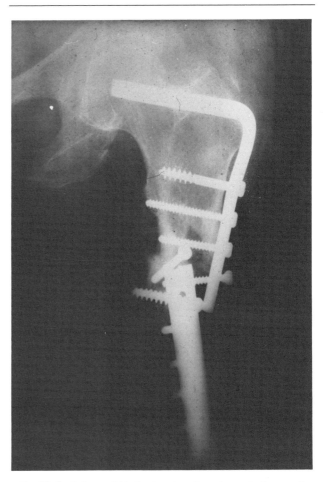

Fig. 24-2 Failure of blade-plate in subtrochanteric fracture because of unstable medial buttress.

of any long bone in the skeleton. This was originally described by Koch[1] in 1917, when he noted that 100 lb of force applied to the femoral head resulted in 1,000 to 1,300 lb of stress per square inch in the proximal femoral shaft. More recent investigators have confirmed Koch's work and have further noted that these stresses may be increased threefold because of the pull of powerful muscle groups controlling the proximal femur.

The trochanteric medullary canal proximal to the fracture is short and wide, affording little fixation for

standard intramedullary nails designed for the midshaft. The use of nail plates designed for routine hip fractures is fraught with the hazard of stresses beyond the strength capacity of the plates. This is particularly a problem when comminution of the medial cortex is present (Figs. 24–1 to 24–3). Mechanical failures of devices in subtrochanteric fractures have been described previously.[2-4] The goal of internal fixation should be to create a load-sharing relationship between the device and the bone itself. Intramedullary fixation, when used properly, can create such a load-sharing relationship. For intramedullary fixation to be consistently successful, it should maintain an anatomic or valgus reduction of the fracture. Subtrochanteric fractures frequently include intertrochanteric fractures that may not be apparent initially, requiring that intramedullary devices, if used, have adequate fixation into the femoral

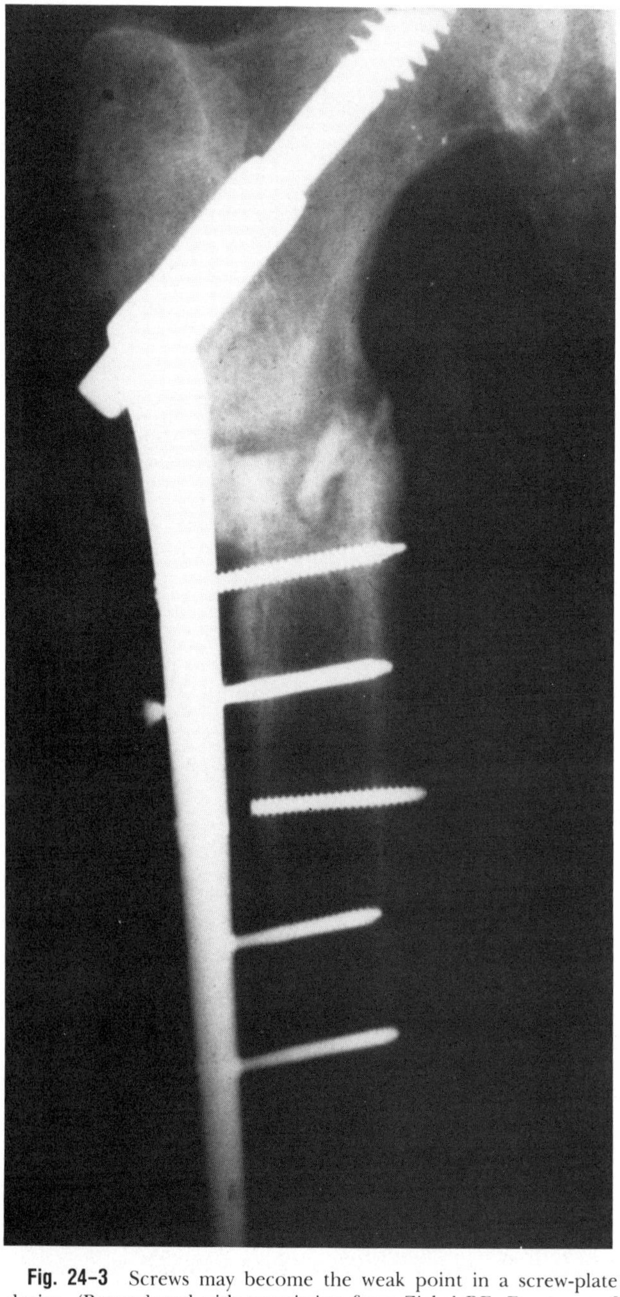

Fig. 24–3 Screws may become the weak point in a screw-plate device. (Reproduced with permission from Zickel RE: Fractures of the adult femur excluding the femoral head and neck: A review and evaluation of current therapy. *Clin Orthop* 1980;147:93–114.

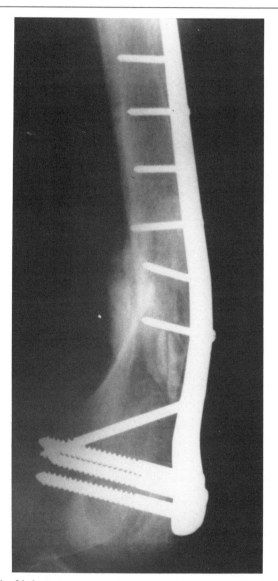

Fig. 24–4 Deformation of supracondylar plate in delayed union of supracondylar fracture.

head and neck. In 1964, the Zickel subtrochanteric nail was designed to meet these criteria.[5] Since that time, other devices have been added. The multiple pins of Ender, which in theory provide the required fixation, sometimes back out of the head and neck of the femur, losing internal fixation. This is in part the result of the difficulty of placing these nails in the good bone of the inferior part of the femoral head and neck. Because of this, Ender pins used in subtrochanteric fractures should probably be augmented by traction for three to six weeks postoperatively.

Interlocking nails anchored by screws in the proximal femur may not provide adequate fixation in the femoral neck in subtrochanteric fractures, particularly those with intertrochanteric components. Breakage of the proximal screws and the nails was shown in one series where mechanical failure approached 30%.[6] For intramedullary fixation to be consistently successful, strong anchorage to the femoral head and neck is required with a load-sharing relationship maintained.

Distal Third of the Femur

The anatomic and biomechanical characteristics of the distal third of the femur differ from those of the proximal third. Here the stresses are considerably less and, as in the proximal shaft, the blood supply is excellent. Proximity to the knee joint, poor bone stock, a truncated widening canal, and the pull of gastrocnemius muscles are anatomic characteristics of this area that make both closed and open management difficult. In the past, many of these fractures were treated with traction and casts. Investigators who reviewed large series of supracondylar fractures managed at their institutions warned surgeons of the hazards of internal fixation and recommended skeletal traction.[7,8] With the development of better fixation devices, more of these fractures have been treated with internal fixation (Fig. 24–4). Most of these devices have been special bone plates contoured to match the distal shaft and condylar areas of the femur, the ends of which provide condylar fixation with nail, blade, screw, or bolt. The supracondylar plates depend on adequate bone stock. This bone stock can, however, be poor in this area, particularly in elderly patients. Intramedullary pins such as those designed by Rush and Ender provide internal alignment of these fractures, but often cannot deal with intracondylar fractures and may be too flexible to provide secure fixation. The Zickel supracondylar nail, modeled after the Rush pin concept, was designed to provide more substantial fixation than its predecessor and to provide transcondylar fixation with large compression screws placed through tunnels in the condylar ends of the nails. Interlocking nails may be appropriate in some infraisthmic fractures, but probably have little place in low supracondylar fractures. The surgeon should insert these nails so that the transfixation holes are well distal to the fracture, as breakage of the nails has occurred through the distal holes when at or near the level of the bone fracture.

A pseudarthrosis (Fig. 24–5) of a supracondylar fracture is difficult to immobilize because of its proximity to the knee joint. Attempts to flex the knee usually result in flexion at the pseudarthrosis rather than at the knee joint itself, making immobilization difficult.

Salvage

In 1968, ZumBrunnen and Brindley,[9] in an analysis of 149 nonunions of long bones, listed four necessary

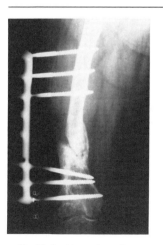
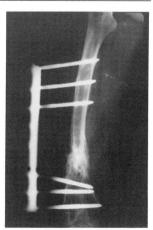

Fig. 24–6 Nonunion of supracondylar fracture. **Left:** External fixator treated with indirect electrostimulation. **Right:** Progression to successful union.

Fig. 24–5 Pseudarthrosis of a supracondylar fracture, showing that knee flexion occurs at pseudarthrosis site.

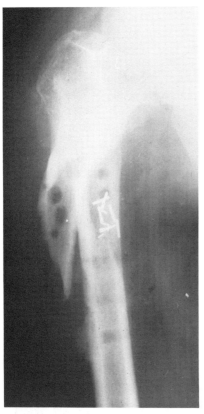
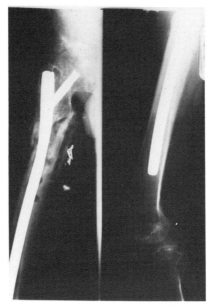
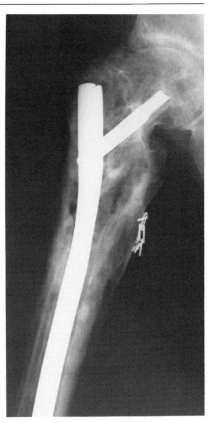

Fig. 24-7   Infected nonunion. **Left**: Six months after removal of nail plate. **Center**: Salvage operation with Zickel subtrochanteric nail and autogenous bone grafts. **Right**: Five years later.

criteria to effect union: (1) apposition of fragments; (2) adequate immobilization; (3) healing of soft tissue; and (4) stimulation of osteogenesis. When these criteria were met, the authors reported an 85% rate of successful salvage. In femoral nonunions these rules still remain the basis of successful salvage.

Salvage methods may be classified as noninvasive, semi-invasive, and invasive.

Noninvasive Procedures

Casts or braces may have some place in the treatment of delayed unions, but have little place in the treatment of an established nonunion. Increased muscle atrophy and joint stiffness result, with little chance of bone healing (Fig. 24–6).

The most popular noninvasive choice in recent years has been the use of indirect electrical stimulation. A comparison of results from two centers recognized for their work with electrostimulation found a marked variation in the treatment of femoral nonunions. One center had a success rate of approximately 80% (C.A.L. Bassett, personal communication, 1986), whereas the other was successful in less than 50% of cases (C.T. Brighton, personal communication, 1986). This discrepancy may be attributed to difference in case selection and the type of stimulating device used, but cer-

tainly the results raised concern about the efficacy of this form of treatment for established nonunions of the femur.

Semi-Invasive Methods

External fixators or direct electrostimulation are currently used semi-invasive methods. External fixators have little or no place in subtrochanteric fractures because of the proximity of the fracture to the hip joint but are probably of value in the management of femoral nonunion as a temporary measure to permit soft-tissue healing and wound care. External fixators used in the femur for prolonged periods are often complicated by pin-tract infections and inadequate fixation of the fracture. In one study, direct electrostimulation with implanted electrodes produced a 58% success rate in the proximal femur and only a 43.7% success rate in the distal femur (C.T. Brighton, personal communication, 1986).

Invasive Procedures

Internal fixation with bone grafting still remains the most reliable choice in an established pseudarthrosis. Careful dissection of scar tissue with strong internal fixation to achieve good bone contact is essential. The addition of autogenous bone grafts circumferentially

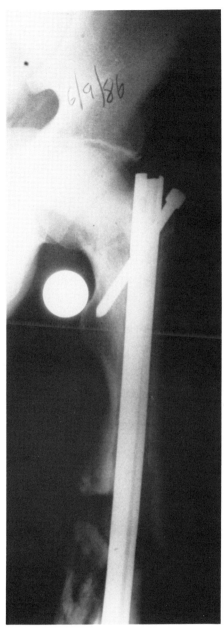

Fig. 24–8 Nonunion of a femoral shaft fracture treated unsuccessfully with interlocking nail after open reduction.

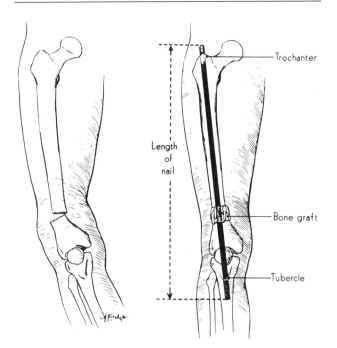

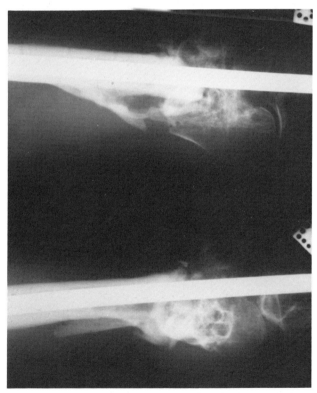

Fig. 24–9 Transarticular fixation. **Top:** With bone grafting as described by Beall and associates.[12] **Bottom:** Example of pseudarthrosis.

around the pseudarthrosis site should stimulate osteogenesis.

In the subtrochanteric area, strong intramedullary fixation with adequate proximal anchorage is the preferred method. The Zickel subtrochanteric nail achieved union in 14 of 15 subtrochanteric pseudarthroses (Fig. 24–7). One successful salvage occurred in a femur that had undergone 15 previous operations with a variety of devices over a 20-year period, all of which had failed. Heiple and associates[10] reported a 100% success rate with the Samson fluted intramedullary rod in 25 femoral nonunions, three of which were in the proximal shaft and six of which were distal (Fig. 24–8). Com-

minuted fractures that failed to unite after treatment by methods that do not restore femoral anatomy because of obliteration and distortion of the medullary canal preclude the use of intramedullary fixation. Various strong nail-plate and screw-plate devices have been used in such cases but the surgeon should protect the

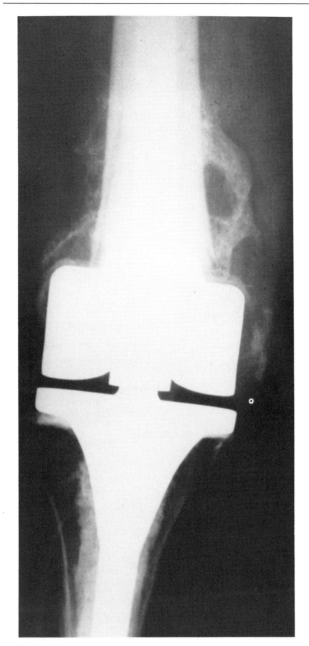

Fig. 24–10 Special knee replacement for nonunion of supracondylar fracture.

limb by traction or cast immobilization for two to three months postoperatively until there is good radiographic evidence of osteogenesis.

Replacement of the proximal femur by custom-designed prostheses remains a final choice after multiple attempts to heal the fracture have failed. The prosthesis must fit well and maintain stabilization. Replacement can be a primary salvage choice in some elderly patients who require early mobilization and who cannot tolerate the treatment and prolonged care necessary to achieve union of the fracture.

The nonunion of the supracondylar fracture is par-

ticularly challenging. Knee joint stiffness transfers fixation to the pseudarthrosis site, making immobilization difficult. In such cases it may be necessary to restrict knee motion to obtain successful salvage. In 1952, Scuderi and Ippolito[11] treated ten supracondylar nonunions successfully with inlay-outlay bone grafts and blade-plate fixation. The blade plate used would be considered inadequate by today's standards. In describing the total management of these cases, they noted that postoperative traction in bed was used for as long as three months. This prolonged immobilization was probably responsible for their success.

More recently, Beall and associates[12] (Fig. 24–9) treated 11 supracondylar nonunions by transarticular fixation and bone grafting. They inserted a Küntscher nail across both the nonunion and the knee joint, achieving purchase in the proximal tibia. After union was achieved, the nail was removed in eight patients with an average return of motion of only 40 degrees. Again, their success in achieving union must be attributed to knee joint immobilization. Although such methods may seem undesirable at a time when great emphasis is placed on joint function, it may become the only way to heal a difficult pseudarthrosis. Once union is achieved surgically, mobilization of the knee followed by continuous passive motion can be performed. Quadriplasty and capsulotomy can achieve motion up to 90 degrees in a stiff knee, a reasonable goal in many of these cases.

Joint replacement with a special prosthesis in elderly patients (Fig. 24–10) may be a reasonable choice in low supracondylar nonunions. Again, preoperative planning to ensure the proper prosthesis is critical.

Summary

Subtrochanteric and supracondylar fractures of the femur are challenging, and specific anatomic and mechanical problems make fixation precarious. With careful selection of devices and techniques, nonunions may be avoided.

Nonunion treatment requires strong immobilization and osteogenesis stimulation with bone grafts. Noninvasive and semi-invasive salvage systems are not as effective as invasive procedures.

The first goal of salvage is union. Joint function and muscle strength are secondary goals to be achieved later.

References

1. Koch JC: The laws of bone architecture. *Am J Anat* 1917;21:177–298.
2. Boyd HB, Anderson LD: Management of unstable trochanteric fractures. *Surg Gynecol Obstet* 1961;112:633–638.
3. Watson HK, Campbell RD, Wade PA: Classification, treatment

and complications of the adult subtrochanteric fracture. *J Trauma* 1964;4:457–480.

4. Fielding JW, Magliato HJ: Subtrochanteric fractures. *Surg Gynecol Obstet* 1966;122:555–560.

5. Zickel RE: An intramedullary fixation device for the proximal part of the femur: Nine years' experience. *J Bone Joint Surg* 1976;58A:866–872.

6. Moncade N: Les fractures hautes du femur. Presented at the Tenth Anniversary Meeting of Grosse-Kempf Nailing, Strasbourg, April 1984.

7. Stewart MJ, Sisk TD, Wallace SL Jr: Fractures of the distal third of the femur: A comparison of methods of treatment. *J Bone Joint Surg* 1966;48A:784–807.

8. Neer CS II, Grantham SA, Shelton ML: Supracondylar fracture of the adult femur: A study of one hundred and ten cases. *J Bone Joint Surg* 1967;49A:591–613.

9. ZumBrunnen C, Brindley H: Nonunion of long bones (analysis of 144 cases). *JAMA* 1968;203:637.

10. Heiple KG, Figgie HE III, Lacey SH, et al: Femoral shaft nonunion treated by a fluted intramedullary rod. *Clin Orthop* 1985;194:218–225.

11. Scuderi C, Ippolito A: Nonunion of supracondylar fractures of the femur. *J Int Coll Surg* 1952;17:1–18.

12. Beall MS Jr, Nebel E, Barley RW: Transarticular fixation in the treatment of non-union of supracondylar fractures of the femur: A salvage procedure. *J Bone Joint Surg* 1979;61A:1018–1023.

Arthroscopic Surgery

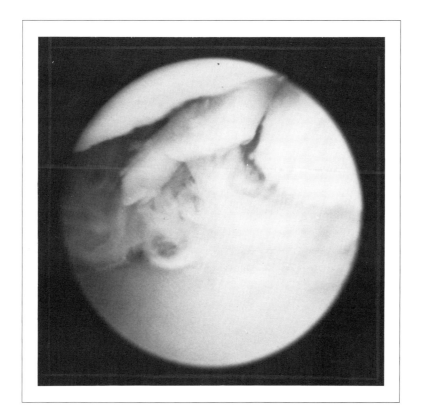

Arthroscopic Surgery of the Wrist

James H. Roth, MD, FRCS(C)

Gary G. Poehling, MD

Terry L. Whipple, MD

Introduction

The arthroscope has dramatically changed the diagnosis and management of knee injuries.[1-5] More recently, arthroscopy has been used to advantage in the shoulder,[6] ankle,[7] and even the temporomandibular joint.[7]

The precise diagnosis of internal derangements of the wrist can be elusive despite careful history-taking, complete physical examination, and many noninvasive and invasive investigations. Even at arthrotomy, exact pathologic documentation can be difficult. A "negative arthrotomy" often produces resistant stiffness and pain. For these reasons, many hand surgeons believe that wrist injuries are among their most difficult and often frustrating cases. In many aspects, the problems related to diagnosis and treatment of wrist conditions today are similar to those encountered in knee conditions in the 1960s before the introduction of arthroscopic knee surgery.

This chapter presents the technique of wrist arthroscopy, reviews the principles and strategy of arthroscopy, describes arthroscopic wrist anatomy, compares wrist arthroscopy and arthrography, and illustrates several surgical cases.

Preparation and Instruments

The procedure is performed in the operating room with the patient under general or regional anesthesia. Most procedures are performed on an outpatient basis.

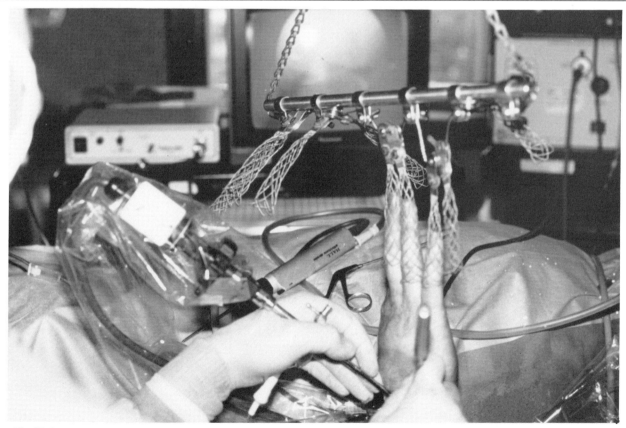

Fig. 25–1   The long, ring, and little fingers are placed in finger-traps. The hand-holder consists of a bar with nine finger-traps. There are three large, three medium, and three small traps so that any hand can be suspended. The entire hand-holder is autoclavable. In this case, the holder is suspended from a ceiling hook. Note that the arthroscopy equipment, including the light source, television monitor, and power source, are on the far side of the patient. The surgeon sits comfortably, directly facing the dorsum of the wrist, and visualizes the procedure on the monitor.

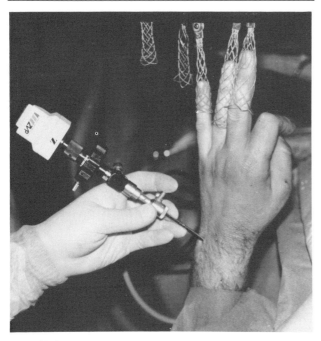

Fig. 25-2 A lightweight "chip camera" is attached to an arthroscope with an outside diameter of 3 mm and a 30-degree angle. The arthroscope is in the 6R portal.

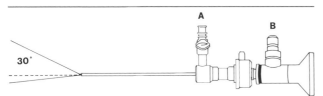

Fig. 25-3 An angled arthroscope is recommended. The single portal (A) on the arthroscope allows insertion of an intravenous line to provide constant gravity-feed irrigation fluid. The light source is connected to the attachment (B) on the arthroscope. The authors prefer an arthroscope which has an outside diameter of 3 mm, is angled at 30 degrees, and is 6 mm long.

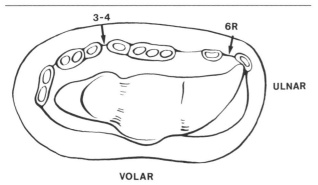

Fig. 25-4 The arthroscopic portals can best be thought of in relation to the six extensor tendon compartments. The most commonly used portals are located between the third and fourth compartment (3–4 portal) and just radial to the sixth compartment (6R).

The room must be arranged to ensure the surgeon's comfort and to provide easy access to equipment and instruments. The patient is positioned supine on the operating table. The torso on the side to be operated on is placed close to the edge of the table so that when the shoulder is abducted 30 degrees the arm hangs free from the table. A hand-holder, incorporating many finger-traps of different sizes, is suspended from either a ceiling hook or an overhead boom (Fig. 25–1). The hand-holder and traps have been sterilized previously.

For primarily ulnar abnormalities, the long, ring, and little fingers are inserted into the finger-traps. For primarily radial abnormalities, the index and long fingers and, occasionally the thumb, are inserted. A 7-lb weight is attached to a sling over the arm. This counterweight provides some distraction of the carpus and helps stabilize the wrist so that it is less mobile during the procedure. Above-elbow tourniquet pressure is increased to 250 mm Hg. The authors prefer to perform arthroscopic procedures, of both the knee and wrist, with proximal tourniquet pressure increased to prevent hemorrhages that might hinder visualization.

The surgeon must be comfortable when performing wrist arthroscopy. A chair with adjustable arm supports is recommended. The arm supports are adjusted so that the surgeon's hands are in a working position while the elbows are resting comfortably. Without such support, neck and shoulder discomfort from fatigue may affect the surgeon's ability to persevere with a difficult or prolonged case. The chair is draped with sterile sheets. The surgeon wears a plastic bib or impermeable gown to prevent soakage from the irrigation fluid. The chair is positioned directly facing the dorsum of the wrist. The height of the patient's hand is adjusted so that the surgeon can use the instruments comfortably.

Most of the arthroscopic equipment is positioned on the far side of the patient. This includes the light and power source, video cassette recorder, and television monitor. The authors recommend viewing arthroscopy on a monitor. This adds to the surgeon's comfort, enhances sterility, improves the morale of operating room personnel, and makes it possible to document and record the pathologic disorders and procedure. A small, lightweight "chip" camera is attached to the arthroscope (Fig. 25–2). An irrigation bag is connected by intravenous tubing to the arthroscope. The bag is elevated on an intravenous pole to maintain constant gravity-feed irrigation and provide some joint distension.

The authors believe that the ideal wrist arthroscope should be angled at 25 to 30 degrees (Fig. 25–3). The angle allows vision around and into the many concavities and convexities of the wrist. With a straight arthroscope, the articular cartilage of the proximal row may be traumatized when visualization of the volar ligaments is attempted. The angled arthroscope allows the surgeon to place the arthroscope into the scaphoid or

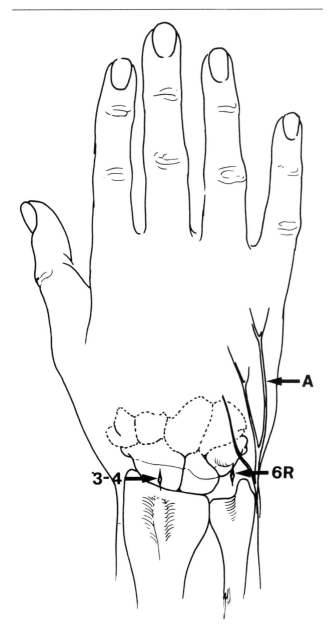

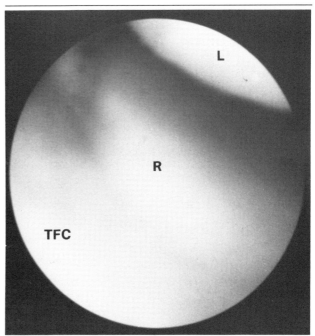

Fig. 25–6 This is a left wrist. The arthroscope is in the 6R portal. The articular cartilage of the lunate (L) and lunate facet of the radius (R) is intact. The triangular fibrocartilage complex (TFC) and its attachment to the ulnar border of the radius are well visualized.

Fig. 25–5 The 3–4 portal is located just distal to Lister's tubercle. The 6R portal is located just proximal to the triquetrum. Longitudinal stab incisions minimize the chance of injury to the extensor tendons, posterior interosseous nerve, and dorsal sensory branch of the ulnar nerve (A).

lunate fossa of the radius and, by rotating the arthroscope, to see the volar ligaments atraumatically.

Before the development of the shorter and smaller arthroscopes, wrist arthroscopy was performed with arthroscopes designed for the knee. It is possible to perform wrist arthroscopy with this larger equipment, but the authors prefer the smaller equipment. An outside diameter of 2.5 to 3.0 mm seems to be ideal for the wrist arthroscope. This is small enough to allow easy maneuverability in the wrist, but stout enough not to be easily damaged. Arthroscopes with smaller outside diameters are available and may be desirable in some

cases. At times, we return to the larger knee arthroscopes when performing wrist procedures. The ideal length for the wrist arthroscope is in the range of 50 to 60 mm.

Many hand instruments for wrist arthroscopy are available. A small hook probe approximately 2.0 mm in diameter is required. Basket forceps 40 to 60 mm long and 2 to 3 mm in diameter are desirable. They should be square at the tip and have a strong but shallow lower cutting jaw. Grasping forceps with the same dimensions as the basket forceps are recommended. They should have thin jaws that open adequately but do not displace a great deal of space. Straight grasping forceps are most useful, but curved instruments are advantageous in some cases.

The authors often use a power end-cutting tool with suction. The ideal outside diameter for this tool is 2 to 3 mm. The cutting should be efficient but not aggressive. The suction attachment allows rapid removal of joint debris.

It is not our purpose to compare and evaluate the many pieces of equipment and the instruments available for wrist arthroscopy. The companies specializing in arthroscopy instrumentation have a wide range of equipment that is evolving and changing rapidly. The authors believe that the most important decision in choosing the company from which to purchase equipment is its record of servicing equipment. Arthroscopy is an equipment-dependent procedure, so any equipment or instrument failure must be corrected quickly.

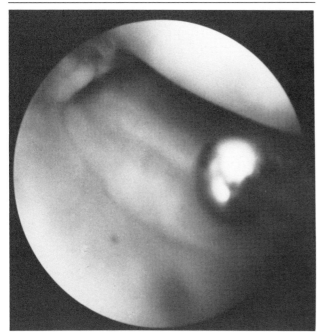

Fig. 25-7 This is the same wrist and orientation as shown in Figure 25–6. The hook probe has been inserted through the 3–4 portal. The tip of this probe is in a more radial portal than the arthroscope and the arthroscope has been rotated until the probe is seen in the 3 o'clock position. This allows appropriate orientation. Knowing the size of the probe allows determination of the size of the structures seen on the monitor. They are always magnified. The degree of magnification depends on how close the arthroscope is to the object being visualized. The hook probe is the "palpating finger" of the arthroscope, allowing differences in texture to be appreciated. In this instance, the distal radius felt smooth and firm. The triangular fibrocartilage felt smooth but rubbery.

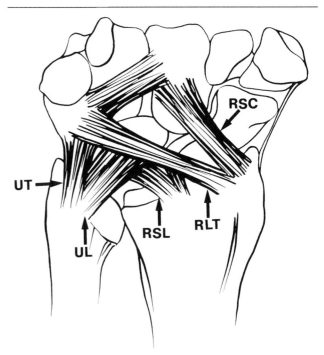

Fig. 25-8 Diagrammatic representation of the volar radiocarpal ligaments seen from the volar aspect. This is a right wrist. From most radial to most ulnar, the ligaments attached to the radius are the radioscaphocapitate (RSC), the radiolunotriquetral (RLT), and the radioscapholunate (RSL). The two ligaments attached to the distal ulna, from radial to ulnar, are the ulnolunate (UL) and ulnotriquetral (UT). These ligaments are difficult to visualize from a volar approach, even in a fresh cadaver specimen.

Principles

The principles of arthroscopy include obtaining a view into the joint, seeing the entire space, determining the characteristics of the abnormality, and, finally, modifying the abnormality. To obtain a view in the wrist, we use a combination of distension and distraction with an angled arthroscope. Multiple small views make up the whole. It is important to see the entire space.

The arthroscope gives a magnified view. We recommend using the hook probe to determine size and orientation. Placing the probe beside a visualized defect allows accurate determination of its size and helps determine its significance.

Orientation can be difficult in the wrist, since most structures are white. Visualizing the hook probe allows for proper orientation of the arthroscope. If the arthroscope is in an ulnar portal site and the hook probe in a central portal, the hook should always be at the 9 o'clock position on the monitor. The probe also allows the surgeon to appreciate differences in texture, such as between the firm distal radius and the rubbery triangular fibrocartilage complex. The hook probe becomes the "palpating index finger" of the arthroscopist.

Contouring ensures that the entire space is visual-

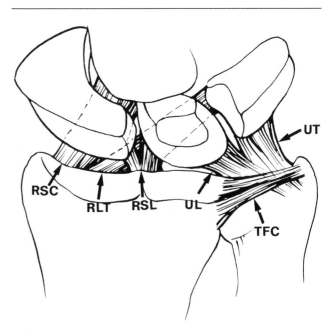

Fig. 25-9 Diagrammatic representation of the volar radiocarpal ligaments seen from the dorsum as in arthroscopy. This is a right wrist. The triangular fibrocartilage (TFC) is also illustrated. The radiocarpal ligaments are readily visualized from a dorsal approach. However, a dorsal arthrotomy must be extensive for these structures to be visualized. They are readily seen arthroscopically.

ized. For example, the volar aspect of the radius is visualized. The entire volar edge of the radius can be seen by following its border radially and ulnarly. Contouring establishes the boundaries of each part and the relationship between parts.

The characteristics of the abnormality are determined by visualization and use of the probe. The probe is positioned in front of the arthroscope by a triangulation technique. The instruments are placed in the portal sites. The surgeon imagines positioning the instruments to form a triangle with the tips of the two instruments at the apex. If this is difficult, one of the instruments can be made to touch and cross the other. The instrument is then directed along the arthroscope until the end is reached and the instrument visualized.

The strategy of arthroscopy involves several steps. The first step is to get into the joint with a clear view. Next, identify a familiar landmark and orient yourself to the local area. Expand the focal area by contouring to get a view of the entire space, to establish the limits and relationships of the joint, and to define the characteristics of any abnormality. A decision must be made on how to modify the abnormality. Finally, an appropriate instrument is positioned at the point of attack and the procedure carried out.

When performing arthroscopic surgery of the knee, the surgeon has the advantage of multiple safe portal sites. This allows one to grasp with an instrument in one portal, visualize through another portal, and cut

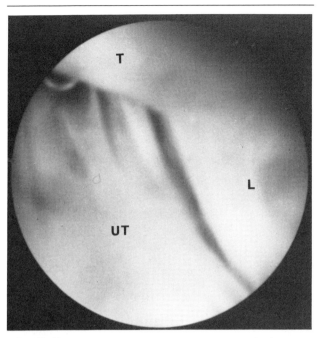

Fig. 25–11 This is a left wrist. The arthroscope is in the 6R portal. The articular cartilage of the triquetrum (T) and lunate (L) is intact. The triquetrolunate ligament is intact. The ulnotriquetral (UT) ligament is well visualized. Superiorly adjacent to the triquetrum is a small air bubble.

with an instrument in a third portal. Portals can be widely separated, making the procedure easier. This is not the case in the wrist. The surgeon is confined to using two closely positioned portals. One portal is required for visualization and the other for operating. Techniques and instrumentation must be developed and used accordingly.

Before attempting arthroscopy of the wrist, the surgeon should attend a hands-on instructional course and practice on wrist models or cadaver wrists. A thorough knowledge of wrist anatomy and internal derangements is a prerequisite. The arthroscopist must be familiar with all the equipment and with basic arthroscopic techniques.

Technique

The arthroscopic portals can best be thought of in relation to the six extensor tendon compartments (Fig. 25–4). The two usual portal sites are located between the extensor pollicis longus and extensor digitorum communis tendons (3–4 portal) and just radial to the extensor carpi ulnaris tendon (6R portal). The 3–4 portal is located 1 cm distal to Lister's tubercle (Fig. 25–5). In creating this portal, the operator's thumb is placed on Lister's tubercle and rolled over into the "soft spot" between the third and fourth extensor compartments.

An 18-gauge needle attached to a saline-filled syringe is inserted at this point and advanced into the radiocarpal joint. It must be remembered that the normal

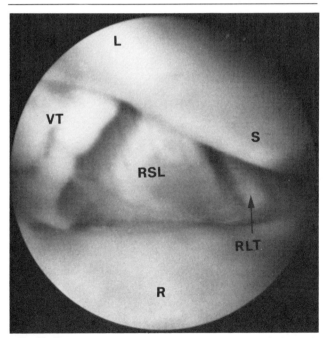

Fig. 25–10 This is a left wrist. The arthroscope is in the 3–4 portal. The articular cartilage of the distal radius (R), scaphoid (S), and lunate (L) are intact. The scapholunate intercarpal ligament is intact. The radioscapholunate (RSL) intercarpal ligament is well visualized. Note the vascular tuft (VT) of tissue associated with the ligament. The radiolunotriquetral ligament (RLT) can be partially seen just radial to the radioscapholunate ligament.

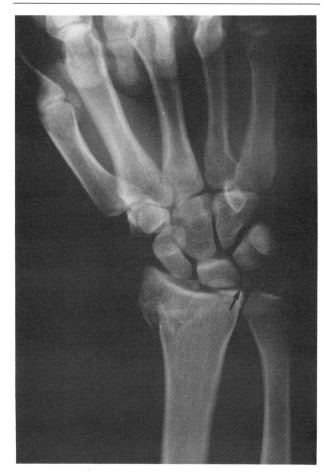

Fig. 25-12   Posteroanterior radiograph of the wrist of case 1. There is a displaced impacted distal radius fracture. There is a free osteochondral fracture fragment (arrow). There is an undisplaced fracture at the base of the ulnar styloid process.

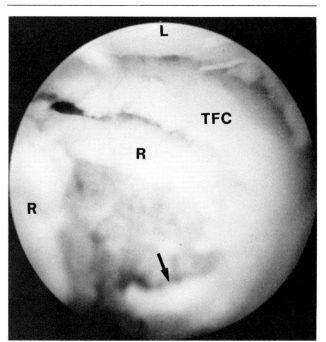

Fig. 25-13   The arthroscope is in the 3–4 portal. This is a right wrist. The intra-articular fracture through the ulnar aspect of the distal radius (R) remains displaced. The free osteochondral fracture fragment has been removed. Note that the complete detachment of the triangular fibrocartilage has avulsed a small fragment of bone from the radius (arrow). The articular cartilage of the lunate (L) is intact.

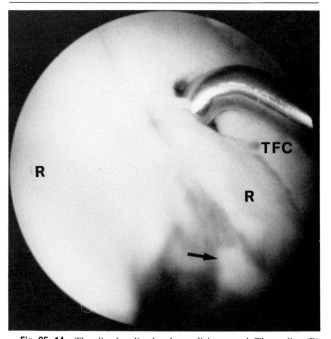

Fig. 25-14   The distal radius has been disimpacted. The radius (R) fracture has been reduced under arthroscopic control. The hook probe is between the ulnar aspect of the radius volarly and the detached triangular fibrocartilage (TFC). The defect that remains after reduction is the donor site of the free osteochondral fracture fragment removed from the joint. The small fragment of dorsal radius (arrow) attached to the triangular fibrocartilage has been reduced.

tilt of the distal radius is 10 degrees apex dorsal. The needle, therefore, must be directed volarly but also proximally. When the radiocarpal joint has been entered, the needle tip seems to be free in a space. The joint is distended with saline. If this does not go easily, the needle is not properly placed and should be repositioned. Once the joint is distended, the needle is removed.

At the same point of entry and with the same angulation as the needle, a No. 15 or No. 11 blade is used to create a longitudinal stab incision through the skin. A longitudinal incision minimizes the risk of damage to the extensor tendons and to the posterior interosseous nerve. A small capsulotomy is created in the dorsal capsule. This is signaled by the return of saline previously injected into the joint.

The surface landmark for the 6R portal is the proximal border of the triquetrum (Fig. 25–5). The distal ulna should not be used to determine the position of this portal, as the triangular fibrocartilage has varying depths and the distal ulna has varying lengths with respect to the radius. In contrast, the relationship between the triquetrum and triangular fibrocartilage

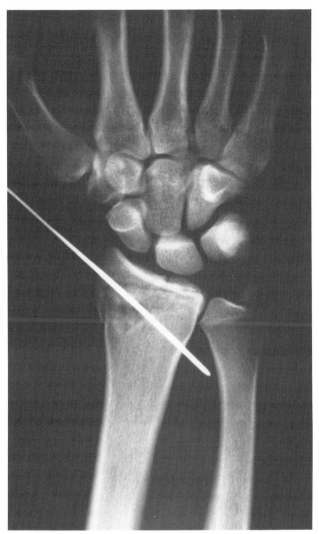

Fig. 25-15 Intra-operative posteroanterior radiograph demonstrating satisfactory reduction of the distal radius fracture and positioning of the nonthreaded pin. Note that the free osteochondral fracture fragment has been removed. An intra-operative radiograph is strongly recommended for all arthroscopic bone procedures.

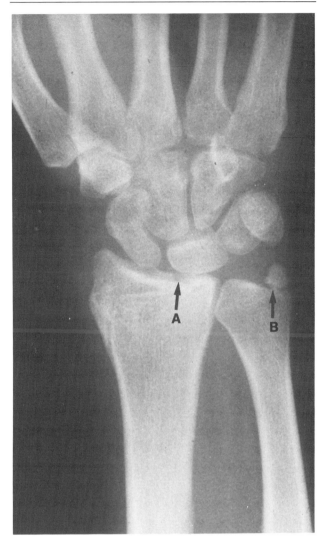

Fig. 25-16 Posteroanterior radiograph taken four months after arthroscopic reduction and internal fixation. The nonthreaded pin has been removed. The fracture has united without collapse. Note the persistent defect in the distal radius (arrow A), which was the donor site of the free osteochondral fracture fragment. Note that the ulnar styloid process fracture appears to be progressing to nonunion (arrow B).

complex is consistent. The proximal border of the triquetrum just radial to the extensor carpi ulnaris tendon is palpated. A longitudinal stab incision through the skin and dorsal capsule is created. Saline returns once the capsulotomy has been made.

The blunt-tipped trochar is placed into the sheath of the arthroscope and the sheath introduced through the 6R portal. The authors advise against using sharp trochars, because these may result in articular cartilage damage. The trochar is removed from the sheath and the arthroscope inserted. The irrigation line is attached to the arthroscope and opened. A hook probe is placed through the 3–4 portal. The arthroscope is oriented to the hook probe and the arthroscopic inspection and procedure performed.

At the conclusion of the procedure, the joint is injected with 0.5% bupivacaine hydrochloride to diminish postoperative discomfort. A bulky hand dressing, incorporating volar and dorsal plaster splints, is applied and the tourniquet released. The dressing is removed five to seven days postoperatively and an appropriate rehabilitation regimen begun.

Arthroscopic Radiocarpal Anatomy

The radiocarpal joint includes the articular arch of the proximal carpal row, the distal radius, and the triangular fibrocartilage complex. The distal radius has a scaphoid and a lunate facet separated by a ridge. The triangular fibrocartilage connects the radius to the base of the ulnar styloid (Figs. 25–6 and 25–7). It is thick on the edges and thin in the center.

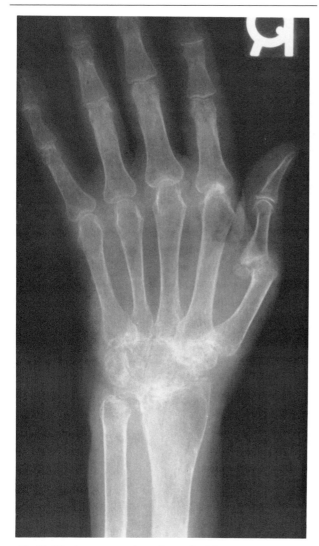

Fig. 25-17 Anteroposterior radiograph of the wrist in case 2. Note the erosions and loss of cartilage space. This patient has long-standing wrist synovitis without extensor tenosynovitis.

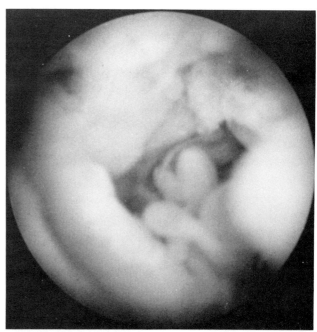

Fig. 25-18 Radiocarpal arthroscopy demonstrated hypertrophic synovium. The arthroscope is in the 3–4 portal. This is a right wrist. This synovium is located volar ulnarly in the region of the prestyloid recess. The entire radiocarpal articulation was filled with similar synovium.

The volar radiocarpal ligament (Figs. 25–8 and 25–9) can be visualized arthroscopically. The most radial volar ligament is the radioscaphocapitate. The second volar ligament on the radial side is the radiolunotriquetral and the third is the radioscapholunate (ligament of Testur). This ligament is Y-shaped with a central tuft of vascular tissue (Fig. 25–10). The ulnolunate ligament is next and is a part of the triangular fibrocartilage complex. The most ulnar volar radiocarpal ligament is the ulnotriquetral, which is also a part of the triangular fibrocartilage complex (Fig. 25–11).

The intercarpal ligaments between the scaphoid and lunate and between the lunate and triquetrum are readily visualized arthroscopically (Figs. 25–10 and 25–11). It is important to "feel" the intercarpal ligaments with the hook probe, as differentiating between carpal bones by visualization alone can be difficult because both appear white and smooth when normal.

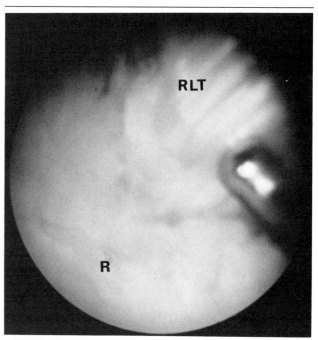

Fig. 25-19 After arthroscopic synovectomy, the radiolunotriquetral (RLT) ligament is clearly visualized. It is being palpated by the hook probe. The articular cartilage of the distal radius (R) demonstrates erosions and irregularity. Access to the volar aspect of the wrist in such patients is easier arthroscopically than it would be through a dorsal arthrotomy.

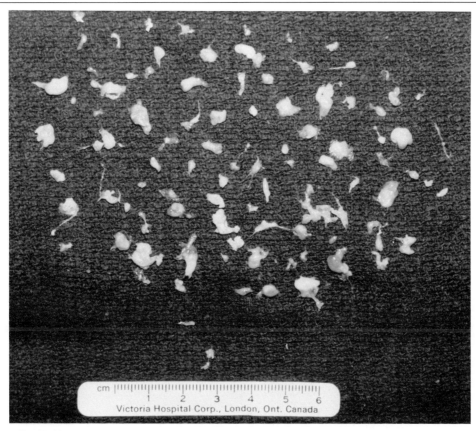

Fig. 25-20 Surgical specimen obtained from arthroscopic radiocarpal synovectomy in case 2. The procedure was performed with an avulsion technique using a small rongeur.

Comparison of Arthrography and Arthroscopy of the Radiocarpal Joint

A prospective study of patients with undiagnosed wrist pain was undertaken to compare radiocarpal arthrography and arthroscopy.[7] There were strict entry criteria. To be included in the study, a patient had to have had disabling ulnar wrist pain for more than three months. Routine and stress radiographs had to have been normal. Patients with rheumatoid arthritis were excluded. Thirty-seven patients met the entry criteria.

Sixteen patients had leakage of contrast into the distal radioulnar joint on arthrogram. All 16 had triangular fibrocartilage tears seen arthroscopically. Arthroscopy allowed exact documentation of the size and type of tear, as well as determination of whether or not there was associated chondromalacia of the lunate or synovitis. These arthroscopic findings could not be visualized on the arthrograms even when they were examined with these findings in mind.

Seven patients had leakage of contrast into the midcarpal articulation. Only two of these had an intercarpal ligament disruption identified arthroscopically.

Seventeen patients had normal arthrograms. Nine of these also had normal findings on arthroscopic examination but seven had triangular fibrocartilage complex perforations and one had isolated lunate chondromalacia.

On the basis of this study, the authors believe that radiocarpal arthroscopy allows better recognition and documentation of abnormalities than radiocarpal arthrography in patients with undiagnosed chronic ulnar wrist pain.

Selected Cases

Arthroscopic surgery techniques can be used to manage internal derangements of the wrist. The techniques and instrumentation have been borrowed and modified from those used in knee arthroscopy. The two major differences between wrist and knee arthroscopic procedures are the smaller joint size and limited number of portal sites in the wrist. The smaller size necessitates smaller instrumentation. Safe portal sites are confined to the dorsum of the wrist. In the knee, three or more portal sites can be used safely, allowing techniques involving multiple instruments. This is not the case in the wrist. In most cases, the arthroscopist must work through two portals only. One of these must contain the arthroscope, leaving only one operating instrument portal.

The authors stress that the procedures performed

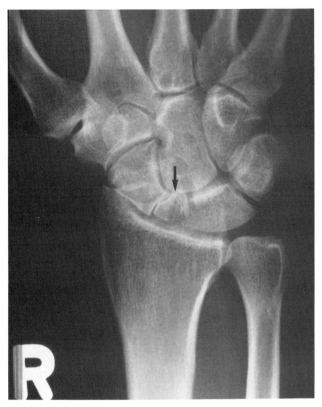

Fig. 25-21 Posteroanterior radiograph demonstrating a long-standing proximal nonunion of the scaphoid (arrow) with radioscaphoid arthritis.

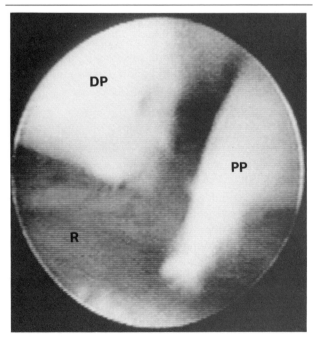

Fig. 25-22 This is a right wrist. The arthroscope is in the 3–4 portal. The wrist has been ulnarly deviated to "open" the nonunion of the scaphoid. The proximal pole (PP) and distal pole (DP) of the scaphoid are clearly visualized. There is erosion to subchondral bone involving the radius (R).

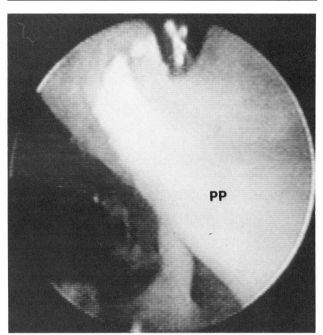

Fig. 25-23 This is the same wrist shown in Figure 25–22. The arthroscope has been moved to the 6R portal. A rongeur has been inserted into the 3–4 portal. The rongeur has been positioned to remove a portion of the proximal pole (PP) of the scaphoid.

arthroscopically are not new procedures. The operations have been done previously through arthrotomies. The authors emphasize that the procedures are not new; they merely use different techniques and instrumentation. What is described is anecdotal. Long-term follow-up and comparative studies are required. However, considering the success of arthroscopic surgery in the treatment of internal derangements of other joints, there is reason to believe the results of arthroscopic surgery of the wrist will be as good, if not better than results of open procedures.

Three illustrative cases are presented.

Case 1

A 24-year-old athlete fell onto his outstretched hand. He sustained a displaced intra-articular fracture of his distal radius (Fig. 25–12) with a loose osteochondral fracture fragment.

Arthroscopy of the radiocarpal joint demonstrated a displaced intra-articular distal radius fracture with much more articular surface involvement and displacement than was suspected radiographically. The triangular fibrocartilage complex had been avulsed from the ulnar aspect of the radius (Fig. 25–13). The loose osteochondral fracture fragment was located and removed arthroscopically. The distal radius fracture was disimpacted arthroscopically and reduced (Fig. 25–14). The fracture was percutaneously pinned with a non-threaded wire (Fig. 25–15). The pin was removed eight weeks later in the clinic (Fig. 25–16). The arthroscope allowed direct visualization of the articular fragments,

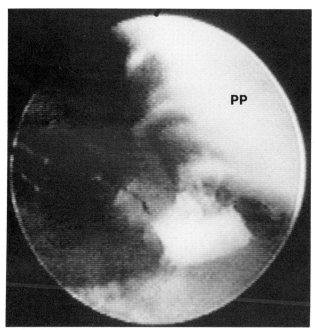

Fig. 25-24 This is the same wrist shown in Figures 25–22 and 25–23. A portion of the proximal pole (PP) of the scaphoid has been grasped and separated by the rongeur. It will be removed from the joint.

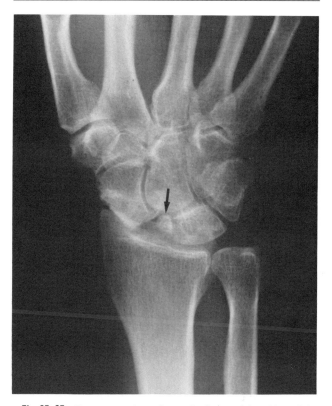

Fig. 25-25 Posteroanterior radiograph after partial excision of the proximal pole of the scaphoid. Note that a portion of the scaphoid remains attached to the lunate (arrow). This emphasizes the importance of obtaining intra-operative radiographs to ensure that you have resected all that you had planned.

ensuring as accurate a reduction as possible. The combination of an ulnar styloid process fracture and complete detachment of the triangular fibrocartilage complex from the radius is an interesting combination of injuries that would not have been recognized without arthroscopy.

The authors believe that arthroscopy will delineate many previously unrecognized pathologic conditions and normal anatomic variations of the wrist. As opposed to an open reduction and internal fixation (ORIF), this technique represents an arthroscopic reduction and internal fixation (ARIF).

Case 2

A 55-year-old woman had long-standing rheumatoid arthritis. She had disabling radiocarpal synovitis and arthritis resistant to prolonged nonoperative management (Fig. 25–17). She did not have significant extensor tenosynovitis. Radiocarpal arthroscopy demonstrated hypertrophic synovium (Fig. 25–18). An arthroscopic radiocarpal synovectomy was performed (Figs. 25–19 and 25–20).

In patients with rheumatoid and degenerative arthritis, the joint appears very narrow, suggesting that arthroscopy will be difficult. This, however, is not the case. The radiocarpal space opens widely with distraction. Arthroscopic procedures performed on such patients are often the most easily performed.

Case 3

A 42-year-old man had disabling wrist pain. Radiographs demonstrated a long-standing proximal scaph-

oid nonunion with radioscaphoid degenerative arthritis (Fig. 25–21). Radiocarpal arthroscopy confirmed the degenerative arthritis and established nonunion of the scaphoid (Fig. 25–22). The proximal pole of the scaphoid was excised by arthroscopic surgery (Figs. 25–23 to 25–25).

Comments

Our present techniques and instruments limit wrist arthroscopic surgery to removal procedures. As the three illustrative cases show, loose bodies, synovium, and portions of carpal bones can be removed. Triangular fibrocartilage perforations are also amenable to arthroscopic treatment. The authors perform partial excisions if the centrum of the perforated complex is mobile.

The distal ulna can be partially excised arthroscopically. In cases of triangular fibrocartilage tears with ulnar plus variance and degenerative changes of the ulna, the "seat" of the ulna can be excised arthroscopically to "level" it with the distal radius. In cases of marked distal radioulnar arthritis with disruption of the triangular fibrocartilage complex, a hemiresection of the distal ulna can be performed arthroscopically.

Arthroscopic joint irrigation for gout, pseudogout,

or infection of the radiocarpal articulation can be performed easily.

Summary

This article has presented the technique of wrist arthroscopy, reviewed the principles and strategy of arthroscopy, described arthroscopic wrist anatomy, compared wrist arthroscopy and arthrography, and illustrated several cases of arthroscopic wrist surgery. We have not discussed indications. More cases and careful follow-up studies must be performed before definite recommendations can be made. The authors are encouraged by their early achievement and believe that the future of arthroscopy of the wrist is exciting. The hand surgeon who performs wrist arthroscopy considers wrist patients to be among the most interesting. The authors believe that arthroscopic surgery will become as important diagnostically and therapeutically in the wrist as it has in the knee.

References

1. McGinty JB, Freedman PA: Arthroscopy of the knee. *Clin Orthop* 1976;121:173.
2. Poehling GG, Bassett FH III, Goldner JL: Arthroscopy: Its role in treating nontraumatic and traumatic lesions of the knee. *South Med J* 1977;70:465–469.
3. Jackson RW, Abe I: The role of arthroscopy in the management of disorders of the knee: Analysis of 200 consecutive examinations. *J Bone Joint Surg* 1972;54B:310–322.
4. DeHaven KE, Collins HR: Diagnosis of internal derangements of the knee: The role of arthroscopy. *J Bone Joint Surg* 1975;57A:802.
5. Andrews JR, Carson WG Jr, Ortega K: Arthroscopy of the shoulder: Technique and normal anatomy. *Am J Sports Med* 1984;12:1–7.
6. Pritsch M, Horoshovski H, Farine I: Ankle arthroscopy. *Clin Orthop* 1984;184:137–140.
7. Roth JH, Haddad RG: Radiocarpal arthroscopy and arthrography in the diagnosis of ulnar wrist pain. *Arthroscopy* 1986;2(4):234–243.

Arthroscopy of the Elbow

William G. Carson, Jr., MD

Arthroscopy, although most commonly used to diagnose and treat various disorders of the knee, is now being applied to smaller joints, including the elbow.[1-6] Unlike arthroscopy of the knee, in which instruments pass only through a thin retinacular layer and maintain generous distances from neurovascular structures, arthroscopy of the elbow requires meticulous attention to detail as the instruments must be placed through deeper muscle layers and close to important neurovascular structures.

Indications

Arthroscopy of the elbow is a relatively new advance in the field of arthroscopy and thus the indications for its use are still being developed. However, elbow arthroscopy appears to be appropriate for (1) the extraction of loose bodies; (2) the evaluation and debridement of osteochondritis dissecans lesions of the capitellum; (3) the evaluation or debridement of chondral or osteochondral lesions of the radial head; (4) the debridement and lysis of adhesions of posttraumatic or degenerative processes about the elbow; (5) partial synovectomy in rheumatoid disease; and (6) the evaluation of a chronically painful elbow when the diagnosis is obscure.

These indications most readily apply to chronic disorders of the elbow. Although arthroscopy of the elbow in the acute situation is less clearly indicated, arthroscopy can be used to evaluate subtle fractures of the capitellum or radial head. Contraindications for arthroscopy of the elbow include bony ankylosis and severe fibrous ankylosis that would prevent the introduction of the arthroscope into the elbow joint and previous surgical procedures (such as anterior transposition of the ulnar nerve) that alter the anatomy around the elbow so that the placement of the usual arthroscopic portals might jeopardize the neurovascular structures.

Surgical Technique

General anesthesia is preferred for elbow arthroscopy as it provides complete comfort for the patient and total muscle relaxation. The patient is placed in a supine position on a routine operating table with the affected scapula just at the edge of the operating table to allow the upper arm and forearm to hang freely over

the edge of the table. The hand and forearm are placed in a prefabricated forearm gauntlet connected to an overhead suspension device so that the elbow is flexed to 90 degrees (Fig. 26–1). Just enough traction is applied through a pulley-and-weight system to keep the arm suspended and the elbow flexed at 90 degrees. This position provides access to both the medial and lateral aspects of the elbow and permits the forearm to be pronated and supinated freely throughout the surgical procedure. In addition, this positioning and suspension device eliminates the need for an assistant to hold the arm in a fixed position. I believe that it is extremely important to maintain the elbow in this 90-degree flexed position at all times when examining the anterior structures of the elbow arthroscopically so as to relax the neurovascular structures in the antecubital fossa com-

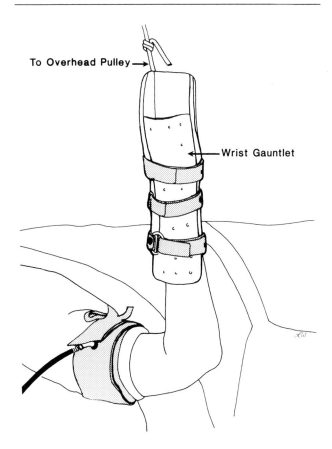

To Overhead Pulley →

Wrist Gauntlet

Fig. 26-1 Position of the arm for arthroscopy of the elbow. (Reproduced with permission from Andrews JR, Carson WG: Arthroscopy of the elbow. *Arthroscopy* 1985;1:97–107.)

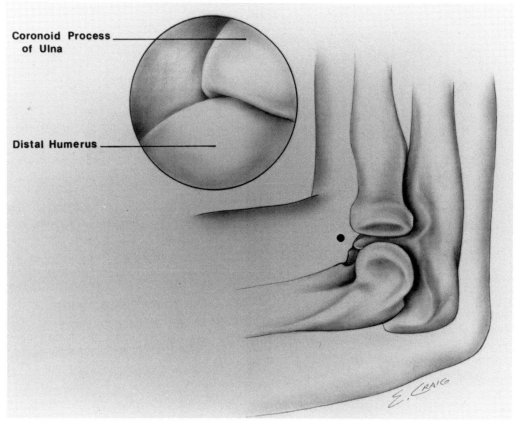

Fig. 26–2 The anterolateral portal is located approximately 3 cm distal and 2 cm anterior to the lateral humeral epicondyle. Areas visible through this portal include the distal humerus and the coronoid process of the ulna. (Reproduced with permission from Andrews JR, Carson WG: Arthroscopy of the elbow. *Arthroscopy* 1985;1:97–107.)

pletely.[1-4] The arm, including the wrist, is then draped in a sterile fashion.

The bony anatomic landmarks are outlined with a marking pin before the initiation of the procedure. As there can be copious amounts of extravasated fluid during the arthroscopic procedure, marking the landmarks beforehand keeps them identifiable throughout surgery. The areas usually marked are the radial head and lateral epicondyle on the lateral side of the elbow and the medial epicondyle on the medial aspect of the elbow. Posteriorly, the olecranon is identified as well.

The three arthroscopic portals most often used for elbow arthroscopy are the anterolateral, anteromedial, and posterolateral portals. Before the arthroscope is inserted into any of the portals, however, the elbow should be maximally distended with fluid via an 18-gauge needle. The most reliable insertion site for the 18-gauge spinal needle is through the triangular area over the lateral aspect of the elbow bordered by the radial head, lateral epicondyle, and olecranon tip. This portal is often used to aspirate the elbow for a hemarthrosis and in this area the needle traverses only skin, a thin subcutaneous layer, the anconeus muscle, and the capsule. After the needle is inserted, the elbow is maximally

distended with a 50-ml syringe. Proper placement is verified by brisk backflow from the 18-gauge needle. Once entry has been verified, the needle is removed and the elbow is left maximally distended. The anterolateral portal is now ready to be established.

Anterolateral Portal

The anterolateral portal should always be the initial arthroscopic portal for elbow arthroscopy; the anteromedial portal should only be established under direct visualization after the anterolateral portal is already established. An 18-gauge needle is placed 3 cm distal and 2 cm anterior to the lateral humeral epicondyle (Fig. 26–2) and aimed directly toward the center of the elbow joint. The needle course is just anterior to the radial head, which can be identified by pronating and supinating the forearm. Once again, verification of entry into the elbow joint is confirmed by free backflow provided by the fluid previously placed into the elbow joint. If this fluid has leaked out, additional fluid may be inserted with intravenous connecting tubing and a 50-ml syringe. Once proper placement of the needle is confirmed and the elbow is maximally distended, the larger instruments such as the arthroscope and cannula system can be introduced.

At this point the surgeon makes a small skin incision, taking care not to injure the underlying subcutaneous nerves. Although a stab incision is usually made in the knee with a No. 11 blade, in the elbow the surgeon can lay the No. 11 blade against the skin and then pull the skin across the blade, using a hemostat to deepen the skin incision and cut through the underlying subcutaneous tissue area.[7] The superficial nerves to be avoided during the insertion of the anterolateral portal include the lateral and posterior antebrachial cutaneous nerves (Fig. 26–3). At this point, rather than the sharp trocar and cannula usually used in the shoulder or the knee, I like to use a blunt cannula initially since it can often be inserted readily through the subcutaneous fat and the muscles. Once resistance is noted, the sharp trocar can be inserted through the deeper fascial and capsule layers and then the blunt trocar can once again be introduced into the elbow joint. Using the blunt trocar as much as possible when inserting the cannula minimizes damage to any neurovascular structures. Superficial or deeper nerves may also be injured less than with the sharp trocar.

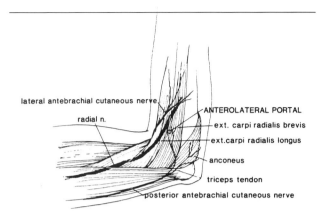

Fig. 26–3   Anterolateral portal anatomy. (Reproduced with permission from Lynch GJ, Meyers JF, Whipple TL, et al: Neurovascular anatomy and elbow arthroscopy: Inherent risks. *Arthroscopy* 1986;2:191–197.)

After the trocar and cannula are inserted, the angle of insertion is carefully monitored. The instrument should be directed toward the center of the elbow as the elbow is kept flexed at 90 degrees. Once the elbow capsule is entered, free backflow will be noted through the cannula and entrance into the elbow joint is thus

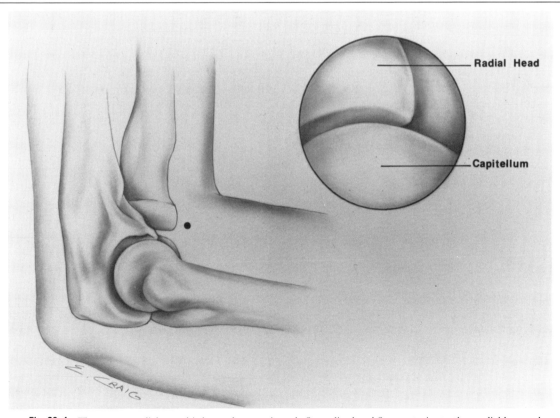

Fig. 26–4   The anteromedial portal is located approximately 2 cm distal and 2 cm anterior to the medial humeral epicondyle. The radial head and capitellum are well visualized from this portal. (Reproduced with permission from Andrews JR, Carson WG: Arthroscopy of the elbow. *Arthroscopy* 1985;1:97–107.

confirmed. At this point the arthroscope is inserted and diagnostic arthroscopy begun.

Continuous distention of the elbow is maintained by overhead bags of normal saline attached to the arthroscope; however, occasionally more pressure is needed to distend the elbow and an additional inflow can be attached to the arthroscopic sleeve with a 50-ml syringe and intravenous tubing. Intermittent suction on the arthroscopic sleeve can be used to remove any cloudy fluid or debris. The arthroscope used on the knee is also used on the elbow and I prefer a 4-mm arthroscope angled at 30 degrees for optimal visualization of the elbow joint. The use of a smaller, 2.7-mm "needle" arthroscope has been described,[6] but since the difference in diameter between this smaller arthroscope and the 4-mm arthroscope is only 1.3 mm, the rationale of using smaller arthroscopes to avoid injury to neurovascular structures is not valid.

Intra-articular structures of the elbow that can be visualized from the anterolateral portal are the distal humerus and trochlear ridges as well as the coronoid process of the ulna (Fig. 26–2). Flexion and extension of the elbow allows the arthroscopist to see the coronoid process of the ulna and extension of the elbow provides a better view of the medial and lateral trochlear ridges and the trochlear notch of the distal humerus. Slowly retracting and angling the arthroscope toward the radial head makes a small portion of it visible from the anterolateral portal.

Dissections of the arthroscopic portals of the elbow in cadavers have revealed that during the establishment of the anterolateral portal, the arthroscope passes anterior to the radial head and through the extensor carpi radialis brevis muscle.[1-7] Although the arthroscope passes beneath the radial nerve when the anterolateral portal is established, Lynch and associates[7] have shown that the instruments pass within 4 mm of the radial nerve, while Andrews and Carson[1] have shown that the instruments pass within 7 mm of the radial nerve. Lynch and associates[7] demonstrated that arthroscopic instruments pass within a mean distance of 4 mm of the radial nerve regardless of the flexion or extension of the elbow when the capsule is not distended with fluid. However, inserting 35 to 40 ml of fluid into the elbow capsule moves the radial nerve an additional 7 mm anteriorly.[7] Thus, maximum distention of the elbow joint should be maintained at all times, particularly during initial insertion of the arthroscopic portals.

Anteromedial Portal

After the anterolateral portal has been established, the anteromedial portal can be safely established by direct visualization intra-articularly. The anteromedial portal is located approximately 2 cm anterior and 2 cm distal to the medial humeral epicondyle (Fig. 26–4).

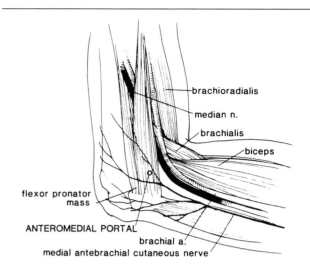

Fig. 26–5   Anteromedial portal anatomy. (Reproduced with permission from Lynch GJ, Meyers JF, Whipple TL, et al: Neurovascular anatomy and elbow arthroscopy: Inherent risks. *Arthroscopy* 1986;2:191–197.)

With the arthroscope in the anterolateral portal, an 18-gauge spinal needle is inserted at this entry point with the elbow flexed at 90 degrees and the elbow maximally distended with fluid. The needle is aimed directly toward the center of the joint. Confirmation of the needle's entry into the joint is provided by direct visualization. The needle passes just anterior to the medial humeral epicondyle and inferior to antecubital structures. A small skin incision is made and the arthroscopic cannula and trocar system are introduced. An interchangeable cannula system permits the surgeon to change at will from the anterolateral to the anteromedial portals with the various instruments. At this point, the inflow can be placed through this anteromedial portal to provide better distention.

The capitellum and radial head are best seen from the anteromedial portal with examination of the radial head facilitated by pronating and supinating the forearm. At times one can visualize the anular ligament coursing over the radial neck. Slowly retracting the arthroscope and directing it toward the ulna makes the coronoid process visible through this portal.

Most arthroscopic surgical procedures in the elbow are performed for pathologic processes located over the lateral aspect of the elbow, such as loose bodies or osteochondritis dissecans of the capitellum. Visualization of these lateral structures through the anteromedial portal is superior to visualization through the anterolateral portal and thus both portals are necessary.

Cadaver studies have shown that when the anteromedial portal is established, the arthroscope enters through the tendinous portion of the pronator teres and penetrates the radial aspect of the flexor digitorum superficialis.[1] As these muscles are penetrated, the median nerve is 1 cm lateral to the arthroscope and the brachial artery is just lateral to the median nerve. As the arthroscope passes deeper and closer to the joint capsule, it comes within 6 mm of these neurovascular structures. These dissections were performed on a non-distended elbow joint, however, and other studies have demonstrated that 35 to 40 ml of fluid in the elbow joint moves the median nerve 10 mm and the brachial artery 8 mm more anterior.[7] Thus, a safe entry for instrumentation from the medial aspect of the elbow requires maximum distention and 90 degrees of flexion (Fig. 26–5).

Posterolateral Portal

Occasionally a third portal, the posterolateral portal, may be required. The entry point for the posterolateral portal is located approximately 3 cm proximal to the olecranon tip, superior and posterior to the lateral humeral epicondyle just off the lateral border of the triceps muscle (Figs. 26–6 and 26–7). This portal is established with the elbow in 20 to 30 degrees of flexion. The 18-gauge needle is directed toward the olecranon fossa. Backflow confirms entry into the elbow joint.

Structures visualized from this portal are the olecranon fossa located over the posterior aspect of the distal humerus and the tip of the olecranon. Flexion and extention of the elbow will help delineate various portions of the distal humerus. Neurovascular structures to be avoided when establishing this portal include the posterior antebrachial cutaneous nerve, which courses over the posterolateral distal humerus (Fig. 26–7), and the ulnar nerve, which lies approximately 2.5 cm medial to the center of the elbow joint.

If a second posterior portal is required, a straight posterior portal may be established under direct visualization approximately 2 cm medial to the first posterolateral portal directly through the triceps tendon. Only 20 to 30 degrees of flexion is needed to relax the triceps muscle. This portal is valuable for the removal of loose bodies from the posterior elbow joint as well as for resection of impinging olecranon osteophytes.[3]

Postoperative Routine

At the completion of the procedure the arthroscopic portals may be closed with suture material or left open,

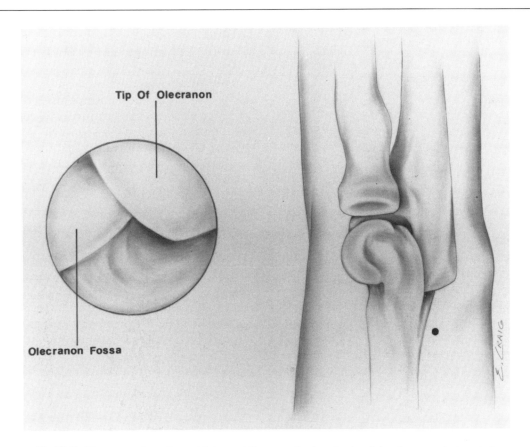

Fig. 26–6 The posterolateral portal is located 3 cm proximal to the tip of the olecranon, just posterior and superior to the lateral humeral epicondyle. This portal is established with the elbow extended so that the tip of the olecranon fossa can be visualized. (Reproduced with permission from Andrews JR, Carson WG: Arthroscopy of the elbow. *Arthroscopy* 1985;1:97–107.)

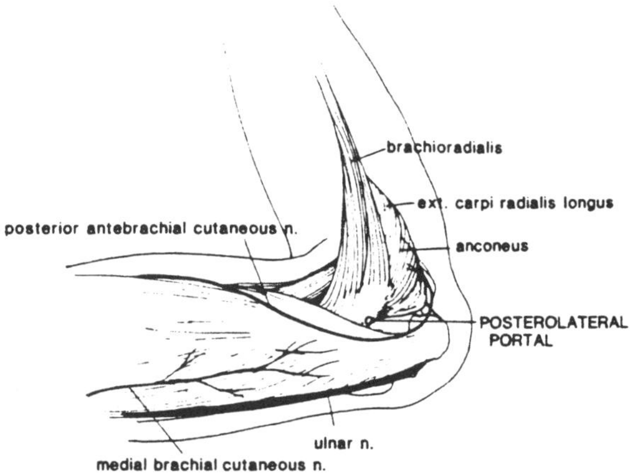

Fig. 26-7 Posterolateral portal anatomy. (Reproduced with permission from Lynch GJ, Meyers JF, Whipple TL, et al: Neurovascular anatomy and elbow arthroscopy: Inherent risks. *Arthroscopy* 1986;2:191–197.)

depending on the preference of the surgeon and the amount of subcutaneous swelling. Soft dressings are applied to the elbow and immobilization is usually not required. Active range of motion of the elbow joint is begun as soon as pain and swelling permit. Once pain and swelling are minimal and the patient's preoperative range of motion has been regained, flexibility and strengthening exercises are initiated.

Complications

Complications of elbow arthroscopy include infection, problems related to the use of a tourniquet, instrument breakage, iatrogenic scuffing of articular surfaces, and neurovascular problems. In a series of 21 elbow arthroscopies, Lynch and associates,[7] reported one transient low radial nerve palsy, a transient low median nerve palsy, and a neuroma formation of the medial antebrachial cutaneous nerve. Casscells[8] reported a case of irreparable damage to the ulnar nerve during an attempt to perform abrasion arthroplasty of the elbow, and Thomas and associates[9] described injury to the radial nerve during elbow arthroscopy. In a series of 45 patients described by Guhl,[5] one patient suffered an injury to the sensory branch of the radial nerve; and in a series of 24 elbow arthroscopies reported by Andrews and Carson,[1] one patient experienced a transient median nerve palsy. This transient nerve injury was probably caused by leakage of the local anesthetic injected into the elbow joint after the arthroscopic procedure, producing a temporary nerve block. (Because of the proximity of the neurovascular structures, I do not recommend using a local anesthetic in the elbow because this kind of temporary nerve block may interfere with the assessment of the patient's postoperative neurovascular status.)

Discussion

Arthroscopy of the elbow is a demanding surgical technique that requires great attention to detail. Unlike knee arthroscopy, in which the portals can be established easily over the anterior aspects of the knee and in which the most demanding part of the procedure is dealing with intra-articular abnormalities, the most demanding aspect of elbow arthroscopy is the establishment of the arthroscopic portals.

Several technical points of the elbow warrant further discussion. Lynch and associates[7] demonstrated the necessity of maintaining maximum distention of the elbow to move neurovascular structures away from the arthroscopic instruments. This also provides better visualization of the elbow and more room in which to manipulate the various instruments. I have had no experience with the infusion pump method of distention and believe that it should be studied further before it can be recommended for routine use. The extracapsular extravasation of fluid needs to be monitored closely. This extracapsular extravasation occurs most often after repeated attempts to establish the arthroscopic portals. The multiple holes in the capsule result in fluid leakage. An inflow cannula should have an opening on the end only and should not have any side vents. If the inflow cannula slips back somewhat during the arthroscopic procedure, the side vents will be outside the joint capsule and fluid will go directly into the subcutaneous tissues.

Another important technical consideration is the actual maneuvering of instruments inside the elbow joint. The distance between the articular surfaces of the elbow and the joint capsule is usually short, making it easy for the instrument to slip out of the capsule. Once this happens, there is further fluid extravasation and reintroducing the arthroscope adds to the risk of damage to neurovascular structures. The arthroscope should be moved slowly, particularly during retraction. The cannula should be stabilized next to the skin with the other hand.

Despite the many technical problems associated with elbow arthroscopy and the risk of neurovascular injury, this surgical procedure effectively treats various disorders. It appears to produce the best results in extracting loose bodies or in removing impinging osteophytes. However, it is less successful for treating certain degenerative processes such as chondroplasties of articular surfaces or intra-articular lysis of adhesions.[1,3]

Summary

Arthroscopy of the elbow is a technically demanding surgical procedure and attention to detail is essential. The surgeon needs a thorough knowledge of the extra-articular portal anatomy to avoid damaging nearby neurovascular structures. Several technical points need to be considered at all times, especially maintaining the elbow at 90 degrees of flexion to relax the neurovascular structures and maximally distended to move them farther away from the entering arthroscopic instruments.

References

1. Andrews JR, Carson WG: Arthroscopy of the elbow. *Arthroscopy* 1985;1:97–107.
2. Andrews JR, Carson WG: Arthroscopy of the elbow, in McGinty JB (ed): *Techniques in Orthopaedics: Arthroscopic Surgery Update*. Rockville, MD, Aspen Systems Corp, 1985, pp 183–190.
3. Andrews JR, St. Pierre RK, Carson WG: Arthroscopy of the elbow. *Clin Sports Med* 1986;5:653–662.
4. Carson WG, Andrews JR: Arthroscopy of the elbow, in Zarins B, Andrews J, Carson WG (eds): *Injuries to the Throwing Arm*. Philadelphia, WB Saunders, 1985, pp 221–227.
5. Guhl JF: Arthroscopy and arthroscopic surgery of the elbow. *Orthopaedics* 1985;8:290–296.
6. Johnson LL: Elbow arthroscopy, in *Arthroscopic Surgery: Principles and Practice*. St. Louis, CV Mosby Co, 1986, pp 1446–1477.
7. Lynch GJ, Meyers JF, Whipple TL, et al: Neurovascular anatomy and elbow arthroscopy: Inherent risks. *Arthroscopy* 1986;2:191–197.
8. Casscells SW: Editor's comment. *Arthroscopy* 1986;2:190.
9. Thomas MA, Fast A, Shapiro D: Radial nerve damage as a complication of elbow arthroscopy. *Clin Orthop* 1987;215:130–131.

Arthroscopic Meniscectomy

Thomas D. Rosenberg, MD

Robert W. Metcalf, MD

Wm. Douglas Gurley, MD

Operative arthroscopy has greatly improved our ability to deal with meniscal pathology. Much greater exposure of the entire meniscus is available by arthroscopy than by arthrotomy. Available options include partial meniscectomy, meniscal repair, and careful observation. Selection of the proper treatment option depends on the type of tear.

Classification of Meniscal Tears

Meniscal tears can be classified by the orientation of tears relative to the three-dimensional structure of the meniscus (vertical, transverse, horizontal, longitudinal, or oblique) (Fig. 27–1). Tears may be complex, simple,

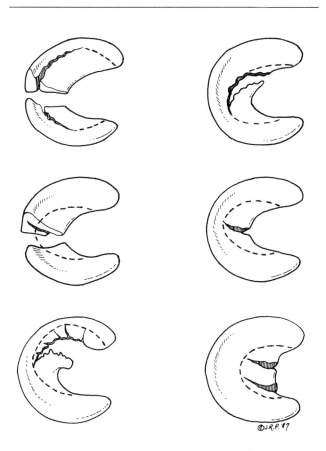

Fig. 27-1 Classification of meniscal tears, with proposed partial meniscectomy shown in dotted lines. **Top left:** Bucket-handle. **Top right:** Flap. **Middle left:** Horizontal. **Middle right:** Radial. **Bottom left:** Degenerative flap. **Bottom right:** Radial tears in a discoid meniscus.

multiple, degenerative, complete, or incomplete. For example, proper classification of a common bucket-handle tear might be a complete tear with both vertical and longitudinal components. Flap tears have vertical and oblique components. Horizontal cleavage tears are horizontal and longitudinal. Radial tears are transverse and vertical.

General Principles of Arthroscopic Meniscectomy

In any surgical procedure, adequate exposure is paramount. Exposure in arthroscopic meniscal surgery requires attention to several details. Iatrogenic abrasions to articular cartilage by arthroscopic instruments must be avoided. They are usually the result of inadequate exposure.

When a meniscal tear is deemed irreparable and unstable, partial meniscectomy is indicated. The goal of arthroscopic meniscectomy is to excise only the unstable, damaged portion of the meniscus while leaving the maximum amount of the stable portion intact. The transition from the area of excision to the remaining meniscus must be tapered or contoured. Sudden transitions may provide an edge or lip for future propagation of the meniscal tear.

Complete muscular relaxation with the patient under general anesthesia provides the best possible circumstances for safe meniscal surgery. We believe that the combination of a secure, low-profile thigh-holding device and a well-trained surgical assistant is necessary for safe, maximal exposure of the medial and lateral compartments. The assistant applies varus or valgus stress at the appropriate range of flexion or extension. Another useful maneuver is to have the assistant apply posterior digital pressure to the joint line. This can deliver a meniscal fragment forward in the joint where it may be more accessible to cutting instruments. Support should also be provided for the uninvolved leg in a position of flexion, abduction, and slight external rotation. A padded lithotomy leg-holder works well for this purpose. Supporting the well leg in this way provides better access to all sides of the affected knee, protects the well leg from femoral nerve palsy, and diminishes lordotic stress on the lumbar spine (Fig. 27–2).

Proper portal placement can greatly facilitate any arthroscopic procedure. The portal sites are located by palpating the joint line with the knee at 45 degrees of

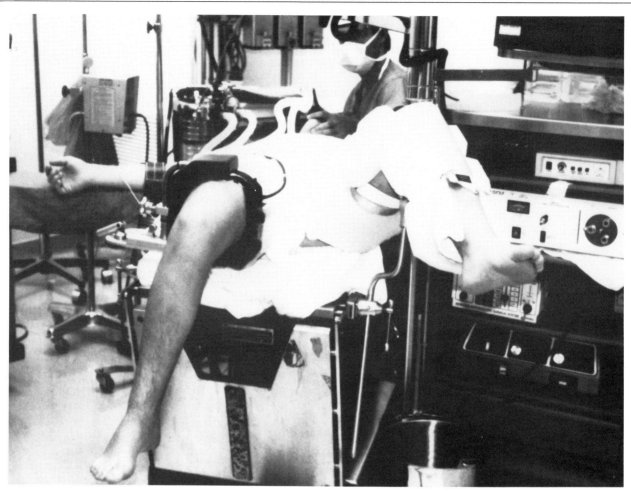

Fig. 27–2 Patient positioning. The well leg is supported in a padded lithotomy leg-holder in a position of hip flexion, abduction, and slight external rotation. The leg to be operated on is held in a low-profile thigh-holder with a tourniquet.

flexion. We place the anterolateral portal 1 cm above the joint line and immediately adjacent to the patellar tendon. The anteromedial portal is placed 1 cm above the medial joint line and slightly medial to the patellar tendon. These positions place the instruments above the bulk of the fat pad and menisci (Fig. 27–3).

Instrumentation

Cutting instruments for arthroscopic meniscal surgery include punch forceps, right-angled rotary punches, arthroscopic scissors, and arthroscopic knives. The safest and most commonly used cutting instrument is the punch forceps. Arthroscopic punches are available in a variety of sizes. To avoid articular cartilage scuffing in tight compartments, smaller but effective 2.75-mm punches have been designed (Fig. 27–4). Knives are useful but must be precisely handled intra-articularly to avoid hyaline cartilage injury.

Motorized instruments are extremely helpful in ad-

vanced procedures. Motorized units are operated by foot or hand controls and work at varying speeds. The cutting tips range from slow, side-cutting blades to high-speed (3,000 rpm) end-cutting, auger-style blades. The full-radius cutter is an excellent all-around blade useful for synovium, cartilage, and meniscus. A high rate of inflow is needed for motorized instruments because they require suction.

Specific Surgical Approaches to Partial Meniscectomy

Flap Tears (Oblique and Vertical)

Meniscal flap tears are among the most common and can occur in several ways (Fig. 27–5). A bucket-handle tear can tear transversely, leaving anterior and posterior flaps (Fig. 27–1, *top left*). A simple radial tear may propagate obliquely to produce a flap. Flap tears are treated by sharp division at the base of the tear, most often by punch forceps. The fragment is removed and the remaining meniscus must be probed to insure sta-

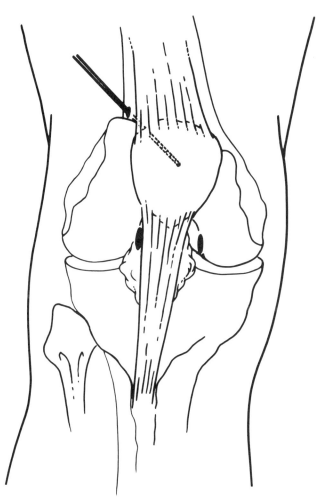

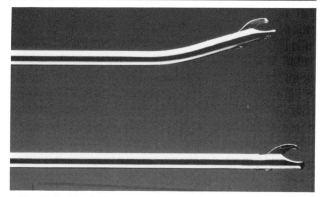

Fig. 27-4 The 2.75-mm straight and upcurved punch forceps are especially useful for meniscectomies in tight compartments.

Fig. 27-3 Placement of standard arthroscopic portals.

bility. The cut edge of the remnant is then contoured to leave a smooth, tapered transition from the area of the meniscectomy to the normal meniscus.

Bucket-Handle Tears (Vertical and Longitudinal)

Bucket-handle tears occur more frequently in younger patients with significant trauma. Very often they occur as part of an anterior cruciate ligament injury. Bucket-handle tears are three times more common in the medial meniscus than in the lateral meniscus. Displacement of the fragment into the notch causes the clinical symptoms of a locked knee. Some of these tears may be only partially displaceable, especially shorter, early tears in the posterior half of the meniscus (Fig. 27–6). In the unstable, irreparable tear, partial meniscectomy is indicated. Smaller, stable, asymptomatic, incomplete tears of less than 1.5 cm may be left untreated.[1,2]

During partial meniscectomy of bucket-handle tears, displaced tears should first be reduced with the probe. The proper varus or valgus stress greatly helps in reduction of the fragment. The fragment is then detached at the posterior horn with small punch forceps or scissors. One useful technique is to leave a small (less than 1 mm) tissue bridge to serve as tether. This keeps the fragment from floating free and obscuring the view of the anterior cut. The anterior extent of the tear is then identified and cut with punch forceps or angled scissors. This can best be performed with the instrument in the ipsilateral portal. The loose anterior edge of the fragment is then grasped with a Schlesinger clamp and the fragment is removed, avulsing the small posterior tether. The remaining meniscal rim is then contoured anteriorly and posteriorly. A motorized meniscal cutter is useful for smoothing the cut surface. The remaining rim must be fully visualized and probed because double and triple longitudinal tears can occur.

Horizontal Cleavage Tears

Horizontal tears occur most often in association with bucket-handle, flap, or degenerative tears (Fig. 27–7). Primary horizontal tears can appear to be "fish-mouthed" and can be associated with meniscal cysts. Any hypermobile portion of superior or inferior leaflets is trimmed. It is not necessary to excise the fragments completely back to the periphery. For horizontal tears in the posterior horns, punch forceps with 15 degrees of upcurve and posterior digital pressure at the joint line can facilitate the procedure.

Radial Tears (Vertical and Transverse)

The most common location for a radial tear is the middle third of the lateral meniscus, presumably because of excessive valgus loading (Fig. 27–8). In anterior cruciate ligament tears there is often a radial tear at the posterior horn of the lateral meniscus.[3] A radial tear of less than 3 mm may be an incidental finding and usually is not symptomatic. Tears of more than 5 mm are usually symptomatic and should be resected. The partial meniscectomy should remove the anterior and posterior lips of the tears only as deeply as the

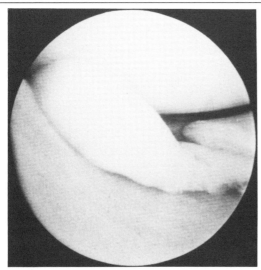
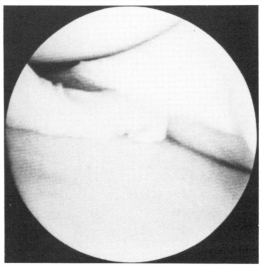

Fig. 27–5   A pedunculated flap tear that has an associated horizontal component.

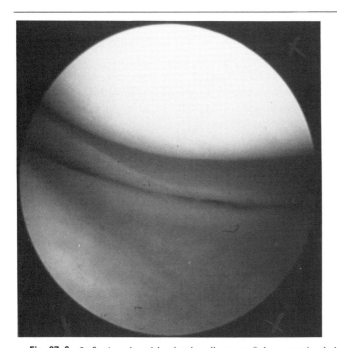
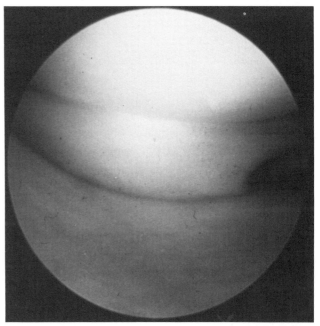

Fig. 27–6   **Left:** A reduced bucket-handle tear of the posterior half of the medial meniscus. **Right:** Displacement by the probe makes diagnosis possible.

apex tear extends. Then, the remnant should be tapered and contoured as previously described. Radial tears can be associated with meniscal cysts (Fig. 27–9). Appropriate treatment of the intra-articular lesion has been reported to result in meniscal cyst involution, without open cyst excision.[4]

Degenerative and Complex Tears

In chronic tears there is usually a combination of several types of tear components (Fig. 27–10). Degenerative menisci are discolored and fibrillated and can show edema of the meniscus itself. As expected, these are much more common in older patients and usually have associated chondrosis of that compartment.[5] Arthroscopic partial meniscectomy of degenerative tears is a good procedure in which to use a combined technique of motorized shavers and punch forceps. Again, the goal is to leave a stable, well-contoured rim.

Tears of Discoid Menisci

Another indication for partial meniscectomy is a symptomatic tear of a discoid lateral meniscus.[6-8] When

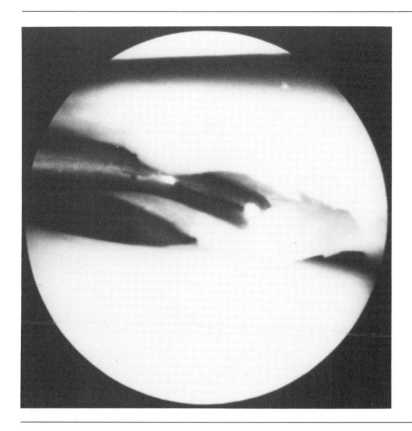

Fig. 27-7 A horizontal cleavage tear with the probe inside the tear.

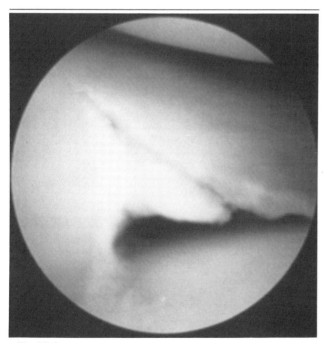

Fig. 27-8 A radial tear with a small horizontal component.

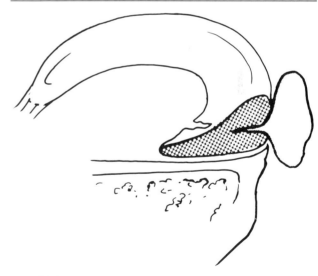

Fig. 27-9 A meniscal cyst, showing its communication with a radial tear.

the peripheral rim is stable, partial meniscectomy of the torn portion and saucerization of the discoid central portion is performed (Fig. 27–1, *bottom right*). The goal here is to change the meniscus into an approximately normal semilunar remnant. Early reports of this procedure in children are encouraging.[8] Because of the bulk of the tissue in the lateral compartment, this procedure may be difficult. Piecemeal excision of the central portion with punch forceps may occasionally be necessary.

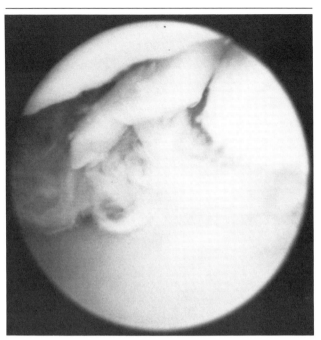

Fig. 27-10 A degenerative meniscal tear. Note the associated chondrosis of the medial femoral condyle.

Results

Our own experience with a five- to eight-year follow-up of 148 arthroscopic partial meniscectomies corresponds well with the studies of others.[9,10] Overall, we found 87% of the results to be good or excellent. Radiographic changes were markedly less than in open, total meniscectomies.[11] In the subgroup of knees with intact anterior cruciate ligaments and no chondromalacia of the condyles, 97% of the results were good or excellent. Results were less gratifying in degenerative tears and in patients with tears of both menisci in the same knee, 57% and 67% good to excellent, respectively.

Summary

Arthroscopic partial meniscectomy is indicated for unstable, irreparable tears. Meniscal repair and partial meniscectomy are not mutually exclusive concepts. These are complementary procedures, with each having specific indications. Larger, more peripheral tears are repaired, whereas smaller, more central irregular or irreparable tears are treated by arthroscopic partial meniscectomy. The emphasis is on leaving a well-contoured stable meniscus while excising only the unstable or damaged portion. The remaining meniscus may still provide some protection for the hyaline cartilage of that compartment.[12]

References

1. Lundberg M, Hamberg P, Lysholm J, et al: The fate of untreated meniscus lesions—A long term follow up study. *Orthop Trans* 1985;9:458.
2. Rosenberg TD, Scott SM, Paulos LE: Repair of peripheral detachment of the meniscus. *Contemp Orthop* 1980;10(3):43–50.
3. Stone RG, Ramsey DC III: Transverse tears of the lateral meniscus. *Contemp Orthop* 1984;9(5):35–40.
4. Ferriter PJ, Nisonsen B: The role of arthroscopy in the treatment of lateral meniscal cysts. Presented at the annual meeting of the Arthroscopy Association of North America, Boston, April 1985.
5. Sprague NF: Degenerative and traumatic flap tears of the meniscus. *Contemp Orthop* 1984;9(4):23–46.
6. Ikeuchi H: Arthroscopic treatment of the discoid lateral meniscus: Technique and long-term results. *Clin Orthop* 1982;167:19–28.
7. Dickhaut SC, DeLee JC: The discoid lateral-meniscus syndrome. *J Bone Joint Surg* 1982;64A:1068–1073.
8. Fujikawa K, Iseki F, Mikura Y: Partial resection of the discoid meniscus in the child's knee. *J Bone Joint Surg* 1981;63B:391–395.
9. McGinty JB, Geuss LF, Marvin RA: Partial or total meniscectomy: A comparative analysis. *J Bone Joint Surg* 1977;59A:763–766.
10. Northmore-Ball MD, Dandy DJ, Jackson RW: Arthroscopic, open partial, and total meniscectomy: A comparative study. *J Bone Joint Surg* 1983;65B:400–404.
11. Fairbank TJ: Knee joint changes after meniscectomy. *J Bone Joint Surg* 1948;30B:664–670.
12. Fahmy NRM, Williams EA, Noble J: Meniscal pathology and osteoarthritis of the knee. *J Bone Joint Surg* 1983;65B:24–28.

Arthroscopic Meniscus Repair With a Posterior Incision

Charles E. Henning, MD

J. Roger Clark, MD

Mary A. Lynch, MD

Robert Stallbaumer, RN

Kim M. Yearout, RPT

Steven W. Vequist, RPT

The importance of the meniscus as both a load-bearing and a stabilizing structure of the knee has been well documented. The ability of this bicondylar joint to have both flexion and extension as well as simultaneous rotation is facilitated by the meniscus, which is slightly concave on the femoral side and nearly flat on the tibial surface. This important part of the knee system has been present in mammals for about 320 million years according to Dye and associates.[1]

Basic Science and Clinical Studies

The menisci are important in load-bearing, transmitting about 50% of the contact force of the medial compartment and an even higher percentage in the lateral compartment according to Walker and Erkman.[2] Seedhom and Hargreaves[3] demonstrated in vitro that removal of only 16% to 34% of the meniscus increased the joint contact forces by about 350%. This much or more of the meniscus is frequently removed during an arthroscopic partial meniscectomy.

The more peripheral portion of the meniscus is an important joint stabilizer. Levy and associates[4] demonstrated that the posterior rim of the medial meniscus is an important stabilizer with respect to anterior translation of the knee.

Degenerative changes occur most rapidly in the knee with a deficient anterior cruciate ligament (ACL) after meniscectomy. Gudde and Wagenknecht[5] in 1973 and Johnson and associates[6] in 1974 reported poor results after meniscectomy in ACL-deficient knees. Lynch and associates[7] demonstrated an 88% incidence of Fairbank's changes at a minimum of three years after meniscectomy in ACL-deficient knees, even when a stable ACL reconstruction was obtained. Lipscomb and Anderson[8] reported a 68% incidence of Fairbank's changes in a group of 13- to 15-year-old adolescents who had ACL lesions after ACL reconstruction and meniscectomy. This group of patients had a shorter follow-up and the patients weighed less than those studied in Lynch and associates' series.

Isolated lateral meniscectomy yielded nearly 50% poorer results in a series of studies by Yocum and associates.[9] Isolated medial meniscectomy yields somewhat better results, but the ten-year follow-up data represent only a small portion of the patients' remaining lives.

This chapter presents a method of arthroscopic repair of the meniscus utilizing a posterior incision. The concept of meniscus repair is not new. In 1885, Annandale[10] reported a repair of a meniscus performed in 1863. King[11] in 1936 concluded that peripheral tears of menisci in dogs would heal provided that there was sufficient vascularity of the peripheral rim. DeHaven and Hales[12] reported their experience with peripheral repair of menisci by a direct suture technique. Ikeuchi[13] first reported a technique of arthroscopically aided meniscus repair in 1976, using a percutaneous approach, guiding the needle through the meniscus arthroscopically and back out to the surface, and tying it over an external bolster.

Scott and associates[14] reported the initial results with the arthroscopic transarticular approach and a posterior incision. The transarticular approach allows suturing of menisci with peripheral white rims of up to 5 mm without excising any of the peripheral white rim.

In our experience, vascularity appears to be essential for healing of the meniscus repairs in humans. From 1980 through 1983 we used a basket forceps to abrade the parameniscal synovium. It is these initial results that were reported by Scott and associates. In November

Table 28-1
Age groups

Ages (Years)	No. of Patients
15 to 18	14
19 to 22	8
23 to 30	24
31 to 35	3
36 or older	5

Table 28-2
Meniscus tears repaired with rasp and clot

Type of Tear	No. of Cases
Single longitudinal	43
Double longitudinal	4
Triple longitudinal	1
Radial	3
Flap	3
Bucket-handle	12

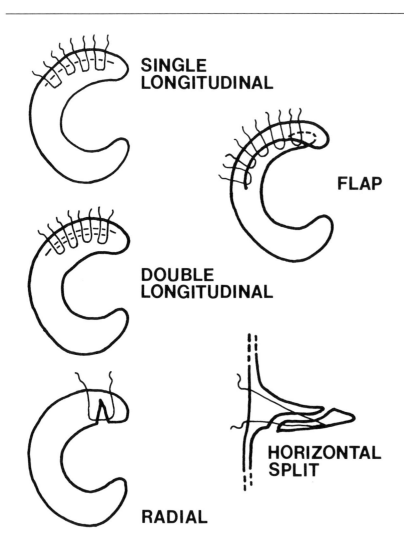

SINGLE LONGITUDINAL

FLAP

DOUBLE LONGITUDINAL

HORIZONTAL SPLIT

RADIAL

Fig. 28-1 Schema shows repair techniques. (Adapted with permission from Scott GA, Jolly BL, Henning CE: Combined posterior incision and arthroscopic intra-articular repair of the meniscus: An examination of factors affecting healing. *J Bone Joint Surg* 1986;68:847–861. Illustrated by Janice LeVine.)

1983, at the suggestion of D. Cannon, MD, we began using a rasp for the parameniscal synovial abrasion. This appeared to improve the healing rates significantly, the overall failure rate decreasing from 22% with the forceps abrasion to 9.5% with the rasp abrasion.[15] Although there was significant improvement in healing, some of the difference in these statistics can be accounted for by the higher percentage of associated ACL reconstructions in the second, rasp group.

Arnoczky and associates[16] reported their experience with the use of the exogenous blood clot to facilitate healing of the meniscus in dogs in 1986. During the last year, we have used the exogenous blood clot and the rasp in combination to stimulate vascularity for healing.

Material

From February 1986 through October 1986, 54 unstable torn menisci were treated with the transarticular arthroscopic suture technique utilizing the posterior

incision. Vascular augmentation was done with the rasp parameniscal synovial abrasion and exogenous blood clot injection. The patients' ages ranged from 15 to 43 years (average, 23 years) (Table 28–1). Ninety-three percent of the tears were associated with an ACL lesion and reconstruction. There were 33 medial and 21 lateral meniscus tears. The numbers of tears less than eight weeks old and more than eight weeks old were approximately equal.

Between November 1983 and February 1986, one primary partial medial meniscectomy was done for a small flap. From February 1986 through October 1986, one primary partial lateral meniscectomy was done for a small flap. The remaining meniscus tears were stable and left alone.

Method

Table 28–2 lists the types of tears in this series. Figure 28–1 shows schematically the repair technique for the tears. The single longitudinal tear is repaired

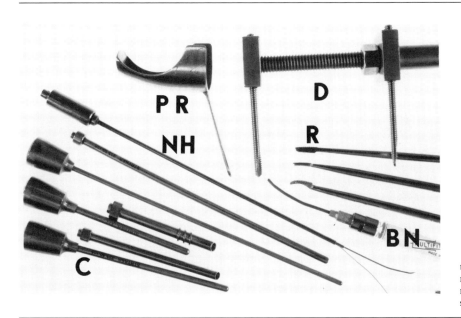

Fig. 28-2 Instruments: PR, popliteal retractor; D, joint distractor; NH, arthroscopic needle holder; R, arthroscopic rasp; BN, blunt needle attached to 2-ml syringe; C, cannula system. Sutures are not shown.

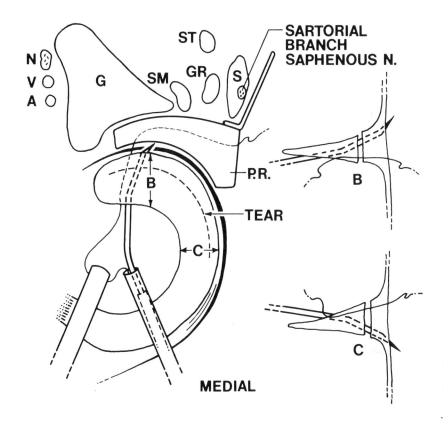

Fig. 28-3 Medial meniscus repair. (Reproduced with permission from Scott GA, Jolly BL, Henning CE: Combined posterior incision and arthroscopic intra-articular repair of the meniscus: An examination of factors affecting healing. *J Bone Joint Surg* 1986;68:847–861. Illustrated by Janice LeVine.)

by placing sutures on the inferior surface at 4-mm intervals. Between these intervals, sutures are placed on the superior surface of the meniscus, thus alternating top and bottom sutures. When a double longitudinal tear is repaired, the needle enters the meniscus closer to the free margin so that both tears will be compressed. A radial split is repaired by placing one end of the double-armed suture on each side of the tear. When the suture is pulled taut, the split is compressed. A long flap is treated like a single longitudinal tear except that the tip is recessed, pulling the thinner tip to the inferior surface of the remaining meniscus material. This avoids stress concentrations right at the tip of the tear. When a tear has a hori-

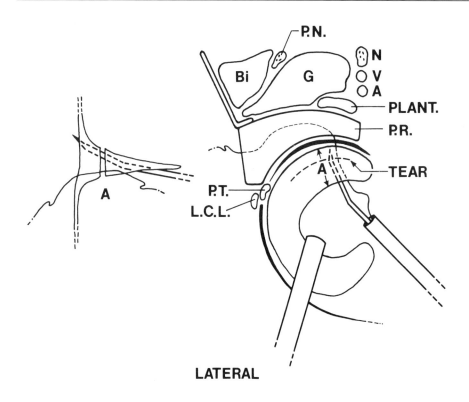

LATERAL

Fig. 28–4 Lateral meniscus repair. (Reproduced with permission from Scott GA, Jolly BL, Henning CE: Combined posterior incision and arthroscopic intra-articular repair of the meniscus: An examination of factors affecting healing. *J Bone Joint Surg* 1986;68:847–861. Illustrated by Janice LeVine.)

zontal component, we expect to get bonding in the more peripheral element. This provides a load path for the mobile fragment to the perimeter of the rim. The horizontal element is compressed by the femoral condyle and becomes asymptomatic.

Figure 28–2 shows the instruments used. One of the most important is the popliteal retractor. It is used throughout the parameniscal synovial abrasion and suturing procedures. The other instruments include the distractor, rasps, and arthroscopic needle holder. A 2-ml syringe and blunt needle are used to inject the blood clot.

Posterior Incisions

The posterior approach begins with a 4-cm incision posteromedially or posterolaterally. Medially, the sartorius along with the sartorial branch of the saphenous nerve, all the medial hamstrings, and the medial half of the medial head of the gastrocnemius are retracted posteriorly (Fig. 28–3). The most difficult portion of the medial dissection involves the very tight insertion of the semimembranous to the posterior capsule and the slip to the oblique popliteal ligament.

When a lateral meniscus repair is associated with an ACL reconstruction, the lateral utility incision exposes the posterolateral corner. In an isolated lateral meniscus repair a 4-cm incision is made over the fibular collateral ligament. Lateral exposure is achieved by spreading between the anterior and middle thirds of the biceps (Fig. 28–4). The peroneal nerve passes along the medial side of the biceps and is not protected by retraction of the biceps. The lateral fascial extension of the lateral head of the gastrocnemius is then spread and the blunt dissection directed medially and slightly distally toward the large space between the lateral head of the gastrocnemius and the articulate complex at the level of the joint line. It is the lateral head of the gastrocnemius that protects the peroneal nerve. The popliteal retractor is placed in the posterior incision. The posterior incisions are made before inflation of the tourniquet.

The foot is prepared and covered only with a sterile drape to allow intraoperative monitoring of peripheral pulses and foot temperature. A specimen should be used to help the surgeon visualize the relationship of the popliteal neurovascular structures.

Portals

The arthroscope is in the anterolateral portal. The anteromedial cannula is used for suturing the posterior third of the medial meniscus. The middle third of the medial meniscus is sutured through an anterolateral cannula, parallel to the arthroscope. The lateral meniscus is sutured through the long anteromedial cannula. This cannula is intentionally long enough to restrict the travel of the arthroscopic needle holder, thus minimizing risk to the popliteal neurovascular structures if the needle misses the popliteal retractor.

The tear is probed to determine the starting point, the stopping point, and the rim width of the tear. In

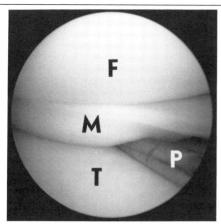

Fig. 28–5   Probing the meniscus while applying a strong high-load anteromedial rotary instability test in the ACL-deficient knee. F, femur; M, meniscus; T, tibia; P, probe.

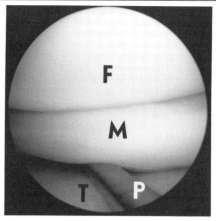

Fig. 28–6   Probing the meniscus in the ACL-deficient knee without applying the strong anteromedial rotary instability test load. F, femur; M, meniscus; T, tibia; P, probe.

the ACL-deficient knee, the combination of the probe plus a strongly applied anteromedial rotary instability test may demonstrate the instability of the medial meniscus tear when probing alone is less effective (Figs. 28–5 and 28–6).

Joint Distractor

The medial distractor is applied by inserting the skeletal pins 3 to 4 cm above and below the joint line. The distractor is progressively tightened with the knee at 20 to 30 degrees of flexion, taking advantage of progressive creep of the collateral ligament. The pins are small enough to bend, reducing the risk of harm to the collateral ligament. (The pins can be straightened and reused more than ten times.)

Vascularity for Healing Parameniscal Synovial Abrasion

Parameniscal synovial abrasion is begun by using a posterior portal. It is helpful to place a small K-wire through the capsule inferior to the meniscus. The me-

dial portal is made at the posterior margin of the medial collateral ligament (Fig. 28–7). The posterolateral portal is made just anterior to the fibular collateral ligament to gain entry anterior to the popliteal tendon. The edge-cut rasp is placed through the portal. Frequently the rasp cannot be seen well arthroscopically, especially in a tight knee, so it is important to put a finger in the space of the popliteal retractor and to palpate the progress of the rasp. The surgeon should note that the posterior capsule is much thinner on the posterior rim of the lateral meniscus and care must be taken to avoid perforating the capsule and passing the rasp into the popliteal space. The double convex rasp can then be placed through this posteroinferior portal and rotated to abrade the parameniscal synovium further.

Using a similar technique, a portal is made on the superior surface of the posterior third of the coronary ligament and the superior parameniscal synovium abraded with a single convex rasp (Fig. 28–8).

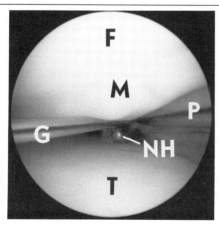

Fig. 28–7   Posteromedial portal for parameniscal synovial abrasion. A guidewire (G) has been placed through the capsule on the inferior surface of the meniscus (M) to guide the entry of a plastic needle holder (NH) that dilates the portal. F, femur; T, tibia; P, probe.

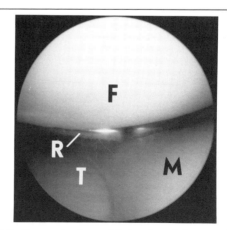

Fig. 28–8   Parameniscal synovial abrasion of the posterior third, superior surface. The single convex rasp (R) has been brought through a posteromedial portal and will be directed posteriorly. The progress of the rasp is monitored by a finger in the space of the popliteal retractor.

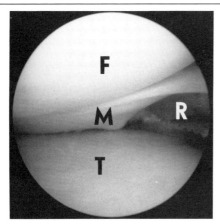

Fig. 28-9 Parameniscal synovial abrasion of the middle third, inferior surface. The edge-cut rasp (R) enters through an anteromedial portal. F, femur; M, meniscus; T, tibia.

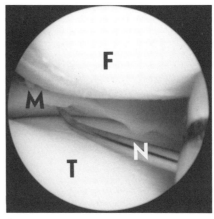

Fig. 28-10 Suturing the posterior third of the medial meniscus. The first tapered needle (N) enters the inferior surface of the meniscus (M) 4 mm from the tear margin. The needle holder is rotated to direct the tip of the needle superiorly to cross near the femoral surface of the tear margin. F, femur; T, tibia.

The inferior and superior parameniscal synovial abrasion of the middle third of the menisci is done with rasps through the anteromedial portal (Fig. 28–9). Parameniscal synovial abrasion should be done 2 to 3 mm anterior to the end of the tear.

The inferior parameniscal synovial abrasion is the most important in stimulating vascularity for meniscal healing. Almost all the visible vascularity proliferates from the inferior parameniscal synovium. It is especially important that no part of the peripheral white rim be removed. This would alter the cross-sectional area of the meniscus and reduce its ability to transmit load. Partial meniscectomy was not combined with any of the repairs.

Many displaced menisci become plastically deformed but recover after reduction and suturing once the distractor is removed and condylar pressure is applied. One must be sure that a displaced bucket-handle tear

is not twisted after reduction, giving the appearance of a degenerative meniscus.

Meniscus Suturing

The suturing technique is shown schematically in Figure 28–3. The tapered needle is placed in the arthroscopic needle holder with a 10-degree bend 4 mm from the tip and a second 10-degree bend 20 mm from the tip. The arthroscope is backed up to give a panoramic view of the knee, including the opening of the cannula. The needle is introduced through the cannula and directed through the inferior surface of the mobile handle fragment 3 to 4 mm from the tear margin (Fig. 28–10). The needle holder is rotated to direct the first needle superiorly to oppose the tear margin at the femoral surface. The greatest difficulty lies in recovering the needle from the most posterior sutures of the medial meniscus. After the needle is directed across the

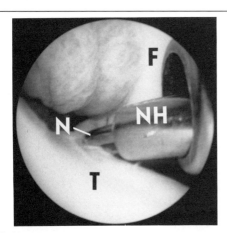

Fig. 28-11 Additional bend in the needle aids in recovery of the posteromedial meniscus sutures. After the tapered needle (N) has crossed the tear margin, the needle holder (NH) is directed toward the medial tibial spine to add an additional bend just as the needle exits its holder. This helps direct the tip of the needle into the space of the popliteal retractor. F, femur; T, tibia.

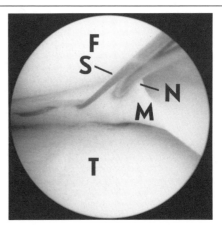

Fig. 28-12 The second tapered needle (N) of the double-armed suture (S) enters the meniscus (M) 4 mm from the tear margin. The needle holder is rotated to direct the tip of the needle inferiorly to cross near the tibial surface of the tear margin. F, femur; T, tibia.

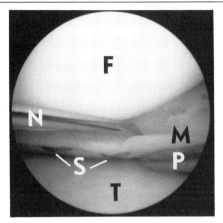
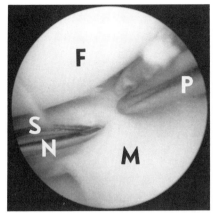

Fig. 28-13 Suturing the middle third of the medial meniscus. **Left:** The first tapered needle (N) is directed into the meniscus (M) 4 mm from the tear margin. The needle holder is rotated to direct the tip of the needle inferiorly to cross the tear margin near the tibial surface. **Right:** The second tapered needle (N) of the double-armed suture (S) enters the meniscus 1 mm from the first suture. The needle holder is rotated to direct the tip of the needle superiorly to cross the tear margin near the femoral surface. The probe (P) can be used to manipulate the meniscus and aid in directing the needle. F, femur; T, tibia.

tear margin and the bends in the needle are directed superiorly and medially, the needle holder is pushed toward the medial tibial spine (Fig. 28–11). This creates an additional bend in the needle just as it leaves the arthroscopic needle holder and better directs the tip of the needle into the space of the popliteal retractor.

The second needle enters the mobile fragment and the needle holder is rotated to direct the needle inferiorly to oppose the tibial margin of the tear (Fig. 28–12). Three to four sutures are placed in the posterior third of the medial meniscus from the anteromedial cannula. The sutures on the superior surface enter the meniscus in the same spot and are separated by rotation of the needle holder (Fig. 28–3).

The middle third of the medial meniscus is sutured from the anterolateral cannula. The first needle is directed superiorly and the second needle, entering right beside the first, is directed inferiorly (Fig. 28–13). All sutures in the lateral meniscus are placed through the long anteromedial cannula. The "outside in" needle and loop system is used for the rare tear that extends into the anterior third.

Blood Clot Preparation

A minimum of 50 ml of blood is obtained for the clot. In an isolated meniscus repair, this must be done by sterile venous puncture. With an associated ACL reconstruction, the blood can usually be collected from bleeding vessels encountered while the 20-mm lateral synovial incision is made or by intentionally dividing a branch of the anterior tibial recurrent or superolateral genicular vessels before inflation of the tourniquet. If the blood is obtained by venous puncture,

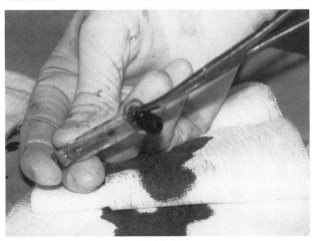

Fig. 28-14 Blood clot preparation. The prepared clot is loaded in a 2-ml glass syringe just before injection.

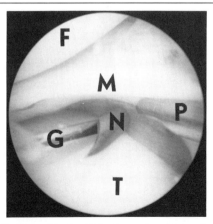

Fig. 28-15 The guidewire (G) has been placed through the capsule on the inferior surface of the meniscus (M), 5 mm anterior to the anterior limit of the tear. This portal is enlarged with a sharp 14-gauge needle (N). F, femur; T, tibia; P, probe.

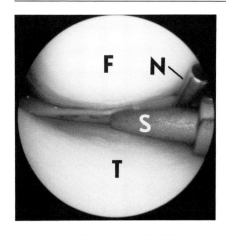 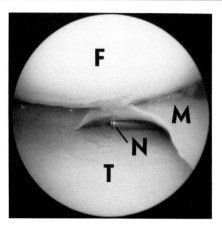

Fig. 28-16 **Left:** The blunt needle (N) has been inserted on the guidewire, the guidewire removed, and the small suction tip (S) used to remove the irrigating solution. **Right:** When the knee is dry, the needle is directed into the meniscus tear and the blood clot injected while the needle is withdrawn slowly. F, femur; M, meniscus; T, tibia.

careful skin preparation and sterile technique must be observed.

The clot is prepared by allowing the blood to clot in a plastic or glass container wetted with Ancef irrigating solution in a water bath at 37 C. A glass stirring rod, glass container, or even glass beads may be required to obtain a firm clot. The clot is placed on a sponge and then washed in an Ancef-containing saline irrigating solution. The sponge is gently wrung out and the clot placed on dry sponges. The clot is compressed between the sponges to remove additional serum. The remaining clot can then be lifted or scraped and loaded into a 2-ml glass syringe (Fig. 28–14). This should be done right before the clot is going to be used because it tends to stick to the plunger in the syringe. The 0.032-inch K-wire is then passed by arthroscopic control through the capsule inferior to the meniscus. From outside in, the hole is enlarged slightly with a sharp 14-gauge needle (Fig. 28–15). The blunt 14-gauge needle has been bent slightly to facilitate passage into the meniscus tear. The needle is introduced via the guidewire and the guidewire is then removed.

The joint is then sucked dry (Fig. 28–16, *left*). The clot must be injected in an air or gas medium. The blunt needle is then passed into the most posterior aspect of the meniscus tear and the clot injected (Fig. 28–16, *right*). For a meniscus tear 20 to 30 mm long, 1.5 to 2 ml of clot is required. The needle is progressively moved through the space of the tear and the clot is progressively injected.

Meniscus and ACL Surgery

When meniscus repair is associated with ACL reconstruction, the blood clot injection is done at the time of meniscus repair. The sutures are kept somewhat compressed with a 5-cm length of small intravenous extension tubing which is placed over each suture pair and held with a clamp. The distractor is required on both the medial and lateral sides, and the distractor is moved to the appropriate side during the procedure. A lateral meniscus repair is done at this time. It is more

difficult to obtain satisfactory clot retention in the more mobile lateral compartment and the clot is not injected at this time. After it has been confirmed that the ligament reconstruction tracks properly from full extension to 105 degrees of flexion, the proximal ACL graft sutures are tied. The medial meniscus sutures are then tied and the clot injected into the lateral meniscus. The lateral meniscus sutures are then tied. This procedure may minimize premature washing out of the clot. Graft tension is obtained with the knee flexed approximately 30 degrees and the distal ACL graft sutures tied to the tibial fixation.

Postoperative Care

The isolated meniscus repair is splinted for three days and then continuous passive motion (CPM) is begun. This begins at 10 to 90 degrees in the first week and progresses to 0 to 110 degrees by four weeks. A repair associated with ACL reconstruction is treated with CPM on the first postoperative day. Range of motion is 10 to 80 degrees for ten minutes, 5 to 90 degrees for ten minutes, and 0 to 100 degrees for ten minutes. The knee is then straightened out on the bed for one hour. This protocol can be used to avoid the incomplete extension associated with ACL reconstruction and resulting from either capsule contracture or filling-in of the surgically formed notch. Ambulation (crutches with toe-touch weightbearing) is continued through the first month. At one month, patients begin 40 to 50 lb of weightbearing; this is increased progressively through weeks 8 to 12. At 12 weeks, full weightbearing with crutches is allowed. The crutches are used less and less during the next two weeks.

Leg lifts with the knee flexed at least 45 degrees and hamstring isometrics are begun on the second postoperative day. Short-arc hamstring curls begin one month postoperatively and 90-degree quadriceps isometrics two weeks postoperatively. Straight leg raises, full knee extensions, and short-arc quads are avoided because of the quadriceps-ACL interaction at less than 60 degrees of knee flexion.

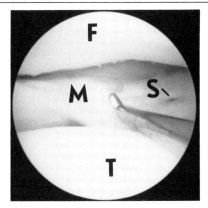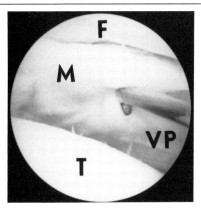

Fig. 28-17 Six-month follow-up of a lateral meniscus repair associated with ACL reconstruction. Initially there was a single longitudinal tear in the posterior third opposite the popliteus hiatus. There was a 2-mm white rim. **Left:** Superior surface of the meniscus (M) is smooth, showing complete healing. The dark spot to the right of the probe is one of the sutures (S). These sutures apparently did not cut into the meniscus or cause long-term problems. **Right:** The inferior surface is also smooth, showing complete healing. The prolific vascular pannus (VP) is seen only as a slightly darker shadow peripheral to the tip of the probe. This area is adjacent to the popliteus hiatus. Vascular pannus was present only on the inferior surface. F, femur; M, meniscus; T, tibia.

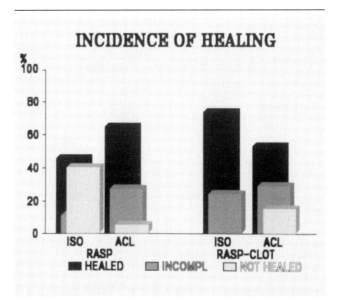

Fig. 28-18 Comparison of rasp treatment and rasp-clot treatment of isolated tears and tears with ACL reconstruction. There were 195 cases in the rasp group and 54 cases in the rasp-clot group.

The patient begins bicycling two months postoperatively. Patients must use toe clips and there must be no resistance on the bike. They should gradually increase to 30 minutes daily. Jogging in place begins at five months, straight-ahead running starts at six months, and figure-8 and carioca drills are initiated at eight to nine months.

Patients must attend two ACL injury-prevention clinics at 11 and 12 months after surgery. If they complete the clinics, the ACL reconstruction is stable, and the menisci are healed, then they can return to competitive sports at one year.

Results

Our method of evaluation has been described by Scott and associates.[14] The subjective evaluation consists of assessment of pain, effusion, catching, locking, and giving way.

A clinically stable bond was obtained in 98% of the group treated with the rasp alone and in 100% of the group treated with the rasp and clot. Medial and lateral meniscus repairs are evaluated by arthrography. If the meniscus had healed over 90% or more of its vertical height it was classed as healed (Fig. 28–17). If the meniscus had healed over 50% to 90% of its vertical height it was classed as incompletely healed. Meniscus tears with healing over less than 50% of the vertical height or with any full-thickness defects were classified as not healed. Figure 28–18 compares the results for rasp alone (November 1983 to February 1986) with those for rasp and clot (February to October 1986). The numbers are too small to draw statistically significant conclusions but there is a trend toward better healing.

Incidence of Healing by Rim Width

It is most meaningful to compare healing in a single classification of tears as a function of rim width. Single longitudinal tears are analyzed in Figures 28–19 through 28–22. Figure 28–19 shows healing of different rim widths in medial meniscus tears associated with ACL reconstruction with rasp parameniscal synovial abrasion alone (*left*) and with the addition of the exogenous blood clot (*right*). There was no significant difference between these groups until the rim width reached 4 mm.

Figure 28–20 demonstrates healing in isolated medial meniscus repairs with a rasp parameniscal synovial

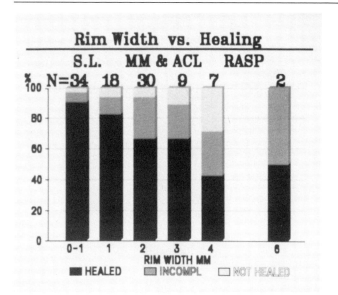

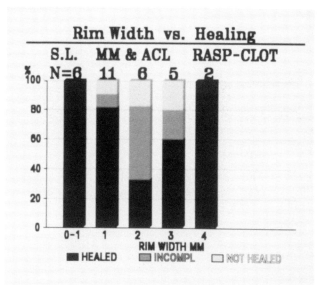

Fig. 28–19 Effect of rim width on healing of single longitudinal medial meniscus tears and tears associated with ACL reconstruction. **Left:** In tears treated with rasp alone, healing rate begins to decline when rim width reaches 3 mm. **Right:** In tears treated with rasp and clot, healing also begins to decline at 3 mm but both cases in which the rim width was 4 mm healed.

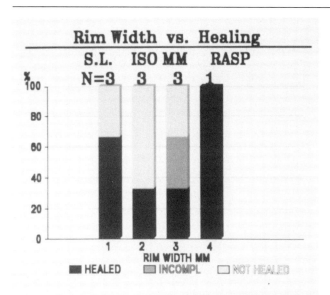

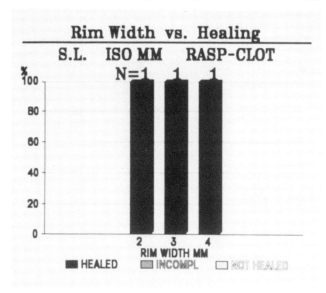

Fig. 28–20 Effect of rim width on healing of isolated longitudinal (medial meniscus) tears. **Left:** In tears treated with rasp alone, six of ten cases healed (40% failure rate). **Right:** In tears treated with rasp and clot, all three cases healed.

abrasion alone (*left*) and with the addition of the exogenous blood clot (*right*). Although the numbers were small in the rasp-clot group, there appeared to be a significant difference in healing rates with all rim widths.

Figure 28–21 shows the healing rate for single longitudinal lateral meniscus tears associated with ACL reconstruction with rasp parameniscal synovial abrasion alone (*left*) and with the addition of the exogenous blood clot (*right*). There was a significant improvement in healing rates in rims measuring 2 mm or more. When these cases were evaluated with follow-up arthroscopy,

there was significantly greater vascular pannus on the inferior surface of the meniscus from the parameniscal synovium in the rasp-clot group, particularly in the area opposite the popliteus hiatus.

Figure 28–22 shows healing of different rim widths in isolated single longitudinal lateral meniscus tears with rasp parameniscal synovial abrasion alone (*left*) and with the addition of the exogenous blood clot (*right*). Since only one tear was available in the rasp-clot group, the only observation was a trend towards better vascularity opposite the popliteus hiatus.

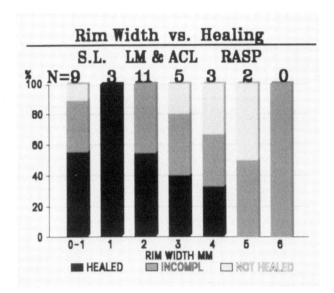 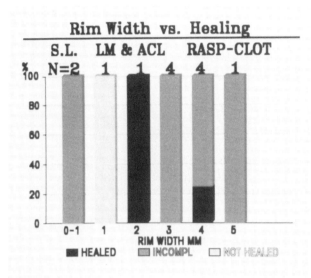

Fig. 28–21   Effect of rim width on healing of single longitudinal lateral meniscus tears and tears associated with ACL reconstruction. **Left:** In tears treated with rasp alone, there is a gradual trend toward decreased healing rates when rim widths are greater than 2 mm. **Right:** In tears treated with rasp and clot, there was no significant change in healing rate. All cases healed.

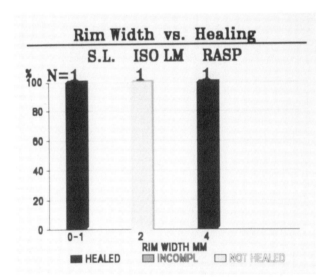 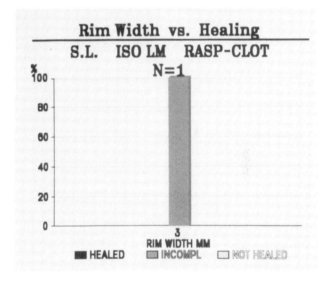

Fig. 28–22   Effect of rim width on healing of isolated single longitudinal lateral meniscus tears. **Left:** In tears treated with rasp alone, one of three cases failed to heal. This tear had a 2-mm rim. **Right:** The only tear treated with rasp and clot healed. It had a 3-mm rim.

Tear Length and Healing

Figure 28–23 demonstrates a gradual decrease in healing rates with tears of more than 30 mm, probably because the longer tears were associated with chronicity. Length alone was apparently less significant. The surgeon must be aware that approximately 2 ml of blood clot is needed for adequate injection of longer tears.

Tear Class and Healing

Figure 28–24 demonstrates healing as a function of classification in tears eight weeks or less old treated

with rasp parameniscal synovial abrasion alone (*left*) and with the addition of the exogenous blood clot (*right*). There was a significant improvement in healing rate in these early tears.

Figure 28–25 shows healing rate as a function of classification in tears of more than eight weeks' duration treated with rasp parameniscal synovial abrasion alone (*left*) and with the addition of the exogenous blood clot (*right*). The healing rates were similar. A possible explanation is the difficulty of retaining clots in more chronic and ill-fitting tears in which the seam of the tear often does not coapt uniformly and smoothly. Us-

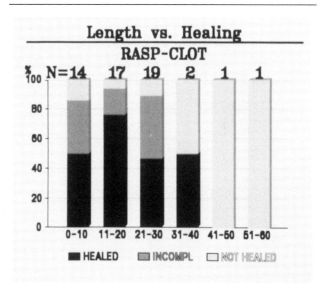

Fig. 28-23 Effect of tear length on healing. Healing rate gradually decreases in tears longer than 30 mm. This probably resulted from the tears' chronicity rather than their length.

ing a paratenon sheath over a large radial split has been successful in one of our cases. It is our impression that developing better ways of obtaining clot retention in the area of the tear will provide the answer. We are now reinjecting additional blood clot material in lateral meniscus tears after completion of the ACL reconstruction. This may prevent washing some of the clot out during wound irrigation and motion of the knee while proper tracking is checked with an isometer.

Complications

In the group treated with the rasp alone, there were two retears of medial menisci, both in isolated repairs.

One was treated elsewhere by partial medial meniscectomy, and the second tear was treated by repeat repair (before the blood clot injection series) by the senior author. It failed to heal on arthrogram but was clinically stable at two years. There was one case of numbness over the infrapatellar branch of the saphenous nerve distribution in this group. The most serious complication occurred in August 1983, before the start of either of these series. This was a popliteal artery laceration associated with a combined medial meniscus repair, lateral meniscus repair, and ACL reconstruction. It is the senior author's opinion that the laceration of the artery occurred during preparation of parameniscal synovium of the lateral meniscus with a basket forceps. A posterior incision had been made but the Doane retractor was used only during suture retrieval. Immediately after that complication, the popliteal retractor was designed and this retractor is now used at all times throughout the procedure. As previously noted, it is still possible to pass an instrument past the medial lip of the retractor, so it is important to monitor the posterior rim preparation with a finger in the space of the popliteal retractor.

There is still substantial confusion about which menisci are repairable and which are not. One of the ways to determine indications is to repair all unstable menisci and see which ones work. We have taken essentially this approach. A careful review of healing rates in terms of rim width, tear classification, and time since tear will help the surgeon define the proper indications.

Summary

The transarticular arthroscopic approach with a posterior incision provided a method of repairing more

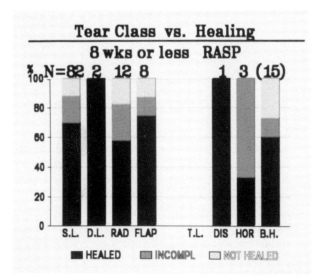

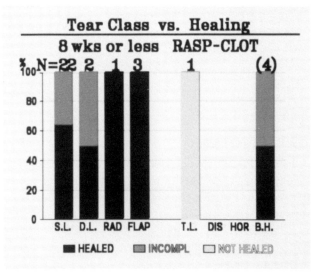

Fig. 28-24 Effect of tear class on healing of tears less than eight weeks old. Comparison of treatment with rasp alone (**left**) and treatment with rasp and clot (**right**) shows a trend toward improved healing in the second group. S.L., single longitudinal tear; D.L., double longitudinal tear; RAD, radial tear; FLAP, flap tear; T.L., triple longitudinal tear; DIS, discoid tear; HOR, horizontal cleavage; B.H., bucket-handle tear.

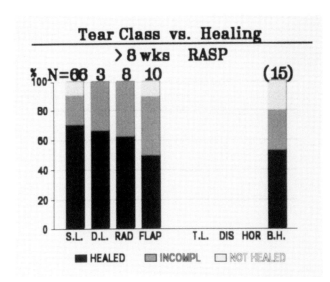
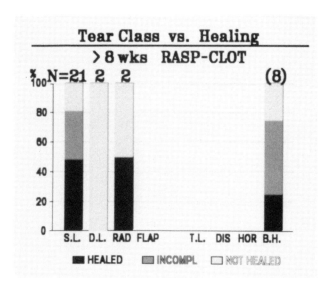

Fig. 28-25 Effect of tear class on healing of tears more than eight weeks old. Comparison of treatment with rasp alone (**left**) and treatment with rasp and clot (**right**) shows no significant difference, perhaps because of the difficulty of clot retention in poorly fitting chronic tears. S.L., single longitudinal tear; D.L., double longitudinal tear; RAD, radial tear; FLAP, flap tear; T.L., triple longitudinal tear; DIS, discoid tear; HOR, horizontal cleavage; B.H., bucket-handle.

than 98% of unstable meniscus tears encountered between November 1983 and November 1986. A clinically stable bond was obtained in most of these tears with a subjective failure rate of 2% or less. There was a trend towards better healing of isolated meniscus repairs and lateral meniscus tears less than eight weeks old associated with ACL reconstruction when a blood clot injection was used to supplement the rasp abrasion of the parameniscal synovium. Healing of rim widths to 5 mm can be obtained with these methods.

Indications for meniscus repair include all lateral meniscus tears and all medial meniscus tears except when repair of a stump would not replace 25% or more of the missing area. In our experience, this includes more than 98% of all unstable meniscus tears.

Contraindications to meniscus repair include short (10 mm or less) stable tears, partial thickness (less than 50% of vertical height), and shallow radial tears (3 mm or less in depth). The posterior incision and popliteal retractor are necessary to protect the popliteal neurovascular structures.

References

1. Dye SF, Via MW, Andersen C: An evolutionary perspective of the knee. *Orthop Trans* 1986;10:70.
2. Walker PS, Erkman MJ: The role of the menisci in force transmission across the knee. *Clin Orthop* 1975;109:184–192.
3. Seedhom BB, Hargreaves DJ: Transmission of the load in the knee joint with special reference to the role of the menisci: Part II. Experimental results, discussion and conclusions. *Eng Med* 1979;8:220–228.
4. Levy IM, Torzilli PA, Warren RF: The effect of medial meniscectomy on anterior-posterior motion of the knee. *J Bone Joint Surg* 1982;64A:883–888.
5. Gudde P, Wagenknecht R: Untersuchungsergebnisse bei 50 Patienten 10–12 Jahre nach der Innenmeniskusoperation bei gleichqeitig vorliegender Ruptue des vordren Kreuzbandes. *Z Orthop* 1973;111:369–372.
6. Johnson RJ, Kettelkamp DB, Clark W, et al: Factors affecting late results after meniscectomy. *J Bone Joint Surg* 1974;56A:719–729.
7. Lynch MA, Henning CE, Glick KR Jr: Knee joint surface changes: Long-term follow-up meniscus tear treatment in stable anterior cruciate ligament reconstructions. *Clin Orthop* 1983;172:148–153.
8. Lipscomb AB, Anderson AF: Tears of the anterior cruciate ligament in adolescents. *J Bone Joint Surg* 1986;68A:19–28.
9. Yocum LA, Kerlan RK, Jobe FW, et al: Isolated lateral meniscectomy: A study of twenty-six patients with isolated tears. *J Bone Joint Surg* 1979;61A:338–342.
10. Annandale T: An operation for displaced semilunar cartilage. *Br Med J* 1885;779.
11. King D: The healing of semilunar cartilages. *J Bone Joint Surg* 1936;18:333–342.
12. DeHaven KE, Hales W: Peripheral meniscus repair in a young athlete. *Orthop Consultant* 1983;4:7–12.
13. Ikeuchi H: Surgery under arthroscopic control, in *Proceedings of the Société Internationale d'Arthroscopie, Copenhagen, Denmark, 1975. Rhumatologie* [Basel] (special issue), 1976, pp 57–62.
14. Scott GA, Jolly BL, Henning CE: Combined posterior incision and arthroscopic intra-articular repair of the meniscus: An examination of factors affecting healing. *J Bone Joint Surg* 1986;68A:847–861.
15. Henning CE, Lynch MA, Clark JR: Vascularity for healing of meniscus repairs. *Arthroscopy* 1987;3:13–18.
16. Arnoczky SP, McDevitt CA, Warren RF, et al: Meniscal repair using an exogenous fibrin clot—An experimental study in the dog. *Orthop Trans* 1986;10:327–328.

Hip Arthroscopy Using the Lateral Approach

James M. Glick, MD

When my colleagues and I first reported on the arthroscopic lateral approach to the hip,[1] we concluded that, with further experience and continued improvement in surgical instrumentation and technique, hip arthroscopy would benefit patients and surgeons. The lateral approach allows the lateral insertion of the arthroscope over the greater trochanter[2,3] (Fig. 29–1). The direct lateral approach is reproducible, provides easy orientation of the hip anatomy, and facilitates instrumentation for surgical procedures.

Technique

Like arthroscopy of the shoulder, the procedure is performed with the patient on his or her side and with the hip abducted (Fig. 29–2). We initially failed to appreciate the importance of distracting the hip. We applied skin traction straps below the knee, holding the leg abducted with attached weights hung from fixed overhead pulleys (Fig. 29–3). We used 25 to 50 lb of traction, depending on the size of the leg. We later learned that some extremely tight hips could not be distracted enough for the instrument to be inserted.

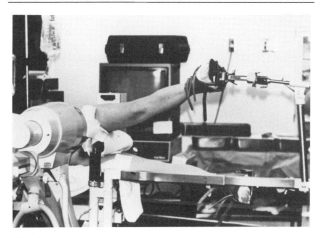

Fig. 29-2 The position of the leg for arthroscopy of the hip on a fracture table. The hip is abducted 30 degrees. The foot is strapped into a footpiece with a crank to apply traction. Note the well-padded crotch post and the position of the image intensifier.

Eriksson and associates[4] reported that adequate visualization of the hip joint in an anesthetized patient required 300 to 500 N of force. After our first report, we began using a fracture table for this operation. The crank on the footpiece of the fracture table is used to apply the traction. We now use a fracture table to provide adequate distraction of the hip joint in all such operations.

The patient, who is under general anesthesia, is placed in the lateral decubitus position with the hip to be treated on top (Fig. 29–2). Place one foot in the foot holder to apply traction. The amount of abduction is not critical. I have abducted the hip as little as 20 degrees and as much as 45 degrees with equal success in entering the hip joint. Most available fracture tables can be modified to position the hip in this manner. The hip should be in the extended position and not flexed because flexion stretches the sciatic nerve and makes anterior insertion of the instrument difficult. Apply traction sufficient to create space to accommodate a 5-mm arthroscope and arthroscopic instruments (Fig. 29–4). Use an image intensifier to verify the amount of hip distraction (Figs. 29–2 and 29–4). The post placed between the legs should be well padded to prevent pressure areas created by the traction (Fig. 29–2). Prepare and drape the hip in a routine sterile manner. Make sure the footpiece can be turned to rotate the femoral head.

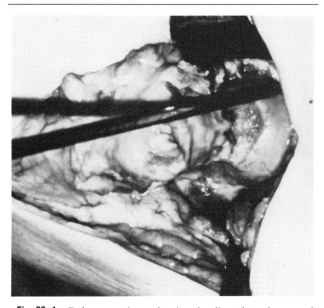

Fig. 29-1 Cadaver specimen showing the direct lateral approach to the hip joint. (Reproduced with permission from Glick JM, Sampson TG, Gordon RB, et al: Hip arthroscopy by the lateral approach. *Arthroscopy* 1987;3:4–12.)

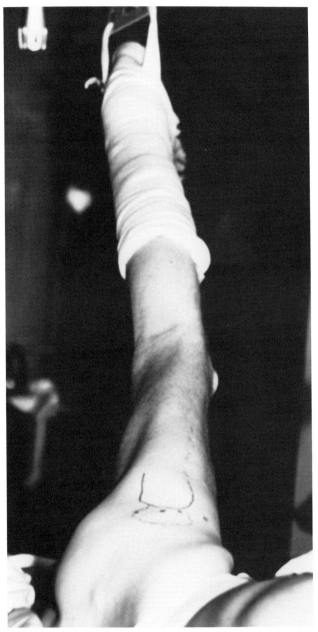

Fig. 29–3 Overhead pulley traction maintaining hip position for arthroscopy. The leg is held in traction by pulleys placed overhead.

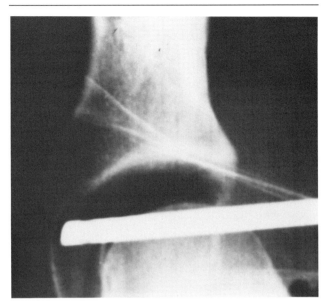

Fig. 29–4 Roentgenogram of a distracted hip with a 5-mm arthroscope in the joint taken from an image intensifier.

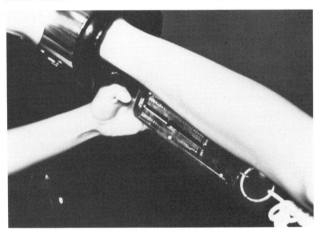

Fig. 29–5 A spring-loaded scale attached between the footpiece and the crotch post to measure the amount of pull for distracting the hip.

Attach a 100-lb spring scale to measure the poundage necessary to distract the hip (Fig. 29–5). Connect the hook end to the footpiece and the other end to the crotch post. About 25 to 30 lb of traction is adequate to distract a loose, abnormal hip but 50 to 65 lb of traction is needed to distract a tight, normal hip.

Make two portals directly over the greater trochanter and a third portal anteriorly (Fig. 29–6). An anterior portal is necessary to visualize the anterior corners of the hip joint. At the anterior point over the superior edge of the greater trochanter, insert a 6-inch 18-gauge spinal needle and maneuver it into the

hip joint, using the image intensifier if necessary. Distend the joint with 30 to 50 ml of irrigating solution. The reverse flow of the fluid signals entrance into the joint. Next, make a stab incision at the needle site and direct the arthroscope sheath in the same direction as the needle into the hip joint. Special extra-long cannulas and sheaths (5¼ inches) have been developed to facilitate insertion and to maintain the instrument's position (Fig. 29–7). The trocar must be sharp to pass smoothly through the abundant tissues about the hip joint. After the capsule has been penetrated, replace the sharp trocar with a blunt one and direct the sheath as far into the joint as possible. An arthroscope of regular length is used. However, the connector por-

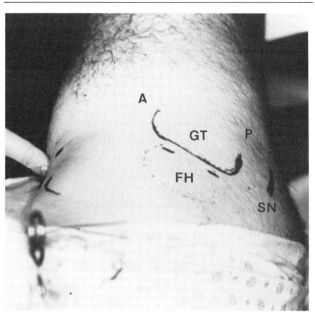

Fig. 29–6   The direct lateral approach. The greater trochanter, femoral head, and sciatic nerve are marked on the right thigh. The small marks are the portals of entry. A finger points to the position of the anterior portal. GT, greater trochanter; FH, femoral head; SN, sciatic nerve; A, anterior; P, posterior.

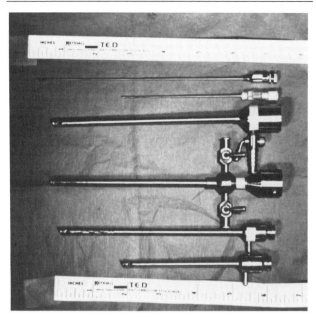

Fig. 29–7   Comparison of extra long instruments used for hip arthroscopy with those of the regular size. (Reproduced with permission from Glick JM, Sampson TG, Gordon RB, et al: Hip arthroscopy by the lateral approach. *Arthroscopy* 1987;3:4–12.)

tion on its sheath (the bridge) should be shortened to provide a relative increase in the length of the arthroscope. This permits deeper penetration into the joint (Fig. 29–8). Keep the joint clear for visualization by instilling irrigating solution through the arthroscope sheath, using either hand pressure via syringe and extension tubing or an irrigation pump. Gravitational inflow does not provide enough pressure to keep the joint distended. Remove the blunt trocar and insert the arthroscope.

Next, insert an inflow-outflow cannula through a direct anterior approach (Fig. 29–9).[5] Introduce the spinal needle at a point where a sagittal line through the anterior superior iliac spine meets a horizonal line from the proximal tip of the greater trochanter. To approach the joint, angle the needle about 45 degrees in the cephalic direction and 20 degrees medially, or triangulate the needle toward the arthroscope. Watch the needle enter the joint either with the arthroscope or on the image intensifier. Make a small stab incision at the needle site and insert a 5¼-inch inflow-outflow cannula. Connect the appropriate tubing to the cannula for inflow or outflow of the irrigating solution. Branches of the lateral femoral cutaneous nerve are close to this portal (Fig. 29–10). The nerve can be avoided by making a shallow incision just through the skin. The sheath and trocar push the nerve to the side as they are directed through the underlying tissues. The femoral vessels and nerves are far medial and safely away from the anterior insertion site. To avoid

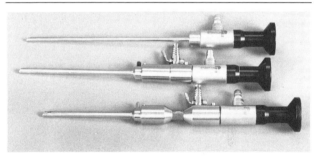

Fig. 29–8   An arthroscope of regular length is shown on top. The shaft of the sheath is elongated by shortening the bridge connector as shown in the middle. The arthroscope can then penetrate deeper into the joint. The regular-length sheath is shown on the bottom.

the femoral artery, palpate and mark it before positioning and draping the patient.

The inflow-outflow cannula and surgical instruments may be interchanged among any of the portals. Removable cannula systems and switching rods make changing portals easier. Extra portals can be made between the initial portals, but instrument crowding may become a problem. A complete view of the hip joint can be achieved by rotating the leg to visualize the femoral head and transferring the arthroscope to each portal.

Anatomy

The lateral approach provides a safe route for the arthroscope. The vital structures are away from the

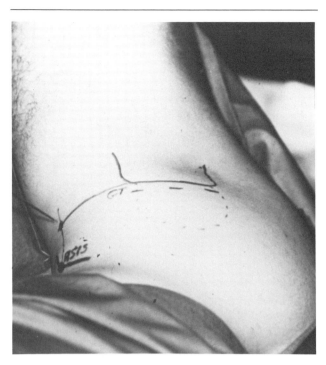

Fig. 29-9 Direct anterior approach. One line is drawn down from the anterior superior iliac spine (ASIS); another line is drawn over from the top of the greater trochanter (GT). The incision is made at the point where the two lines cross. A spinal needle marks the point. (Reproduced with permission from Glick JM, Sampson TG, Gordon RB, et al: Hip arthroscopy by the lateral approach. *Arthroscopy* 1987;3:4–12.)

actual insertion sites and are in jeopardy only if the bony landmarks are not recognized (Fig. 29–10). The palpable bony landmarks are the greater trochanter and the anterior superior iliac spine. The deep bony landmarks are the neck and head of the femur and the acetabulum. These are palpated with the spinal needles and the trocars as the joint is approached. The instruments pass through the gluteus medius and minimus muscles as they are directed into the hip joint. A definite "give" is felt as the capsule is pierced and the instrument is stopped by the bony floor of the acetabulum. If bone is not struck, the joint has not been entered. If bone is struck before the capsule appears to be penetrated, the instrument may be placed too superior, striking the outer wall of the acetabulum, or too inferior, hitting the head of the femur. The vital nearby structures include the sciatic nerve posteriorly and the lateral femoral cutaneous nerve anteriorly. The femoral artery and nerve anteriorly and the superior gluteal nerve are far removed from the portals of entry,[3] but their locations should be kept in mind.

With the surgeon in the posterior position, the video camera is oriented to provide the same image that the surgeon sees through the arthroscope. Thus, on the video screen, the head of the femur is on the same side as the side being operated on (for example, in

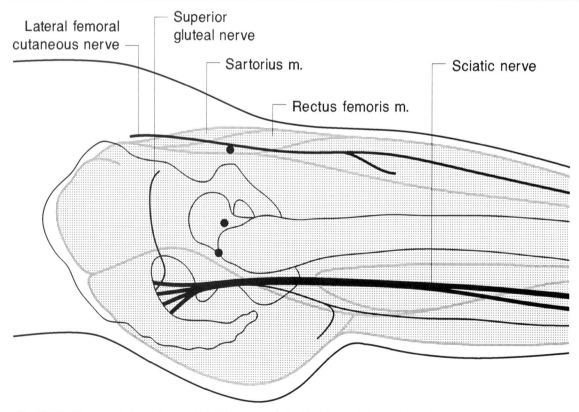

Fig. 29-10 Diagram of the arthroscopic incisions around the hip joint and their relationship to the nerves in the vicinity. The femoral nerve is too medial to depict in this diagram.

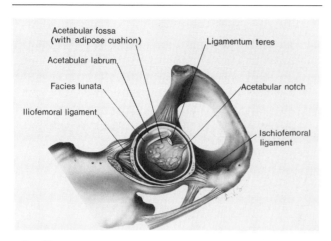

Fig. 29-11 Diagram of a right acetabulum. Note the increased thickness of the anterior hip capsule caused by the iliofemoral ligament. (Reproduced with permission from Glick JM, Sampson TG, Gordon RB, et al: Hip arthroscopy by the lateral approach. *Arthroscopy* 1987;3:4–12.)

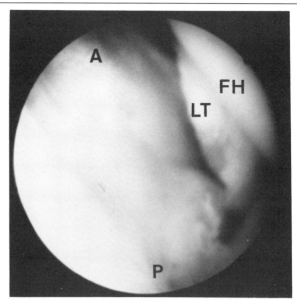

Fig. 29-12 Deep interior of a right hip joint demonstrating the ligamentum teres. FG, femoral head; LT, ligamentum teres; A, anterior; P, posterior. (Reproduced with permission from Glick JM, Sampson TG, Gordon RB, et al: Hip arthroscopy by the lateral approach. *Arthroscopy* 1987;3:4–12.)

the right hip the femoral head is on the right and in the left hip the femoral head is on the left; anterior is up and posterior is down in both right and left hips).

The entire acetabulum can be seen by the direct lateral approach. Figure 29–11 is a diagram of the acetabulum in relation to the arthroscope. Figures 29–12 and 29–13 are arthroscopic views of a normal hip joint. Note the orientation and the position of the ligamentum teres. This structure is best seen with the arthroscope directed to the medial area of the joint.

Clinical Cases

Between February 1985 and August 1987, 29 hips in 28 patients underwent arthroscopy by the lateral approach with a standard 5-mm arthroscope. Sixteen patients were women and 12 were men. They ranged in age from 16 to 70 years. One patient had two arthroscopic debridements, a year apart. Surgical in-

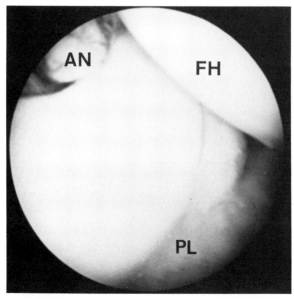

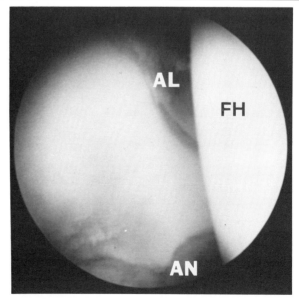

Fig. 29-13 The right hip joint. **Left:** Posterior aspect. FH, femoral head; AN, acetabular notch; PL, posterior labrum. **Right:** Anterior aspect. FH, femoral head; AN, acetabular notch; AL, anterior labrum.

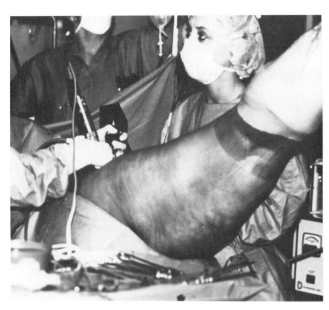
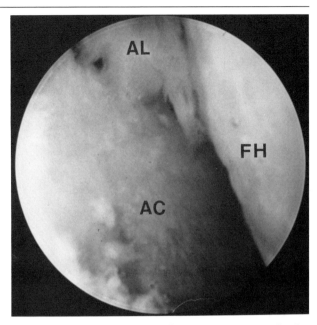

Fig. 29-14 Hip arthroscopy in a 33-year-old, 250-lb woman with severe degeneration of the right hip. **Left:** The leg is in 45 lb of pulley traction. The view is from the posterior side. **Right:** Arthroscopic view. Note the irregular anterior labrum (AL), the denuded acetabulum (AC), and the irregular femoral head (FH). (Reproduced with permission from Glick JM, Sampson TG, Gordon RB, et al: Hip arthroscopy by the lateral approach. *Arthroscopy* 1987;3:4–12.)

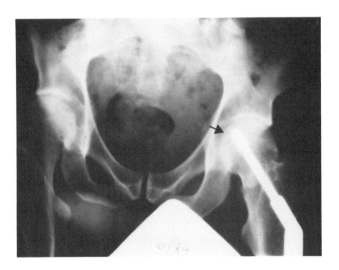
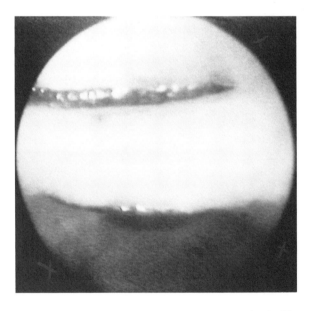

Fig. 29-15 The left hip of a 28-year-old man who had sustained a subcapital fracture in a motorcycle accident one year previously. The fracture was fixated with a nail. **Left:** Roentgenogram shows avascular necrosis (arrow). **Right:** Arthroscopic view. Note the metallic nail protruding through the head of the femur.

dications included unexplained pain (12 cases), osteoarthritic and rheumatoid arthritic pain (ten cases), pain secondary to avascular necrosis (three cases), loose bodies (two cases), and synovectomy and osteochondritis dissecans (one case each).

Visualization of the entire hip joint was achieved in

27 of the 29 hips. In contrast to our failure to obtain full visualization in two of the first 12 hips by means of pulley traction, using the fracture table provided full visualization of the last 17 hips. There was a correlation between hip abnormality and hip laxity. Abnormalities within the hip joint may stretch its capsule

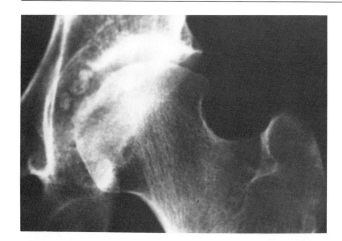

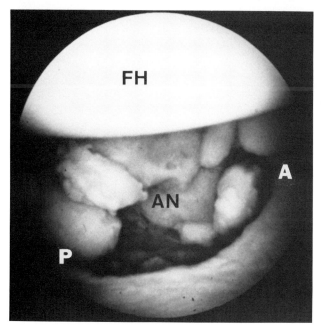

Fig. 29–16 Loose bodies in the left hip of a 40-year-old woman. **Top:** Roentgenogram shows loose bodies. **Bottom left:** Loose bodies in the acetabular notch. FH, femoral head; AN, acetabular notch; A, anterior; P, posterior. **Bottom right:** The loose bodies after removal. Note the broken piece of the grasper below the knife handle. (Bottom left and right reproduced with permission from Glick JM, Sampson TG, Gordon RB, et al: Hip arthroscopy by the lateral approach. *Arthroscopy* 1987;3:4–12.)

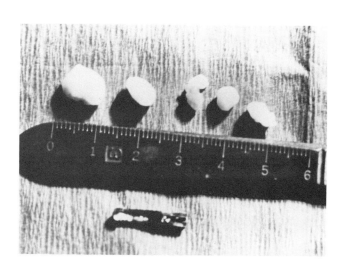

and ligaments. In one such case, that of a 33-year-old, 250-lb woman with severe degeneration of the hip joint, I obtained a complete view of the hip using only pulley traction (Fig. 29–14). I find that it takes 25 to 30 lb of traction to distract the hip 5 mm or more when the hip is known to be lax but at least 50 lb of traction when the hip is known to be tight.

All hips undergoing arthroscopy for arthritis or avascular necrosis were debrided with motorized shavers, abraders, or both. Four were improved temporarily after the procedure and nine showed no improvement. Seven of the patients subsequently underwent arthroplasty. As expected, the patients who improved were those with only moderate degenerative changes. Those with severe degenerative changes and two of the three with avascular necrosis experienced no improvement. One of the patients was a 28-year-old man with avascular necrosis who temporarily im-

proved following arthroscopy. He previously had a subcapital fracture fixated with a compression hip screw and side plate (Fig. 29–15, *left*). Arthroscopically, the femoral head was extensively destroyed and the screw was protruding (Fig. 29–15, *right*). The femoral head was debrided arthroscopically and the screw removed. Apparently, removal of the screw accounted for the temporary relief. One year later this patient again underwent arthroscopy after his symptoms recurred. The head of the femur was completely devoid of articular cartilage and hip arthroplasty was eventually performed. The two patients with avascular necrosis who did poorly had not been operated on before the arthroscopic procedure. Debridement was the only procedure performed. These findings suggest that debridement is not beneficial in the treatment of avascular necrosis of the hip but may provide temporary relief of arthritis.

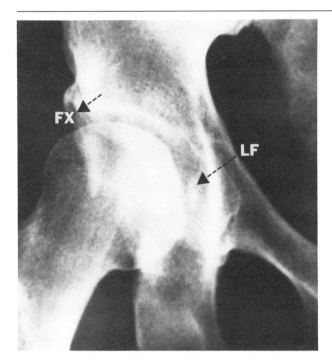 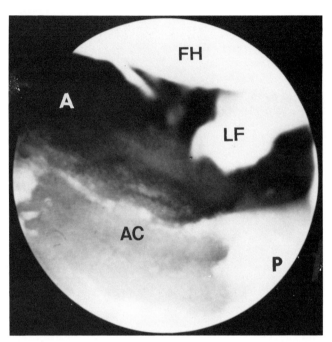

Fig. 29-17 The right hip of a 26-year-old woman after closed reduction of a fracture-dislocation. **Left:** Roentgenogram shows loose fragment (LF) and fracture of the lip of the acetabulum (FX). **Right:** Arthroscopic view. FH, femoral head; AC, acetabulum with articular cartilage damage; A, anterior; P, posterior; LF, portion of loose fragment on edge. (Reproduced with permission from Glick JM, Sampson TG, Gordon RB, et al: Hip arthroscopy by the lateral approach. *Arthroscopy* 1987;3:4–12.)

Arthroscopy of the 12 hips with unresolved pain clarified the diagnosis in three cases. The roentgenographic, computed tomographic, and magnetic resonance imaging findings were all within normal limits. The arthroscopic diagnosis included severe arthritic changes in one, a localized chondral defect on the femoral head of another, and synovial debris in the third. All three patients obtained complete relief after debridement. The relief has continued for the three months to one year of follow-up. Arthroscopy disclosed no abnormalities in the other nine hips with unresolved pain.

The most satisfying results can be expected when loose bodies are the cause of hip pain. The first patient with loose bodies was a 40-year-old woman whose left hip had been injured in an airplane accident (Fig. 29–16, *top*). An attempt was made to retrieve the loose bodies arthroscopically by the anterior approach. A grasper could not be manipulated to reach the loose bodies by this approach. Seven months later, all the loose bodies were located and removed arthroscopically via the lateral approach. During the removal, a piece of one of the graspers broke and this too was retrieved arthroscopically (Fig. 29–16, *bottom left* and *bottom right*). The patient's symptoms were relieved and she has remained asymptomatic for 25 months since the operation.

The other patient was a 26-year-old woman who underwent arthroscopy for removal of loose fragments nine days after a closed reduction of a fracture dislocation of the hip (Fig. 29–17). After 13 months of follow-up, the patient was fully active, including participation in aerobics. This suggests that all dislocated hips that undergo closed reduction should also undergo arthroscopy to wash out debris. Epstein[6,7] described the importance of removing loose fragments and debris from fracture-dislocations of the hip.

Synovectomy was performed on an 18-year-old woman with rheumatoid arthritis. She achieved complete relief of her symptoms after the procedure (Fig. 29–18). The patient with osteochondritis dissecans was a 16-year-old athletic youth who experienced hip pain during his activities (Fig. 29–19). The arthroscopic procedure revealed no intra-articular abnormality. The lesion had not caused observable cartilage damage.

Complications

The complications attributable to this procedure are nerve traction palsies and scuffing of the joint surfaces. The vital neurovascular structures, which include the sciatic nerve and femoral nerve and artery, are a good distance from the portals. As long as the anatomic landmarks are observed, the vital structures can be avoided. A sharp trocar is necessary to pierce the tough capsule.

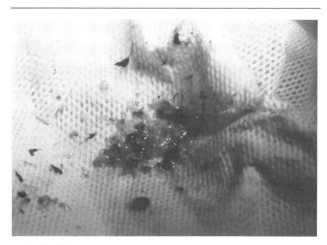

Fig. 29-18 Pieces of inflamed synovium removed with a synovial resector from the hip of an 18-year-old woman with rheumatoid arthritis.

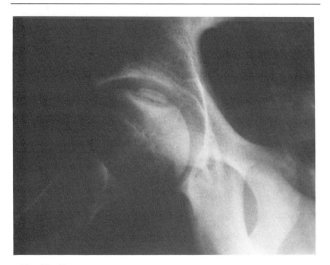

Fig. 29-19 Osteochondritis dissecans in the right hip of a 16-year-old youth.

Care must be taken to keep the sharp trocar from breaking the smooth cartilaginous surfaces.

Three transient neuropraxias occurred. All three procedures were performed on the fracture table and the neuropraxias were thought to be the result of traction. All subsided completely within a few days.

Instrument breakage occurred once. The piece was removed arthroscopically, at the same time of the breakage (Fig. 29-16, *bottom right*). Infections and pressure necrosis of the foot and scrotum were not noted.

Summary

The benefits of hip arthroscopy are apparent. It produces little postoperative morbidity and can be performed on an outpatient basis. The prompt recovery from the operation is also beneficial, particularly for elderly patients. Distraction of the hip by traction on a fracture table is necessary. Suggested indications for this procedure include synovectomy and synovial biopsy; removal of loose bodies; removal of debris after a closed reduction of a fracture-dislocation; evaluation and treatment of osteochondritis dissecans; evaluation for arthroplasty; and unresolved hip pain.

Whether the lateral approach is useful in the following situations is yet to be explored: (1) Evaluation of pediatric conditions such as Legg-Perthes disease and congenital dislocated hip[8-10]; (2) treatment of localized infection[8]; (3) removal of entrapped methylmethacrylate in total hip replacement[11,12]; and (4) reducing and fixating an acetabular fracture (M. Brennan, oral communication, April 6, 1987).

Arthroscopy of the hip joint by the lateral approach is a valuable addition to the evaluation and treatment of hip disorders.

Acknowledgments

Portions of this chapter were adapted with permission from Glick JM, Sampson TG, Gordon RB, et al: Hip arthroscopy by the lateral approach. *Arthroscopy* 1987;3:4–12.

Gary Deaver, arthroscopic technician at Mt. Zion Hospital, constructed the set-up for hip arthroscopy and Dr. Samuel Gordon helped in manuscript preparation.

References

1. Glick JM, Sampson TG, Gordon RB, et al: Hip arthroscopy by the lateral approach. *Arthroscopy* 1987;3:4–12.
2. Edmonson AS, Crenshaw AH: *Campbell Operative Orthopaedics*, ed 6. St. Louis, CV Mosby Co, 1980, pp 65–69.
3. Foster DE, Hunter JR: The direct lateral approach to the hip for arthroplasty. *Orthopedics* 1987;10:274–280.
4. Eriksson E, Arvidsson I, Arvidsson H: Diagnostic and operative arthroscopy of the hip. *Orthopedics* 1986;9:169–178.
5. Watanabe M: *Arthroscopy of Small Joints*. Tokyo, Igaku-Shoin, 1985, pp 97–103.
6. Epstein HC: Posterior fracture-dislocation of the hip: Comparison of open and closed methods of treatment in certain types. *J Bone Joint Surg* 1961;43A:1079–1098.
7. Epstein HC: Posterior fracture-dislocations of the hip: Long-term follow-up. *J Bone Joint Surg* 1974;56A:1103–1127.
8. Parisien JS: Arthroscopy of the hip: Present status. *Bull Hosp Joint Dis* 1985;45:127–132.
9. Gross RH: Arthroscopy in hip disorders in children. *Orthop Rev* 1977;6:43–49.
10. Hogersson S, Brattstrom H, Mogensen B, et al: Arthroscopy of the hip in juvenile chronic arthritis. *J Pediatr Orthop* 1981;1:273–278.
11. Shifrin LZ, Reis ND: Arthroscopy of a dislocated hip replacement: A case report. *Clin Orthop* 1980;146:213–214.
12. Vakili F, Salvati EA, Warren RF: Entrapped foreign body within the acetabular cup in total hip replacement. *Clin Orthop* 1980;150:159–162.

Injuries to Bone and Muscle

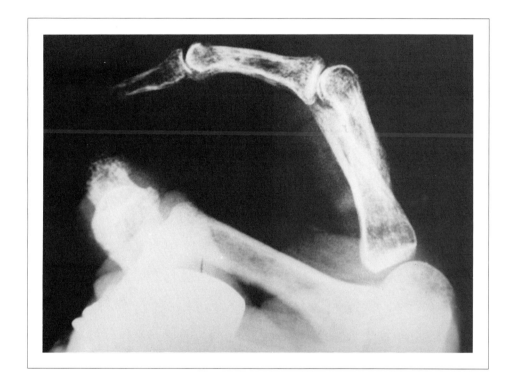

Problem Fractures and Dislocations of the Hand

Norman P. Zemel, MD

Herbert H. Stark, MD

Most fractures of the hand can be treated without surgery, but some are best managed by open reduction and internal fixation. Most of the concepts in our method of evaluating and managing these problem fractures and dislocations of the phalanges and metacarpals are not new; in 1928, Lambotte recommended surgical fixation of certain fractures of the hand, believing this enhanced function by permitting earlier finger motion.[1]

Certain basic principles of treating fractures of the hand are worth emphasizing; if they are followed, the end result usually, but not always, is satisfactory.[2]

(1) Fractures of the hand should be properly reduced and immobilized until they have healed sufficiently not to displace.

(2) Proper reduction includes aligning the fracture and correcting any malrotation. If fractures of the metacarpals and phalanges are not properly aligned and rotated, the fingers deviate or overlap when flexed (Fig. 30–1). Although some dorsal or volar angulation of a finger can be tolerated, if a fracture heals in malrotation, there will be permanent deformity, regardless of the patient's age, and this will compromise finger and hand function.

(3) Displaced intra-articular fractures must be reduced to restore a smooth gliding surface to the joint. If this is not done, the irregular joint surface will abrade the articular cartilage, eventually causing degenerative arthritis and a painful joint.

(4) Most closed fractures of phalanges and metacarpals in adults, if treated conservatively, are sufficiently stable by three weeks to allow protected motion of the joints. Joints completely immobilized for more than three weeks have a tendency to stiffen.

(5) Metacarpophalangeal and interphalangeal joints should be immobilized in semiflexion after the fracture is reduced. The two collateral ligaments stabilize these joints; if these ligaments are splinted in extension, they tend to become bound by scar tissue, and a fixed extension contracture often occurs. This complication can usually be avoided by maintaining the finger in a semiflexed position during the period of immobilization (Fig. 30–2).

(6) Because some of the muscles that move the fingers have tendons that cross the wrist, it is important to immobilize the wrist to maintain reduction of metacarpal and proximal phalangeal fractures. If the wrist is permitted to move, these fractures tend to displace, even when the fingers are splinted. Wrist immobiliza-

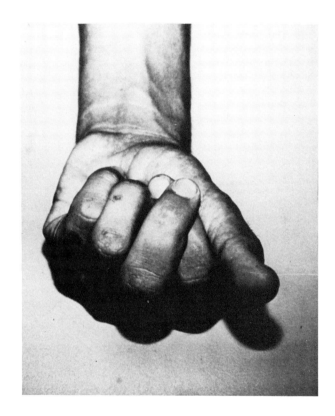

Fig. 30-1 The middle finger is malrotated because of a spiral fracture of the proximal phalanx.

tion is easily accomplished with a short arm cast, and the injured fingers are then immobilized with a wire splint. A sling is fashioned between the two sides of the wire splint with adhesive tape. This sling affords sufficient finger support without forcing the underlying tendons against a fractured bone. This probably lessens the likelihood of the tendons adhering to a damaged bone. The uninjured fingers are unencumbered and free to move.

(7) It is important to obtain posterior-anterior, lateral, and oblique roentgenograms of all injured parts both before and after fracture manipulation and immobilization. Special roentgenographic views may also be necessary for particular injuries.

(8) Many methods of internal fixation of fractures have been reported. Among these are Kirschner wires,

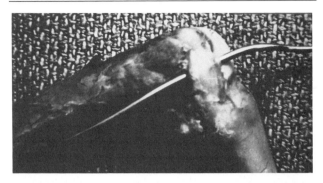

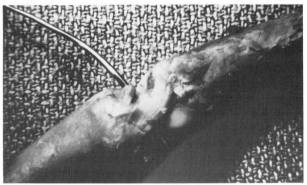

Fig. 30–2 The configuration of the collateral ligament of the metacarpophalangeal joint with the joint flexed (**top**) and with the joint extended (**bottom**).

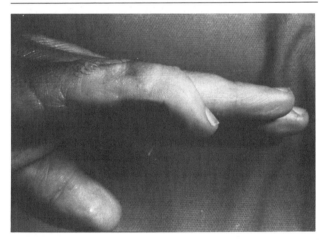

Fig. 30–3 Mallet deformity of a finger can result from rupture of the extensor tendons, an avulsion fracture of the distal phalanx, or a dorsal intra-articular fracture of the distal phalanx.

cerclage wires, screws, plates and screws, tension band wiring, and external fixators.[3] We prefer smooth Kirschner wires inserted with a low-speed power drill. Small fracture fragments can be immobilized with the stylet of an 18- or 20-gauge spinal needle, but 0.028-inch Kirschner wires are now available; these are ordinarily small enough to fix most fracture fragments. We prefer to cut them off beneath the skin. After fracture healing,

they can be easily removed with the patient under local anesthesia.

The best treatment of hand fractures depends on several variables, such as configuration of the fracture, degree of comminution, involvement of the joint surface, whether it is open or closed, the age, occupation, avocation, and handedness of the patient, and the presence of other injuries. Before a particular method of treatment is selected, several of these variables are ordinarily considered.

Certain fractures of the phalanges and metacarpals cannot be adequately reduced by closed methods. These require open reduction and internal fixation to restore maximal function to the digits and hand.

Problem Fractures

Dorsal Intra-Articular Fractures of the Distal Phalanx

Avulsion of the extensor tendon near its insertion or avulsion of the tendon attached to a small bony fragment can produce a mallet deformity of a finger or thumb (Fig. 30–3). This same visible deformity can also occur after an intra-articular fracture of the dorsal lip of a distal phalanx.[4] The extensor tendon, which inserts into the dorsal fragment, and the counterpull of the flexor profundus tendon on the volar aspect of the distal phalanx are responsible for separation of the fracture fragment. This is especially significant when the dorsal fracture fragment involves more than one third of the joint surface, since the dorsal fracture is frequently tilted or rotated, whereas the distal phalanx subluxates in a volar direction. It is usually not possible to obtain an anatomic reduction of this fracture by closed manipulation, and it is almost impossible to maintain an exact reduction by closed splinting. A displacement of the fracture fragment of more than 1 or 2 mm, which disrupts the joint surface, is ordinarily unacceptable. Such a displaced fracture heals with incongruity of the joint surface, eventually making motion limited and painful; with time, the joint becomes arthritic.

This fracture should be treated by open reduction and internal fixation. The dorsum of the joint is exposed by a curved incision, without violating the nail matrix or the extensor tendon. One collateral ligament is divided, permitting a clear view of the joint. If the phalanx is subluxated, it is reduced and immobilized with a transarticular Kirschner wire. The displaced dorsal lip fragment is then replaced into the defect, thereby restoring an almost anatomic joint surface. The fracture is immobilized with two tiny Kirschner wires inserted parallel to the joint. After the collateral ligament is repaired and the skin is closed, the finger is immobilized in a splint with the proximal interphalangeal joint in 30 degrees of flexion. The transarticular Kirschner wire is removed after one month, when guarded

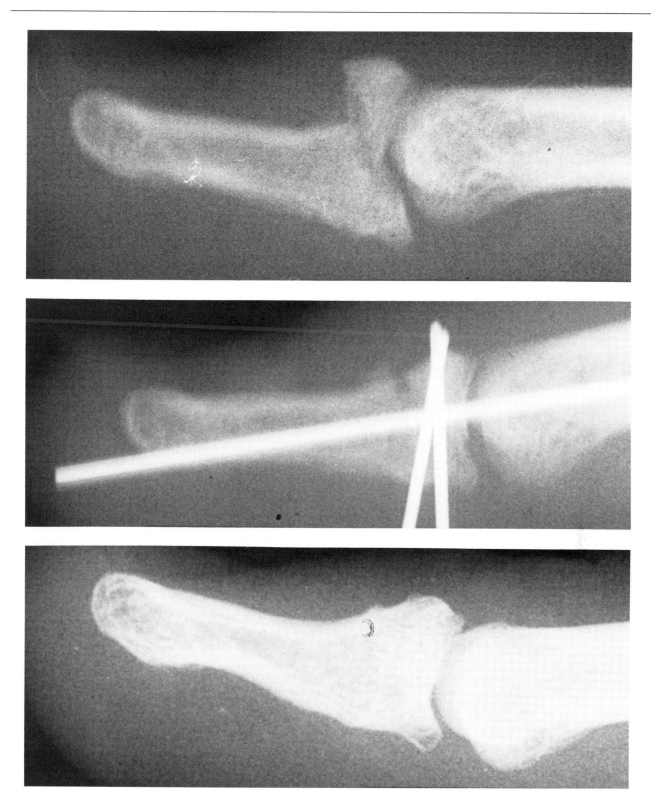

Fig. 30-4 Displaced fracture. **Top:** This fracture occurred during a softball game. **Center:** After open reduction and internal fixation, the joint surface was congruous and the subluxation was reduced. The Kirschner wires (0.028 inch) were inserted parallel to the joint surface. **Bottom:** Six years later, a good joint space was present.

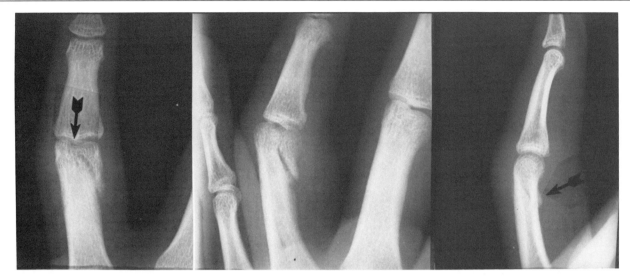

Fig. 30-5 Displaced intercondylar fracture of the proximal interphalangeal joint. The deformity is caused by proximal displacement and tilting of the fracture fragment (arrows).

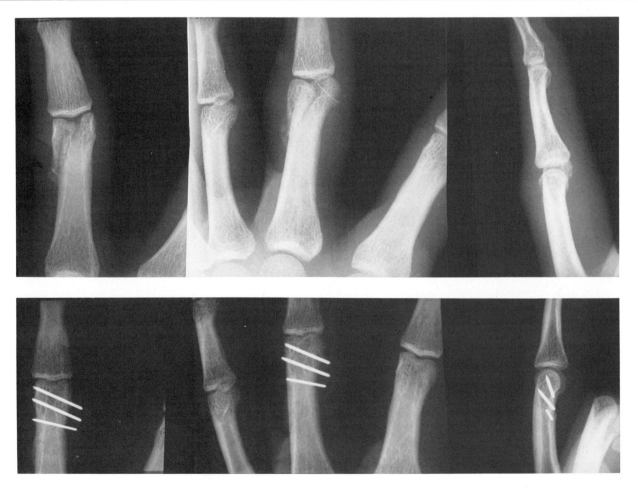

Fig. 30-6 Fracture that was neglected by the patient for three weeks. **Top:** Note early callus (left and central views). **Bottom:** An osteotomy through the fracture site restored the joint surface of the proximal phalanx and corrected the angular deformity of the finger.

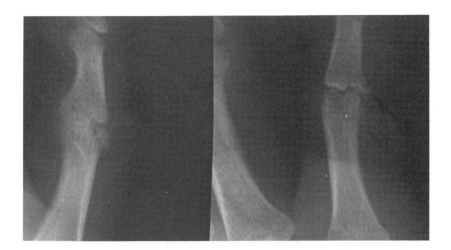

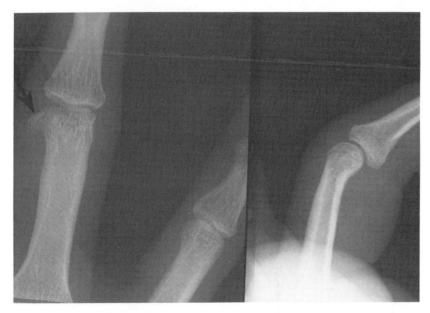

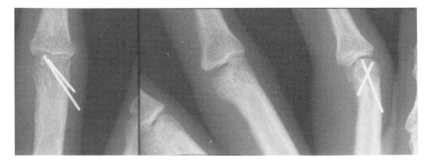

Fig. 30-7 A crush injury to the little finger. **Top:** Intracondylar fracture of the ulnar condyle of the proximal phalanx and an osteochondral fracture of the middle phalanx (arrow). **Center:** There was a small osteochondral fragment from the radial condyle of the proximal phalanx. **Bottom:** The fracture was anatomically reduced and stabilized with Kirschner wires. Because the ends of the Kirschner wires were placed beneath the cartilage surface, finger motion could be started with the pins still in place.

motion of the distal joint can be allowed. When the fracture is healed on roentgenographic examination (usually by eight weeks), the remaining Kirschner wires are removed (Fig. 30–4).

In a study of 36 fractures involving one third or more of the joint surface, followed up for an average of 46 months, 35 joints were either normal or had only minor roentgenographic changes. The average flexion of the distal joint was 71 degrees with an average extension loss of 2 degrees.[5]

If the fracture fragment is very small and the distal phalanx is subluxed in a volar direction, the fracture fragment and the extensor tendon can be reattached to the distal phalanx with a pull-out suture. Before this, the distal phalanx should be reduced and stabilized with a transarticular Kirschner wire.

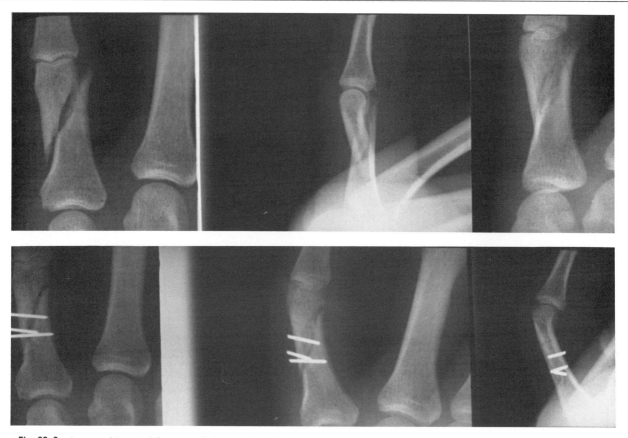

Fig. 30-8 An unstable spiral fracture of the proximal phalanx. **Top:** Shortening, rotation, and angulation of the finger. **Bottom:** Three Kirschner wires were used to fix the fracture. However, the middle pin has started to back out because of poor placement.

Intercondylar and Intracondylar Fractures of the Middle or Proximal Phalanx

A fracture between the condyles (intercondylar and intra-articular) or through a condyle (intracondylar and intra-articular) is a rather common sports injury. Although there may be ecchymosis and swelling, joint motion is often present and the injury may be neglected by the patient, and completely missed if proper roentgenograms are not obtained.

An intercondylar fracture is usually a short oblique fracture that is unstable because of shear forces at the fracture site. The unstable condyle slides proximally, it often rotates, and it may tilt in a dorsal or volar direction. To illustrate this fracture, it is essential to obtain both oblique roentgenographic views of the joint. The offset occurs at the joint surface and, because of this, there may be an angular deformity through the joint (Fig. 30–5). Because the fractured condyle is still attached to the collateral and accessory collateral ligaments, it is usually impossible to reduce the fracture by manipulation. Unless reduction is achieved, the joint surface will be irregular.

Accurate restoration of the joint surface is best done by exposing the joint through a dorsal skin incision. At the distal interphalangeal joint, the extensor tendon can usually be elevated to expose the joint. However, at the proximal interphalangeal joint, it is better to make a longitudinal incision between one lateral band and the central slip. The attachment of the collateral ligament to the fractured condyle is preserved, as this carries the blood supply to the fracture fragment. After anatomic reduction, the fracture is immobilized with two smooth Kirschner wires inserted parallel to the articular surface. It is much better to avoid placing the wires through the articular cartilage, because once the fracture is immobilized, active motion can be allowed as soon as the skin has healed. After the fracture has healed, the Kirschner wires are removed. Some prefer to use small screws or cerclage wires, but we believe the fixation provided by smooth Kirschner wires is adequate in most situations, and they are easier to extract than most other devices. If this fracture is neglected or allowed to heal in a malunited position, better motion can be restored by an osteotomy through the malunion site, providing there is still satisfactory articular cartilage (Fig. 30–6). However, when the joint cartilage has been damaged, a salvage operation (fusion or arthroplasty) is the only viable option to improve the appearance and function of the digit.

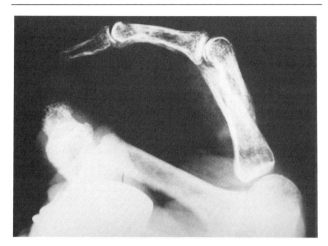

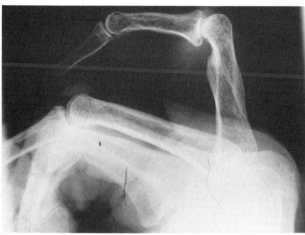

Fig. 30–9 Same fracture shown in Figure 30–8. **Top:** Six months after injury, finger flexion was restricted because of a malunited fracture of the proximal phalanx. **Bottom:** The bone spike in the volar recess was excised, and the joint regained 70 degrees of flexion.

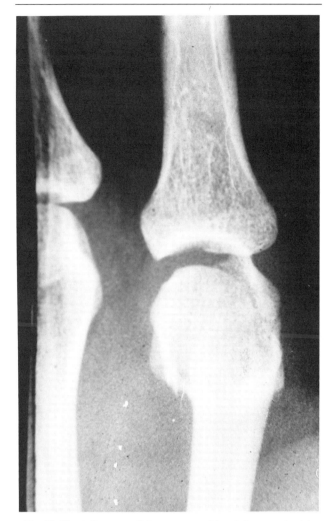

Fig. 30–10 A fracture of the metacarpal head disrupts the joint contour regardless of the degree of displacement.

An intracondylar fracture can result from an impact, hyperextension, or crush injury of the joint (Fig. 30–7, *top*). This produces osteochondral fragments of varying sizes and disrupts the gliding surface of the condyle. If the fragment is small, it is difficult to see on routine roentgenograms. A computed tomographic scan is often helpful. This fracture can be stabilized by small Kirschner wires passed in retrograde fashion through the fragment and buried beneath the cartilage surface of the condyle (Fig. 30–7, *center* and *bottom*). Joint motion can be begun while the Kirschner wires function as an internal splint until the fracture heals.

Spiral or Oblique Fracture of the Middle or Proximal Phalanx

In contradistinction to a stable transverse fracture of a phalanx, an oblique or spiral fracture is always unstable, because it is displaced by the longitudinal pull of the extrinsic and intrinsic muscles. The distal fragment not only slides proximally but also rotates, causing the finger to overlap an adjacent uninjured finger when it is flexed. A rotational deformity does not correct

spontaneously, even in children. In acute fractures, the deformity can be corrected by longitudinal traction, but it is extremely difficult to immobilize such a fracture with a splint or a cast. In the past, various outrigger devices were used for such injuries, but these are awkward, the fracture must undergo frequent roentgenographic evaluation, and the results are all too often unpredictable.[6]

Ordinarily, it is better to obtain an anatomic reduction of this fracture under direct vision. The bone is exposed by an incision that splits the extensor tendon. If possible, the periosteum is incised and elevated along with the extensor tendon to maintain the gliding interface between the tendon and bone. Once the fracture is reduced, two or three smooth Kirschner wires or, as some prefer, bone mini-screws, are used to immobilize the fracture (Fig. 30–8). For proximal phalanx fractures, the wrist as well as the injured finger should be immobilized postoperatively. Because the soft tissues are in immediate proximity to the

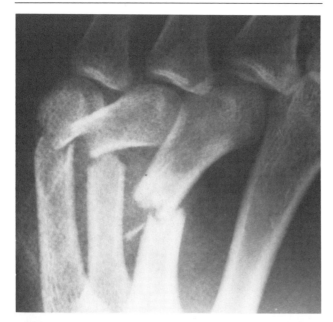

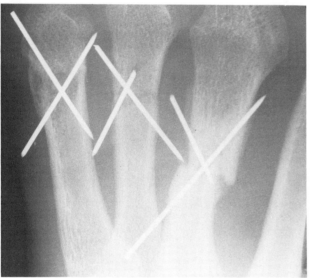

Fig. 30-11   Displaced metacarpal fractures. **Top:** The middle, ring, and little fingers fractured by a crush injury. **Bottom:** The fractures were stabilized with Kirschner wires. Finger motion was started at three weeks.

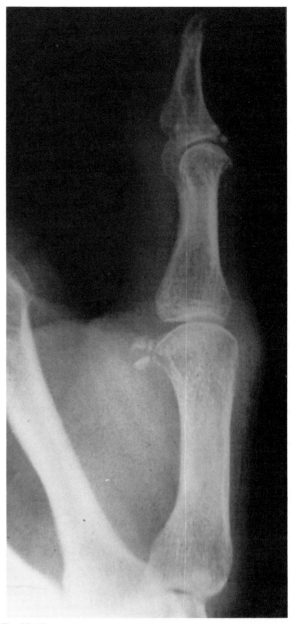

Fig. 30-12   An oblique roentgenogram of the thumb shows a fracture at the sesamoid-metacarpal joint. After immobilization of the thumb for four weeks, the patient was asymptomatic.

fracture, which can involve 50% or more of the bone length, protected finger motion should commence after 14 to 21 days. Adhesions between the tendons and a broken bone are much more common in fractures of the proximal phalanx than in fractures of the middle phalanx.

An oblique fracture through the proximal phalanx sometimes displaces so that a sharp spike of the proximal shaft of bone abuts against the volar recess at the proximal interphalangeal joint. If the fracture heals in this position, there will be a mechanical block on attempted flexion of the middle phalanx. A similar injury

to the middle phalanx limits flexion of the distal interphalangeal joint. When such a malunion occurs, flexion can usually be improved by excising the bony spike and removing the excess bone from the volar recess of the joint, thereby permitting the volar lip of the middle or distal phalanx to glide into the restored volar recess with finger flexion (Fig. 30–9). In children, this deformity sometimes corrects with growth because the deformity is in the plane of motion of the finger. Such spontaneous improvement usually takes two or more years and requires frequent discussions with and reassurance of the child's parents.

Intra-Articular Fracture of the Base of the Proximal Phalanx

Fracture of the proximal articular surface of the proximal phalanx is an unusual injury that occurs most commonly in teenagers who participate in sports. There may be slight spreading of the articular surface but, as long as this does not exceed 1 to 2 mm and the articular surface is not badly depressed, these fractures can be treated by external immobilization of the injured finger and wrist. If the fracture is displaced or malrotated, then open reduction and internal fixation is recommended. Rotation of such a fracture fragment is more common in the proximal phalanx of a thumb than in a finger.

We prefer to approach this fracture through a dorsal incision. The extensor tendon is divided longitudinally. When the joint is flexed, the fracture can be identified easily, reduced anatomically, and immobilized with Kirschner wires without crossing the metacarpophalangeal joint. Motion can be started after three weeks.

A more complicated problem is a comminuted intra-articular fracture of the proximal end of the proximal phalanx. This results from an impact or crush injury of the joint. Posterior-anterior, lateral, and both oblique roentgenographic views are necessary to evaluate the extent of injury accurately. The only hope of achieving a painless, mobile joint is to restore the joint surface by open reduction and internal fixation. The metacarpophalangeal joint, including the entire proximal end of the proximal phalanx, is exposed through a dorsal approach. The multiple fracture fragments must then be restored to their proper place and stabilized with small Kirschner wires. Because fixation of some of the fragments may be precarious, the joint should be immobilized for a full three weeks. Normal joint motion is rarely achieved after such an injury, but reasonable grip and useful motion can be expected for several years. This injury frequently leads to painful degenerative arthritis of the metacarpophalangeal joint, but this can be delayed, if not prevented, by doing everything possible to restore some congruity to the joint by meticulous replacement of the articular fracture fragments.

Fractures of the Metacarpal Head

The head of the metacarpal is entirely covered with articular cartilage, permitting the metacarpophalangeal joint to move in several planes. This large cartilaginous surface overlying the soft cancellous bone makes it especially difficult to treat fractures of the metacarpal head, for even fractures that are not greatly displaced often disrupt the contour and cartilage of a metacarpal head (Fig. 30–10). A Brewerton roentgenographic view of the metacarpal is most useful when such a fracture is suspected.[7-9] In one review of metacarpal head fractures, injuries to the second metacarpal were the most common, followed in decreasing order by injuries to

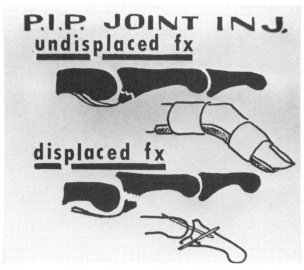

Fig. 30-13 Depending on the force of the injury, either an undisplaced fracture of the volar lip of the middle phalanx or a dorsal fracture-dislocation can occur. The former is treated by immobilization with a gutter splint in semiflexion, whereas the latter usually requires open reduction and internal fixation.

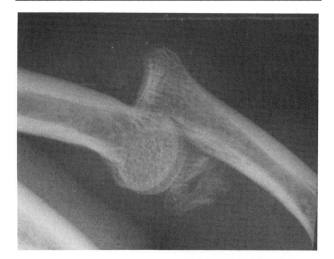

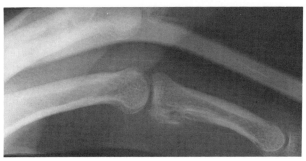

Fig. 30-14 Displaced fracture-dislocation. **Top:** A closed reduction was successful. **Bottom:** A dorsal extension-block splint was used to restrict finger extension while permitting some finger flexion.

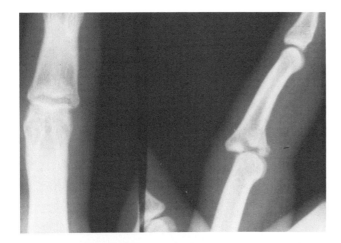

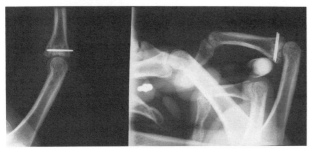

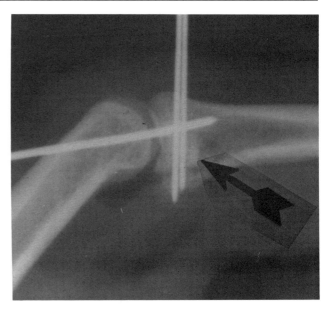

Fig. 30-15   This fracture occurred after an impact-hyperextension injury. **Top left:** The middle phalanx is subluxated dorsally, the central part of the articular surface is depressed, and the volar lip has been fractured. **Top right:** The fracture was reduced and immobilized with Kirschner wires. A bone graft from the radius (arrow) was used to maintain the correct position of the articular surface. **Bottom:** Flexion and extension of the joint eight weeks later.

the fifth, third, fourth, and first metacarpals. They found a variety of fracture types.[7] Proper shape of the head of the metacarpal can usually be restored by open reduction and internal fixation, but often the Kirschner wires have to be passed in retrograde fashion through the articular surface of the metacarpal head. Normal joint motion is seldom obtained, and it is not uncommon for metacarpophalangeal joint motion to remain painful for weeks or even months after such an injury. Sometimes a joint remains significantly painful because of secondary degenerative arthritis; if this occurs, a secondary fusion or arthroplasty may be beneficial.

Metacarpal Shaft Fractures

Single Fractures These fractures are usually transverse, minimally displaced, and stable. Even when there is displacement, most can be manipulated and reduced with the patient under local anesthesia.

Because most are inherently stable, they do well with three or four weeks of plaster immobilization. Occasionally a metacarpal fracture cannot be reduced. A transverse, completely displaced fracture may be caught in an interosseous muscle, or an oblique or spiral fracture may be so unstable that satisfactory reduction cannot be maintained by splinting. Oblique or spiral fractures of the metacarpals can also cause a rotational deformity of a finger. An oblique midshaft fracture of the fifth metacarpal is likely to angulate, and the head of the metacarpal displaces and becomes prominent in

the palm. This displacement can only be discerned on a true lateral roentgenogram, which is difficult to obtain. Prominence of the metacarpal head in the palm limits grip strength because of pain. When "things are just not right," the fracture must be exposed, reduced, and stabilized internally.[10] Finger motion can be started two to three weeks after internal stability has been achieved.

Multiple Fractures Multiple metacarpal fractures are caused by major trauma, and are associated with extensive soft-tissue injury. They may be transverse or oblique; when displaced, they are difficult to reduce by manipulation. A dorsal transverse skin incision provides easy access to the multiple broken bones, lessens the tendency toward extensor tendon adhesions, and minimally interferes with the blood supply of the traumatized skin and soft tissue. Each fracture should be realigned and stabilized, with each finger carefully placed in proper rotation.

Kirschner wires are inserted obliquely across each fracture site without violating joint surfaces (Fig. 30–11). Passing wires through a joint surface, down the medullary canal, and across the fracture site provides poor fixation, does not control rotation, does not allow active finger motion before removal of the wires, and produces additional injury by compromising intact articular cartilage. In such injuries, the internal fixation must not be removed until the fractures are healed, or the fractures will angulate or redisplace.

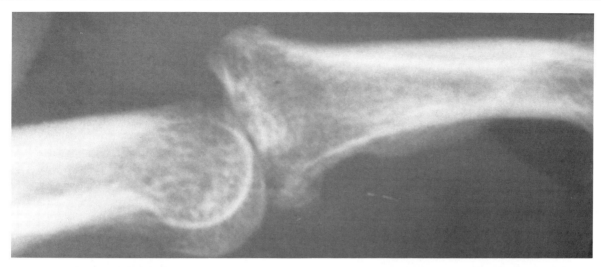

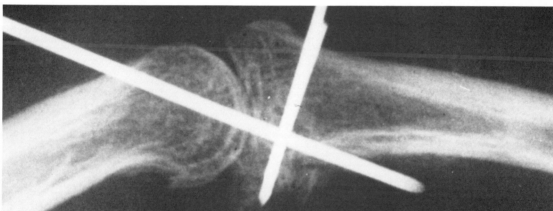

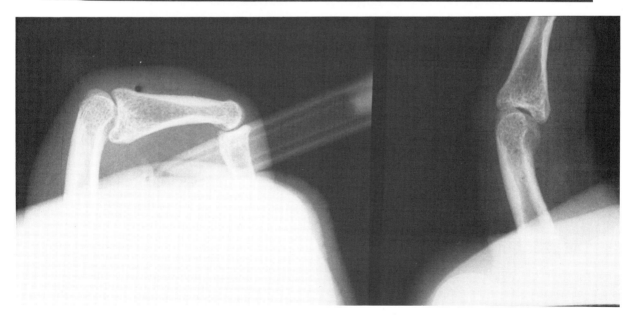

Fig. 30-16   Malunited dorsal subluxation of the proximal interphalangeal joint. **Top:** At six weeks. **Center:** An osteotomy and bone graft were used to restore the volar lip of the middle phalanx. **Bottom:** Four months after surgery, the finger had better motion.

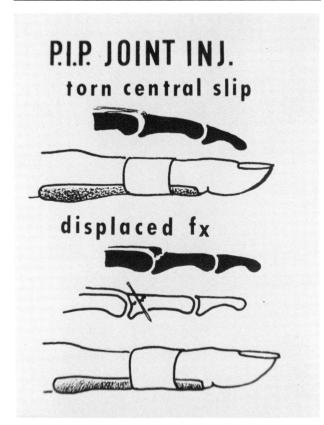

Fig. 30–17   A volar fracture-dislocation of the proximal interphalangeal joint must be splinted in extension.

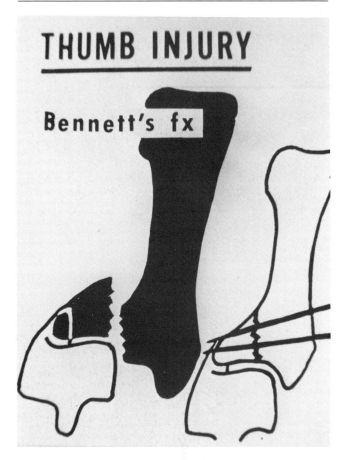

Fig. 30–18   In a Bennett's fracture, the thumb metacarpal is the unstable element, not the small fracture fragment.

Sesamoid Fractures

Pain over the volar aspect of the metacarpophalangeal joint of a thumb, index, or little finger can be caused by fracture of a sesamoid bone, either from direct trauma or from a hyperextension injury. The fracture can involve the articular surface of the sesamoid, which articulates with the metacarpal head. An oblique view of a painful joint usually shows the fracture[11] (Fig. 30–12). Such fractures are usually undisplaced, or minimally displaced, and heal after three or four weeks of cast immobilization.[12] As with any intra-articular fracture, subsequent degenerative arthritis can occur at the sesamoid-metacarpal head joint, necessitating removal of the sesamoid.

Problem Fracture-Dislocations

The three most common fracture-dislocations in the hand are those of the proximal interphalangeal joint of a finger, of the metacarpotrapezial joint of the thumb, and of the fifth metacarpohamate joint.

Fracture-Dislocations of the Proximal Interphalangeal Joint

Dorsal Fracture-Dislocation This is caused by an impact injury of the finger associated with hyperextension of

the proximal interphalangeal joint. As a result, the volar lip of the middle phalanx is fractured, and remains attached to the distal insertion of the volar plate. The central slip of the extensor tendon tends to pull the middle phalanx dorsally and proximally, causing a dorsal subluxation or dislocation of the middle phalanx (Fig. 30–13). Dislocation can occur at the time of injury, but it is more apt to occur several days afterward if the finger is improperly splinted. If a dislocation persists, flexion of the finger is severely compromised and, additionally, flexion of adjacent fingers is often diminished.

A true lateral roentgenogram of the finger is necessary to diagnose this injury.

When the volar lip is fractured and undisplaced, immobilization of the finger with a gutter splint that maintains the proximal interphalangeal joint in 40 degrees of flexion for three weeks assures a satisfactory outcome. When the joint has dislocated, and this is recognized within a few days of the injury, the dislocation can be reduced by manipulating and splinting of the finger with the proximal interphalangeal joint in 30 to 45 degrees of flexion for three weeks. Extension block splinting is an alternative method. Theoretically, it permits earlier joint motion[13] (Fig. 30–14), but there is no evidence that this provides a better result than rigid splinting for three weeks.

If the fractured volar lip compromises 30% to 50% of the articular surface of the middle phalanx and a congruous joint surface cannot be restored by closed reduction, open reduction and internal fixation should be performed.[14,15] The joint is exposed through a mid-lateral incision. The transverse retinacular ligament and collateral ligament are divided and the fracture fragment is identified. The dislocation must first be reduced and immobilized in 45 degrees of flexion with a transarticular Kirschner wire. The fracture fragment can then be replaced in the defect and immobilized with two Kirschner wires placed parallel to the joint surface. Insertion of the Kirschner wires in this manner permits joint motion to be started when the transarticular Kirschner wires are removed three to four weeks after surgery. When the fracture fragment is too small to accept a Kirschner wire, it can be secured with a pull-out suture.

Occasionally, the central third of the articular surface of the middle phalanx is depressed into the subchondral bone. The depressed segment should be elevated to its proper place and a small bone graft from the radius used to hold it in place. The bone graft can be stabilized by a Kirschner wire (Fig. 30–15). The divided collateral ligament and transverse ligaments are repaired before the skin is closed.

If treatment of a fracture-dislocation has been delayed several weeks or months, the dislocation should be reduced and the joint surface improved by an osteotomy through the displaced volar lip fracture. The dislocation is manipulated into a better position and a bone graft is used to hold the tissue in place.[16] Useful and painless joint motion has been restored by this method even several months after injury (Fig. 30–16). This procedure is preferable to fusion or arthroplasty, especially in younger individuals.

Volar Fracture-Dislocation If the dorsal lip of the middle phalanx is fractured, the middle phalanx may dislocate in a volar direction because of the unopposed pull of the flexor digitorum superficialis tendon. The fracture-dislocation is reduced and stabilized through a mid-lateral incision. Postoperatively, the proximal interphalangeal joint should be immobilized in extension for three or four weeks, when gentle flexion exercises can commence (Fig. 30–17).

Bennett's Fracture

Bennett's fracture is an intra-articular fracture-dislocation at the metacarpotrapezial joint. In 1886, Bennett[17] described two clinical cases. This intra-articular fracture occurs at the joint surface of the base of the thumb metacarpal. The small ulnar-volar fracture fragment remains attached to its tethering liga-

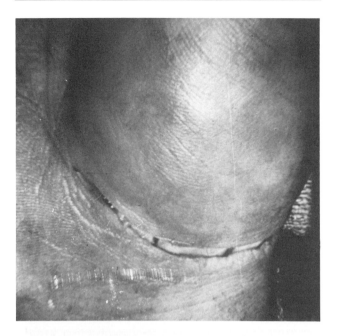
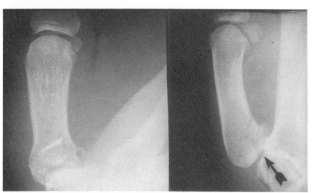
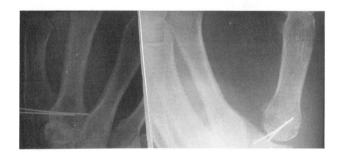

Fig. 30–19 Bennett's fracture. **Top:** A transverse incision gives good exposure of this fracture. **Center:** Bennett's fracture complicated by comminution as seen on a lateral roentgenogram. Offset indicated by arrow. **Bottom:** The joint surface has been restored. Lateral and hyperpronated views show the joint surface very well.

ments, remaining in its normal position. The rest of the thumb metacarpal, which is unstable, slides dorsally and radially because of the unopposed force of the abductor pollicis longus muscle (Fig. 30–18). Because this is an intra-articular fracture-dislocation of a very mobile joint, accurate restoration of the joint surface

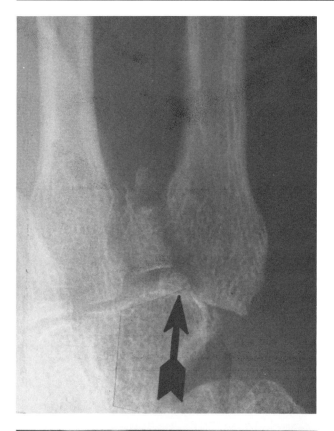

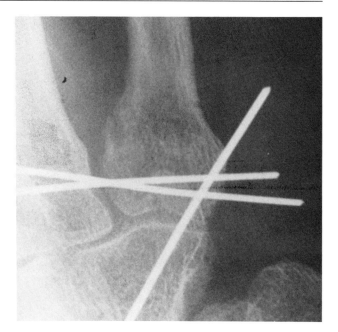

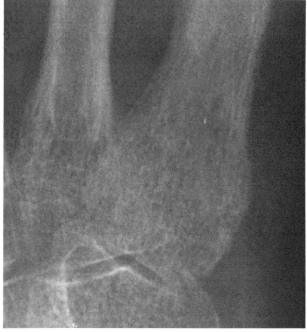

Fig. 30-20 Proximal and lateral displacement of the fifth metacarpal shaft. **Top left:** An articular fracture of the fifth metacarpal bone. **Top right:** After open reduction and internal fixation. **Bottom:** Motion was painless and almost normal after the fracture healed.

provides the best chance for the metacarpotrapezial joint to remain healthy. Although many types of treatment have been described,[18] it is our belief that open reduction and internal fixation is the preferred method.

The metacarpotrapezial joint is exposed through a curved volar and radial incision, as described by Gedda and Moberg.[19] The thenar muscles are elevated from the proximal end of the thumb metacarpal and the metacarpotrapezial joint capsule is divided transversely (Fig. 30–19, *top* and *center*). Reducing the thumb metacarpal onto the trapezium brings the displaced metacarpal to the smaller, undisplaced fracture fragment. After the fracture has been reduced anatomically, it is immobilized with two Kirschner wires placed parallel to the joint surface (Fig. 30–19, *bottom*). We also immobilize the metacarpotrapezial joint with a transarticular Kirschner wire for four weeks, although the thumb should be immobilized with a thumb spica plaster cast for six weeks. Active thumb motion is then permitted, but the Kirschner wires are not removed until the fracture is healed on roentgenographic examination.

A true lateral roentgenogram of the base of the thumb metacarpal[20] and a hyperpronated view of the base of the thumb[21] are extremely useful in diagnosing this fracture-dislocation and in assessing the displacement of the metacarpal on the trapezium.

Fracture-Dislocation of the Base of the Fifth Metacarpal

This injury, somewhat analogous to a Bennett's fracture, occurs when there is a fracture of the radial fourth of the base of the fifth metacarpal bone. The small fracture fragment remains in place, while the remainder of the metacarpal dislocates dorsally and in an ulnar direction because of the pull of the extensor carpi ulnaris muscle. Niechajev[22] believed that this injury is more common than Bennett's fracture, but this has not been our experience. The base of the metacarpal should be reduced and restored to a congruous surface by open reduction and internal fixation (Fig. 30–20). If the joint surface becomes incongruous and deformed, motion will be painful and the patient's grip will be weak. Salvage reconstructive operations are the only remaining choices in this circumstance. Fusion of this joint should be avoided, because fusion restricts grip strength. Resection arthroplasty with an interposition material, however, usually improves function when the joint is painful.

Complications

Even with accurate diagnosis, excellent judgment, meticulous surgical technique, and use of the latest innovative fixation devices, not all fractures heal as we would like them to, and not all joints regain normal painless motion. Certain complications do occur, and the treating surgeon should be prepared to deal with them. These include skin or soft-tissue loss, malunion (angular or rotatory), delayed union, nonunion, joint stiffness, tendon adhesions, tendon rupture, and degenerative arthritis.

References

1. Lambotte A: Contribution to conservative surgery of the injured hand. *Arch Franco-Belges Chir* 1928;31:759–761.
2. Stark HH: Troublesome fractures and dislocations of the hand, in American Academy of Orthopaedic Surgeons *Instructional Course Lectures, XIX.* St. Louis, CV Mosby Co, 1970, pp 130–149.
3. Jones WJ: Biomechanics of small bone fixation. *Clin Orthop* 1987;214:11–18.
4. Stark HH, Boyes JH, Wilson JN: Mallet finger. *J Bone Joint Surg* 1962;44A:1061–1068.
5. Stark HH, Gainor BJ, Ashworth CR, et al: Operative treatment of intra-articular fractures of the dorsal aspect of the distal phalanx of digits. *J Bone Joint Surg* 1987;69A:892–896.
6. Moberg E: The use of traction treatment for fractures of phalanges and metacarpals. *Acta Chir Scand* 1950;99:341–352.
7. McElfresh EC, Dobyns JH: Intra-articular metacarpal head fractures. *J Hand Surg* 1983;8:383–393.
8. Brewerton DA: A tangential radiographic projection for demonstrating involvement of metacarpal heads in rheumatoid arthritis. *Br J Radiol* 1967;40:233.
9. Lane CS: Detecting occult fractures of the metacarpal head: The Brewerton view. *J Hand Surg* 1977;2:131–133.
10. Black D, Mann RJ, Constine R, et al: Comparison of internal fixation techniques in metacarpal fractures. *J Hand Surg* 1985;10A:466–472.
11. Trumble TE, Watson HK: Posttraumatic sesamoid arthritis of the metacarpophalangeal joint of the thumb. *J Hand Surg* 1985;10A:94–100.
12. Hansen CA, Peterson TH: Fracture of the thumb sesamoid bones. *J Hand Surg* 1987;12A:269–270.
13. McElfresh EC, Dobyns JH, O'Brien ET: Management of fracture-dislocation of the proximal interphalangeal joints by extension-block splinting. *J Bone Joint Surg* 1972;54A:1705–1711.
14. Wilson JN, Rowland SA: Fracture-dislocation of the proximal interphalangeal joint of the finger. *J Bone Joint Surg* 1966;48A:493–502.
15. McCue FC, Honner R, Johnson MC Jr, et al: Athletic injuries of the proximal interphalangeal joint requiring surgical treatment. *J Bone Joint Surg* 1970;52A:937–956.
16. Zemel NP, Stark HH, Ashworth CR, et al: Chronic fracture dislocation of the proximal interphalangeal joint—Treatment by osteotomy and bone graft. *J Hand Surg* 1981;6:447–455.
17. Bennett EH: On fracture of the metacarpal bone of the thumb. *Br Med J* 1886;11:12–13.
18. O'Brien ET: Fractures of the metacarpals and phalanges, in Green DP (ed): *Operative Hand Surgery.* New York, Churchill Livingstone, 1982, pp 625–630.
19. Gedda KO, Moberg E: Open reduction and osteosynthesis of the so-called Bennett's fracture in the carpo-metacarpal joint of the thumb. *Acta Orthop Scand* 1953;22:249–257.
20. Billing L, Geeda KO: Roentgen examination of Bennett's fracture. *Acta Radiol* 1952;38:471–476.
21. Lasserre C, Pauzat D, Derennes R: Osteoarthritis of trapezio-metacarpal joint. *J Bone Joint Surg* 1949;31B:534.
22. Niechajev I: Dislocated intra-articular fracture of the base of the fifth metacarpal: A clinical study of 23 patients. *Plast Reconstr Surg* 1985;75:406–410.

Classification of Ankle Fractures: Which System To Use?

Arthur K. Walling, MD

The first etiologic classification of ankle fractures was published by Ashhurst and Bromer[1] in 1922. Lauge-Hansen[2] provided a more detailed "genetic" classification in 1942 based on four major types of injury produced in cadaveric experiments. This classification was later expanded to include ligamentous injuries that can replace fractures in certain stages.[3] Later in that decade Danis[4] introduced a classification system to be applied to surgical treatment. This system has since been modified by Weber[5] and adopted for use by the Arbeitsgemeinschaft für Osteosynthesefragen (AO) group.

Today both the Lauge-Hansen and AO classifications are widely used. Are these classifications synonymous? If not, does one system have a distinct advantage over the other?

The Lauge-Hansen System

Through cadaver experiments Lauge-Hansen was able to produce four major types of injury with characteristic radiographic appearances. These four types were further subdivided into stages based on the dissipation of energy by fracture of the bones and rupture of the ligaments. In this classification the first word refers to the position of the foot at the time of injury and the second to the direction of the injurious force. Supination and pronation describe the position of the foot. Abduction, adduction, eversion, and inversion refer to the force directed against the foot. Eversion describes external or lateral rotation of the foot on the tibia.

Inversion indicates medial or inward rotation on the tibia.

Supination-Adduction

This injury occurs when the foot is fixed in supination and the deforming force adducts the foot on the tibia (Fig. 31–1). There are two stages.

Stage 1 is a transverse fracture of the lateral malleolus at or below the tibial plafond or a rupture of the lateral collateral ligament.

Stage 2 is a vertical fracture of the medial malleolus.

Supination-Eversion

This is a sequential injury occurring when the foot is supinated and the ankle is then subjected to external rotation (Fig. 31–2). There are four stages.

Stage 1 is a rupture of the anterior tibiofibular ligament (occasionally with avulsion of the tubercle of Chaput).

Stage 2 is a spiral oblique (helical) fracture of the fibula beginning at the joint line and running vertically.

Stage 3 is a rupture of the posterior tibiofibular ligament with or without a fracture of the posterior malleolus.

Stage 4 is an avulsion fracture of the medial malleolus or rupture of the deltoid ligament.

Pronation-Abduction

In this injury, a laterally directed force is applied to the foot as it is pronated (Fig. 31–3). There are three stages.

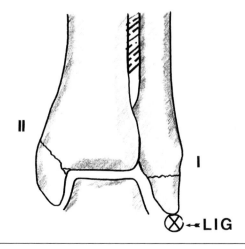
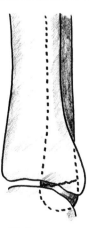

Fig. 31-1 Supination-adduction.

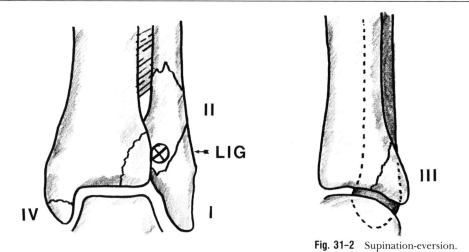

Fig. 31-2 Supination-eversion.

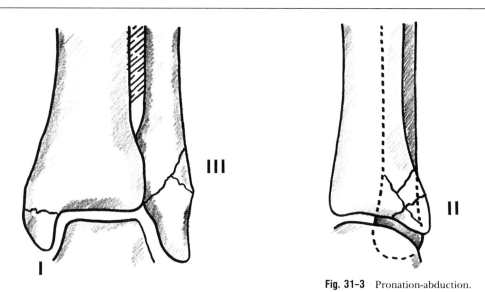

Fig. 31-3 Pronation-abduction.

Stage 1 is an avulsion fracture of the medial malleolus or rupture of the deltoid ligament.

Stage 2 is a rupture of the anterior and posterior tibiofibular ligaments, often with a fracture of the posterior malleolus.

Stage 3 is a short oblique fracture of the fibula beginning at the joint line. There may be lateral comminution.

Pronation-Eversion

This injury occurs when the pronated foot is externally rotated on the tibia (Fig. 31–4). There are four stages.

Stage 1 is an avulsion fracture of the medial malleolus or rupture of the deltoid ligament.

Stage 2 is a rupture of the anterior tibiofibular ligament and interosseous membrane.

Stage 3 is an oblique fracture of the fibula at some

distance proximal to the lateral malleolus (usually 7 to 8 cm).

Stage 4 is a fracture of the posterior malleolus secondary to avulsion by the posterior inferior tibiofibular ligaments.

The practical application of Lauge-Hansen's classification rests on the principle that successful closed reduction is accomplished by reversal of the mechanism of injury. While the Lauge-Hansen system clearly represents a major contribution with its recognition of the role of ligamentous injuries in this scheme, it is complex and not always easily applied to the clinical situation.

Danis-Weber (AO) System

The AO classification is based on the location of the fibular fracture in relation to the syndesmosis and to

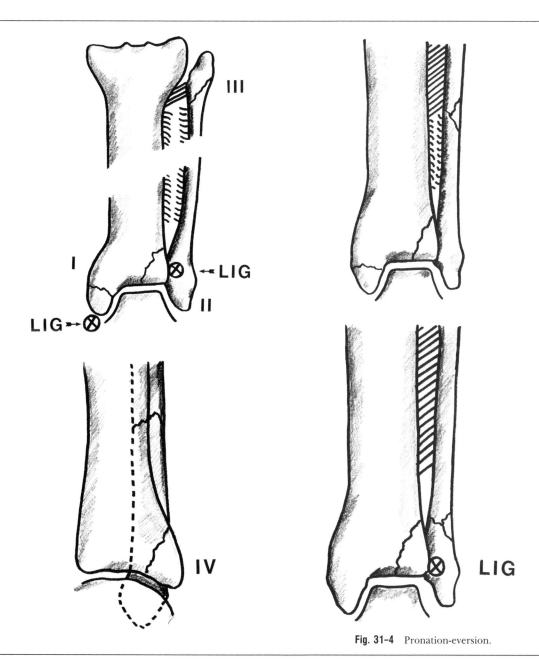

Fig. 31–4 Pronation-eversion.

the horizontal tibiotalar joint. The higher the fibular fracture, the more extensive the damage to the tibiofibular ligaments and the greater the chance of instability of the ankle mortise. This system recognizes three types of fracture.

Type A

Type A fractures are primarily caused by forced supination and result in a fibular fracture below the level of the tibiotalar joint (Fig. 31–5, *left*).

The fibula shows a transverse avulsion fracture at or below the level of the ankle joint or rupture of the lateral collateral ligament.

If the medial malleolus is fractured, the fracture runs in an almost vertical direction.

The posterior edge of the tibia is usually intact.

The tibiofibular ligamentous complex is always intact.

Type B

These fractures occur in the fibula at the level of the syndesmosis and involve a 50% chance of injury to the syndesmosis. The hypothesized mechanism is forced outward rotation of the talus (Fig. 31–5, *center*).

The fibula shows a helical fracture at the level of the syndesmosis.

The medial malleolus is intact or has a horizontal avulsion fracture or rupture of deltoid ligament.

In the tibiofibular ligamentous complex, the interosseous membrane remains intact. The posterior tibiofibular ligament may be disrupted or intact as a result

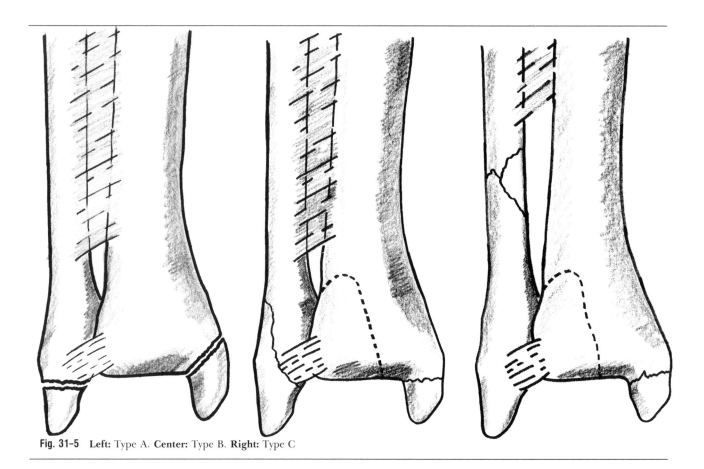

Fig. 31–5 **Left:** Type A. **Center:** Type B. **Right:** Type C

of the avulsion of its attachment to the tibia (Volk-mann's triangle). The anterior syndesmosis remains intact if the spiral fibular fracture begins below the level of the ankle joint. If the fracture begins at the level of the joint, the anterior syndesmosis may be partially or completely torn. The syndesmotic ligament may also be avulsed from either its tibial or fibular attachment.

Type C

Type C injuries are recognized by a fibular fracture above the syndesmotic level with subsequent syndesmosis injury. This is primarily an external rotation injury (Fig. 31–5, *right*).

The fibula may be fractured anywhere from the syndesmosis to the fibular head. Rarely, a proximal tibiofibular joint dislocation results.

The medial malleolus has a horizontal avulsion or a rupture of the deltoid.

At the posterior edge of the tibia, there is an avulsion fracture of the posterior tibiofibular ligament.

The tibiofibular ligamentous complex is always disrupted.

Are the Classification Systems Synonymous?

The classifications are different, but not mutually exclusive. The two systems can be combined, as illustrated by Mast and Teipner.[6] Type A fractures represent Lauge-Hansen's supination-adduction injuries. Type B fractures include both the supination-eversion and pronation-abduction groups. Finally, type C fractures consist primarily of pronation-eversion injuries. Although the two systems seem to overlap nicely, there are those who would point out that this is an oversimplification and that types A, B, and C actually include patterns of other groups depending on the stage of the injury.[7] So, while the two systems do partially overlap, direct translation is not possible in all cases.

Is One System Clearly Superior to the Other?

The main purpose of a classification system is to provide a mental picture of the injury. Both systems certainly provide this. The AO system is the simpler to remember, while the Lauge-Hansen classification provides more information. Neither system can rely on radiographs alone, however, and each must be supplemented by a thorough physical examination to determine ligamentous injury.

A second criterion is that a classification system provide information as to treatment and prognosis. In both systems each group may include fractures that can be treated with either closed or open methods. Therefore, strict recommendations cannot be made on the basis of grouping alone. The Lauge-Hansen system is intended to give information about the mechanism of injury and certainly a knowledge of this makes the principle of reversal of the injury for closed treatment more successful.

With open reduction there is less need to know the mechanism of injury, since treatment is based on open direct reduction of the fracture. In both systems, fractures suitable for open reduction are those in which an unstable injury is susceptible to displacement. However, as long-term studies have attempted to predict the differences in prognosis between closed and open treatment for groups of fractures, a deficiency in the AO classification becomes readily apparent.

Type B fractures include both supination-eversion stage 2 injuries and supination-eversion stage 4 injuries. These two injuries have totally different prognoses. Bauer and associates[8] described 143 patients followed for 29 years after closed reduction (Table 31–1). It should be noted that by the AO classification, 18 patients with type B injuries had radiographic arthrosis of varying degrees. When classified according to Lauge-Hansen principles, only one patient with minimal changes was identified in the stage 2 group whereas 14 with different degrees of arthrosis were found in the stage 4 population.

Therefore, any comparison of treatment methods must distinguish between these supination-eversion injuries to reflect their prognoses accurately. They cannot be evaluated as equivalent groups.

Conclusions

With the increasing use of AO principles in the surgical management of ankle fractures, the Danis-Weber classification system came into wider use. While this system serves well as a simple rule of thumb (the more proximal the fibula fracture, the greater the chance of ligamentous injury and instability), its simplicity makes comparison of treatment alternatives and their results difficult to evaluate.

The Lauge-Hansen system, while more complicated to remember, represents a graded response to injury. This aids not only in the closed treatment of ankle fractures by identifying the direction of the injurious forces so they can be reversed, but also allows better categorization in the analysis of the results of treatment (both open and closed).

Neither system allows classification of ankle fractures by means of the radiographic picture alone. There is no substitute for a careful physical examination that includes manual palpation and testing for stability. For example, an injury to the deltoid ligament changes a

Table 31–1
Ankle fractures: Type and degree of arthrosis at follow-up*

Classification	Degree of Arthrosis					No. of Cases
	0	(*)	*	**	***	
Danis-Weber						
Type A	19	–	1	–	–	20
Type B	85	6	7	3	2	103
Type C	13	3	1	3	–	20
Total	117	9	9	6	2	143
Lauge-Hansen						
Supination-adduction						
Stage 1	10	–	–	–	–	10
Stage 2	4	–	1	–	–	5
Supination-eversion						
Stage 1	1	–	–	–	–	1
Stage 2	48	1	–	–	–	49
Stage 3	10	–	2	–	–	12
Stage 4	24	5	4	3	2	38
Pronation-abduction						
Stage 1	4	–	–	–	–	4
Stage 2	4	1	1	1	–	7
Stage 3	3	–	–	–	–	3
Pronation-eversion						
Stage 1	2	–	–	–	–	2
Stage 2	–	–	–	–	–	0
Stage 3	5	–	1	–	–	6
Stage 4	2	2	–	2	–	6
Total	117	9	9	6	2	143

*Derived from Bauer and associates[8] and Lauge-Hansen.[3]

seemingly innocent supination-eversion stage 2 injury into an unstable stage 4 injury.

Although surgical treatment of ankle fractures has increased, long-term studies have shown only that a better degree of reduction is achieved with open methods.[9,10] As there is a relationship between the degree of reduction and the final result, this has been given as indirect evidence of the superiority of surgical treatment to nonsurgical methods. As yet, clinical trials with direct comparisons have not been able to demonstrate this superiority. This is admittedly a difficult task, and can be achieved only by using the most specific classification system. At present, this continues to be the Lauge-Hansen method.

References

1. Ashhurst APC, Bromer RS: Classification and mechanism of fractures of the leg bones involving the ankle. *Arch Surg* 1922;4:51.

2. Lauge-Hansen N: *Anklebrud: I. Genetisk diagnose og reposition*, thesis. Copenhagen, Munksgaard, 1942.

3. Lauge-Hansen N: "Ligamentous" ankle fractures: Diagnosis and treatment. *Acta Chir Scand* 1949;97:544.

4. Danis R: Les fractures malleolaires, in Danis R (ed): *Theorie et practique de l'ostéosynthèse*. Paris, Masson, 1949, pp 133–165.

5. Weber BG: *Die Verletzungen des oberen sprungelenkes*, ed 2. Bern, Verlag Hans Huber, 1972.

6. Mast JW, Teipner WA: A reproducible approach to the internal fixation of adult ankle fractures: Rationale, technique, and early results. *Orthop Clin North Am* 1980;11:661–679.

7. Lindsjö U: Classification of ankle fractures: The Lauge-Hansen or AO system? *Clin Orthop* 1985;199:12–16.

8. Bauer M, Jonsson K, Nilsson B: Thirty-year follow-up of ankle fractures. *Acta Orthop Scand* 1985;56:103–106.

9. Wilson FC Jr, Skilbred LA: Long-term results in the treatment of displaced bimalleolar fractures. *J Bone Joint Surg* 1966;48A:1065–1078.

10. Bauer M, Bergström B, Hemborg A, et al: Malleolar fractures: Non-operative versus operative treatment: A controlled study. *Clin Orthop* 1985;199:17–27.

Management of Open Fractures in the Multiply Injured Patient

Charles C. Edwards, MD

Introduction

Patients with both open fractures and other major injuries are often difficult to manage. On the one hand, their musculoskeletal injuries are frequently complex and require careful planning. On the other hand, prompt treatment and fixation is needed to maximize survival. This can be a frustrating dilemma for the orthopaedic surgeon unless there is a systematic plan for definitive treatment.

The typical patient with multiple injuries has been thrown from a vehicle, hit by a car, or has fallen from a significant height. The resulting fractures are usually associated with considerable initial displacement, comminution, periosteal stripping, and disruption of soft tissues from the high energy of impact. The resulting compromised soft-tissue envelope and marginal blood supply leave the fracture susceptible to infection and make it slow to heal. Periarticular comminution, tissue loss, and/or other fractures in the extremity frequently complicate orthopaedic management.

There is now substantial evidence to mandate early fracture fixation to permit full mobilization of the patient with multiple injuries. Several investigators have demonstrated better survival rates for such patients with early fracture fixation than for matched populations treated with traction, casts, or other methods that did not permit full mobilization.[1-3] Early fixation appears to reduce fat embolization and improve pulmonary physiology. Stabilization of injured tissues retards the release of substances that trigger fat embolization.[4,5] Early fracture fixation makes it possible for the patient to sit and turn for chest physical therapy. This protects against atelectasis and helps mobilize bronchial secretions. The ability to mobilize the patient early in the course of treatment also facilitates the many transfers needed for diagnostic testing and surgical procedures.

I present a treatment plan for open fractures emphasizing injury patterns frequently seen in patients with multiple injuries. This management plan is based on my published studies of 350 open fractures treated at the University of Maryland Hospital and Trauma Center, as well as recent reports from other similar centers.

Initial Wound Care

At admission, open wounds should be cultured, irrigated, and temporarily dressed and the patient should receive tetanus toxoid and short-term intravenous antibiotics. Cephalosporin, with or without aminoglycoside, is generally recommended. Detailed information on initial wound care and antibiotic selection was presented by Patzakis.[6]

When the patient arrives in the operating room, wound debridement can be performed along with other needed surgical procedures. After hemostasis, thorough debridement, irrigation, and removal of obvious necrotic tissue, a careful assessment of the wound is in order. Are major nerves and arteries intact with sufficient distal flow to support the limb? If not, consider vascular repair or amputation. Is there evidence of soft-tissue crush? If so, consider the possibility of a compartment syndrome.[7,8] The open wound may not provide sufficient decompression for each of the muscle compartments. If an adequate examination was not possible prior to the administration of anesthesia and/or the patient is likely to remain noncommunicative for some time after surgery, measure compartment pressures. What is the extent of injury to the surrounding muscular envelope? Extensive periosteal stripping, muscle loss, and ischemia within remaining muscle suggest a high-energy fracture with a high risk of infection and the need to plan for primary muscle flap coverage.[9]

After irrigation and wound assessment, proceed with the initial debridement. Muscle that does not contract and appears markedly ischemic should be debrided since interstitial edema will render marginal tissues necrotic during the next two to three days. Similarly, necrotic pieces of cortical bone are best removed.[10-12] The extent of debridement should vary inversely with the vascularity of the region. For example, the upper extremity has a dense vascular network that makes it more resistant to infection and delayed union than comparable injuries in the lower extremity. Hence, debridement in the upper extremity can be less aggressive than in the lower extremity. Since the tibia has the least protected blood supply and is, therefore, the most susceptible to infection, debridement here should be the most radical. Thus, questionable muscle or larger pieces of cortical bone that might be initially saved in the upper extremity or even femur are best primarily removed in the tibia.

Fixation of Isolated Open Fractures

Primary rigid fixation of open fractures not only facilitates patient mobilization but also aids the healing process in several ways. Stability appears to improve survival of injured and ischemic tissues.[13-15] It protects against infection by facilitating bacterial phagocytosis.[16-19] Fracture fixation enhances wound access for serial debridements and eliminates potential wound dressing contamination from casts or traction slings. Stable fixation speeds the early stages of callus formation[20] and promotes subsequent calcification by limiting shear forces across the fracture site.[21] Finally, fixation permits early restoration of adjacent joint motion and muscle activity and, thus, provides a more normal vascular and physical environment for the healing fracture.[22] For these reasons, primary rigid fixation is desirable for those severe open fractures classified grade III by Gustilo and Anderson.[23] With current internal and external fixation techniques, it is now possible to effectively stabilize even the most complex fracture patterns.

Forearm Fixation

Grades I or II open fractures[23] in the well-vascularized forearm can usually be treated with primary debridement and plate fixation.[24] Open radial and ulnar fractures are frequently comminuted; thus, Rush or Sage intramedullary nails cannot provide sufficient stability.[25] Forearm fractures with severe soft-tissue injury and/or contamination are best treated with temporary external fixation and delayed plating. Staged fixation approaches will be discussed later.

Humeral Fixation

Early fixation of displaced humeral shaft fractures is generally indicated in the patient with multiple injuries. Effective nonsurgical treatment requires that the patient remain seated with a hanging cast or supine with olecranon pin traction to maintain fracture alignment and stability. Continuous sitting is utterly impractical and continuous supine recumbency can be lethal for such patients. Moreover, open humeral fractures have a high nonunion rate when treated nonsurgically.[26]

Closed intramedullary nailing offers the best results in displaced closed or grades I and II open humeral shaft fractures according to several recent reports.[27,28] In open fractures, flexible nails should be used without reaming to minimize cortical necrosis. A metaphyseal portal of entry can prevent the shoulder and elbow impingement problems formerly associated with humeral nailing. Nails can be inserted just distal to the greater tuberosity or just proximal to the olecranon notch.[28] Several recent studies report no infections when closed flexible nailing was used in low-grade open humeral fractures.[27-29] In contrast, infection often follows plate fixation of open humeral fractures. In recent studies, five of nine platings became infected.[26,30] Thus, plates are best avoided in open humeral fractures.

External fixation is the method of choice for all grade III humeral fractures. External fixation is also indicated for comminuted grade II fractures that may be too unstable for unreamed nailing (Fig. 32–1). Deep infection occurred in only three of 43 severe open humeral and forearm fractures studied by Edwards and associates.[31] Open humeral fractures can be effectively stabilized with three 4-mm half-pins placed in the lateral humerus proximal to the fracture and either posteriorly or laterally distal to the fracture.

Elbow stiffness can be minimized by taking the joint through a full range of motion after trans-triceps pin placement to enlarge the opening in the tendon. Burny and associates[32] reported an average loss of only 9% of the elbow's range of motion after treatment of 100 humeral shaft fractures with trans-triceps external fixation. Triceps tendon impingement can be avoided altogether by placing the distal humeral half-pins into the lateral humeral condyle. With this approach, however, pins must be placed through a small incision under direct vision to avoid the radial nerve.[31]

Foot Fixation

Open injuries about the foot are usually associated with joint and ligamentous disruption. Open reduction with Kirschner wire fixation and posterior splint support will suffice for lesser foot injuries. External fixation is a useful adjunct in cases with bone loss and/or open mid-foot dislocation.[33] The typical foot fixator consists of 3-mm half-pin groupings placed in the distal end of the affected metatarsals or proximal phalanx

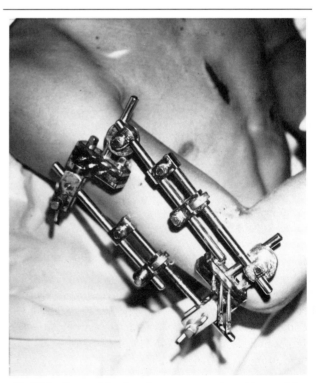

Fig. 32–1 External fixation of open or comminuted humeral fracture.

and a proximal pin group into either the base of the metatarsals or mid-tarsal bones. The half-pin groups can be connected with Hoffmann C-series adjustable rods to maintain foot length and alignment. For particularly unstable injuries, a second unilateral frame can be placed on the lateral aspect of the foot.[34]

Tibial Fixation

Tibial injuries account for about one half of all open fractures encountered in patients with multiple injuries. A windowed cast can be used for grade I or small grade II tibial shaft fractures without compromising patient mobility. Good results using unreamed intramedullary nails for grades I and II open shaft fractures have been reported by several investigators.[35-38] However, with bone loss or major comminution, flexible nails cannot prevent shortening, angulation, or malrotation.

The tibia lacks both a circumferential covering of muscle and a well-collateralized blood supply, thus, open tibial fractures are more susceptible to infection than comparable injuries in other long bones. For this reason, reamed intramedullary nails should not be used in the treatment of open tibial fractures. Reaming further devascularizes the already disrupted intramedullary circulation of bone and leaves a necrotic rim contiguous with the open wound. This exposes the entire length of the tibia to infection. These theoretical objections have been corroborated by several centers that have reported major infections in about 40% of open tibial fractures fixed with reamed nails.[39,40]

Metaphyseal plates can be used to buttress reduction of displaced intra-articular fractures and to fix selected metaphyseal fractures in which no additional periosteal stripping is required for plate application.[13,24] On the other hand, recent reports cite high infection rates when plates are used for grade III tibial shaft fractures.[23,41-43] This may be due, in part, to additional ischemia caused by soft-tissue stripping for plate application, coverage of necrotic and possibly contaminated bone with the plate, and suppression of phagocytosis from metal ions.[44,45]

External fixation can stabilize virtually all patterns of grades II and III open tibial fractures without adding to the risk of infection. Its application does not disrupt the vascular supply to the injured soft tissues or bone. The percutaneous pins can usually be placed away from the site of injury to permit wound care and serial debridement of necrotic bone. The frame can be suspended to protect wound dressings from bedsheet or sling contamination. In addition, current fixators permit alterations of fracture alignment, bone length, and frame flexibility without additional surgery.

Although pin-tract problems offset these advantages to some extent, drainage and loosening can be confined to less than 10% of pins with attention to the details of pin insertion[10,46] and frame design.[10,11] In our study of 202 grade III tibial fractures treated with primary external fixation, we found it particularly important to predrill diaphyseal pins, obtain bicortical fixation, place at least three threaded pins on either side of the fracture, and remove the pins that became loose before they had an opportunity to become infected.[10,12] For metaphyseal fractures, 4-mm transfixion pins through the epiphysis provide excellent fixation with little muscle penetration and few pin-site problems. On the other hand, for diaphyseal fixation, 5-mm half-pins placed through the subcutaneous anteromedial border of the tibia can reduce the incidence of pin-track problems associated with transfixion pins through the distal tibial shaft.[47] By avoiding anterior compartment muscle penetration, half-pins allow greater muscle excursion and ankle motion during treatment.[48]

A single anteromedial bar connecting 5-mm pin groups provides adequate fixation for stable fracture patterns with axial bone contact after reduction. In highly comminuted shaft fractures, comparable stability can be obtained by directing one half-frame anteriorly and one medially and then connecting the two frames proximally and distally with transverse bars to create a triangulated or "delta" frame configuration.[49-51] Recent studies suggested that 5-mm pin delta-frame stability may be approximated with a single rigid Orthofix bar fixed to the tibia with 6-mm half-pins.[52]

Treatment for Anterior Tibial Muscle Loss

Open tibial fractures are often associated with injury to the dorsiflexor muscles within the anterior compartment. Because of the imbalance between the strong ankle plantarflexors and the injured or destroyed dorsiflexors, equinus contracture of the foot occurs unless the foot is held in a neutral position.[53] If equinus deformity is allowed to occur, even the most successful tibial reconstruction will fail to produce normal ambulation.

If anterior compartment injury is not severe and active dorsiflexion is expected within a couple of weeks, a molded thermoplastic or commercial plastic foot splint will maintain foot posture. For more extensive anterior compartment injury, my colleagues and I devised a tibiometatarsal frame extension to maintain the foot in a neutral position.[34,54] We insert 3- or 4-mm half-pins into the dorsomedial aspect of the base of the first and second metatarsals. They are attached to the tibial frame with a plain rod with the foot positioned in slight dorsiflexion (Fig. 32–2). If anterior compartment loss is too extensive for return of active dorsiflexion, tibiometatarsal fixation is maintained for at least 60 days to promote a functional tenodesis with the ankle in neutral position.

Complications with tibiometatarsal fixation have been rare. Pin-tract infection developed in only one of our

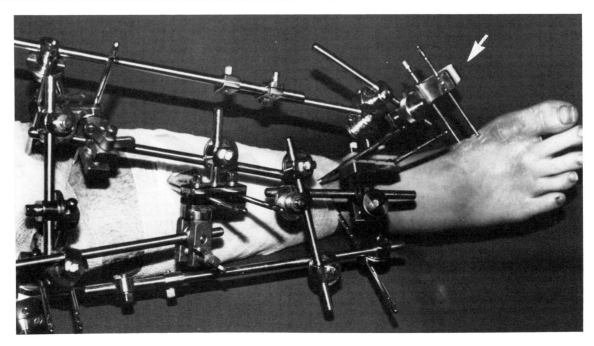

Fig. 32-2 Tibiometatarsal extension (arrow) to maintain foot dorsiflexion when severe injury to the anterior compartment complicates an open fracture of the tibial shaft.

first 127 pins.[47] The tibiometatarsal frame permits sufficient micromotion in the small joints of the foot for survival of articular cartilage and preservation of a reasonably supple foot.

Femoral Fixation

Closed intramedullary nailing is the treatment of choice for most grades I and II open femoral fractures. When the open femoral fracture is the patient's only major injury, the most prudent course of treatment is delayed nailing. The first step is immediate debridement followed by tibial pin traction. Secondary closure is performed if there is no sign of infection at five days or more. Vascular repair is usually sufficient to tolerate closed nailing about two weeks after injury. Using this approach, Chapman and associates[55] reported good results without infections in 49 consecutive cases. Closed reamed nailing with cross-locking for comminuted or infraisthmic fractures can provide good stability for virtually all femoral shaft fracture patterns.

Primary closed nailing or external fixation of grades I and II femoral fractures should be strongly considered for high-risk patients with concomitant head injury, blunt trauma to the chest or abdomen, or multiple pelvic or long bone fractures. Fracture stability and early mobility is particularly important for these patients. Nonreamed closed nailing with Ender pins provides enough stability to mobilize such patients when there is little or no comminution. For such fractures distal to the isthmus, Browner and associates obtained

satisfactory results with an antegrade Ender nailing technique.[56] Infection has not been a problem with primary nonreamed nailing of low-grade open femoral fractures.[56,57]

Grade II open femoral fractures with comminution present a treatment dilemma. Nonreamed nailing often provides fixation inadequate to discontinue traction.[25,56] Primary closed reamed nailing may be possible with a tolerably low infection rate[58] but subjects patients to a greater risk of severe panfemoral infection than either nonreamed nailing or external fixation.

Grade III open fractures of the femur, as well as grade II injuries with moderate comminution or any possibility of contamination, are best treated by primary external fixation. For relatively stable fracture patterns in which axial compression of bone fragments is possible, adequate fixation can be obtained with a lateral half-pin fixator. Widely spaced 5- or, preferably, 6-mm blunt-tipped pins are inserted above and below the fracture near the linea aspera. In unstable femoral fractures with bone loss or major comminution, good clinical results have been reported with 6-mm half-pin fixation with the Orthofix device, the Wagner device, and the original Hoffmann femoral fixator. The last technique uses 4-mm transfixion pins in the distal femoral metaphysis placed between the quadriceps and hamstring muscle groups. Proximal fixation is achieved with triangulated 5-mm half-pins directed from the anterior and lateral surfaces of the femur at the level of the lesser trochanter so as to minimize interference with quadriceps excursion.[59-61]

The effect of distal percutaneous fixation on late knee motion is controversial. Distal femoral pins impale the iliotibial band and poorly placed pins may impale the vastus medialis muscle as well. Knee motion can be improved by taking the knee through a full range of motion in the operating room to split the iliotibial band. In a study of 44 open femoral fractures treated with Hoffmann external fixation, knee motion appeared to recover gradually after fixator removal just as it does after use of a femoral traction pin.[62] In another series of 21 open femurs treated in the same manner, Coppola and Anzel[60] found that patients evaluated more than three years after injury had an excellent (120 degrees) average range of motion.

Overall complications in grade III femoral fractures treated with external fixation are similar to those in open tibias treated with the same method. Infection and nonunion rates were comparable. Drainage or loosening occurred with 10% of femoral pins but was rarely serious[62] (Fig. 32–3).

Pelvic Fixation

For unstable pelvic ring disruptions, prompt external fixation helps slow bleeding, reduces pain, and facilitates patient mobilization.[63] In most injuries, 5-mm half-pins placed in both iliac wings connected with a Slätis "A" frame suffice. For more secure fixation of Malgaigne injuries with complete sacroiliac dislocation, the addition of anterior iliac pin groups with a Pittsburgh-type frame provides more stability.[64]

Open pelvic fractures lead to death in 22% to 50% of cases.[65,66] Most deaths result from hemorrhage or sepsis.[65] To combat these problems, the pelvis should first be reduced and stabilized with external fixation to promote tamponade. In the few cases in which massive bleeding persists, consider arterial embolization,[63] since attempts to control acute bleeding surgically after open pelvic trauma are usually futile and often contribute to fatality.[67] To avoid potential sepsis, a diverting colostomy should be performed if there is any question of bowel or perianal laceration. Pelvic and groin wounds should be treated in an open fashion with frequent surgical debridement. External fixation helps stabilize these wounds while permitting patient mobilization. A split mattress allows the patient to be turned 360 degrees for treatment of posterior pelvic wounds, if necessary.

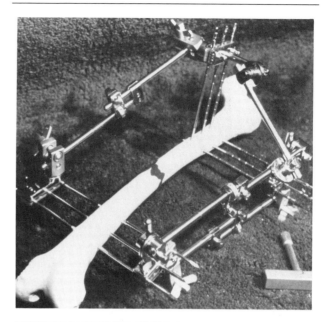

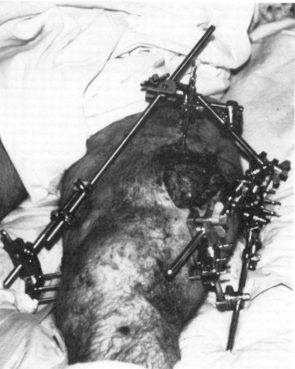

Fig. 32–3   External fixation of grade III femoral shaft fracture.

Stabilization of Multiple Fractures

Floating Knee

For reasons that are not fully understood, patients with ipsilateral fractures of the femur and tibia fare more poorly than those in whom these fractures occur independently.[68-72] When both the tibia and femur are fractured, it is difficult to provide effective stabilization or alignment with traction or cast methods. Accord-

ingly, both delayed union and malunion predominate in patients treated nonsurgically. Indeed, Karlström and Olerud[73] found that their conservatively treated group eventually required more surgical procedures than their group treated with initial fracture fixation. With few exceptions, studies on the treatment of ipsilateral fractures have concluded that overall results are superior when both fractures are rigidly stabilized.[68-72]

Patients with multiple injuries often have an open

tibial fracture and a closed femoral fracture. In such cases it is most efficient to stabilize the open tibial fracture with external fixation first. The tibial frame can then be directly attached to the traction arm of a fracture table. This permits standard closed femoral nailing.[74] Reamed nailing with or without cross locking is preferred for maximum stability of fixation in closed femoral fractures. Open femoral fractures are best fixed with primary nonreamed nailing in patients with multiple injuries or with a period of femoral traction followed by reamed nailing in patients without other major injuries. Patients with grade III open fractures of the femur and tibia should be treated with external fixation for both injuries (Fig. 32–4).

In both my experience and that of Fraser and associates,[68] ligamentous injuries are often associated with a floating knee. Fraser and associates reported a 39% incidence of knee joint laxity. Definitive ligamentous reconstruction is best accomplished early but after life-threatening injuries have been addressed.

Floating Elbow

Ipsilateral fracture of the humerus and both bones of the forearm are, in many ways, analogous to the floating knee. It is difficult to obtain enough control over all four extremity fragments to achieve uniform fracture union and maintain good alignment. Indeed,

Rogers and associates[26] reported humeral nonunions in all six patients with floating elbows treated conservatively but in only two of 13 treated surgically. Similarly, prolonged immobilization of the elbow carries permanent loss of motion, particularly in cases with articular injury. Rogers and associates[26] reported average residual elbow ranges of motion of 58 degrees for patients treated conservatively and 94 degrees for those surgically stabilized. On the basis of these considerations, I recommend early stabilization of both the forearm and humeral fractures in patients with a floating elbow. Depending on the severity of the open fracture, either primary compression plating or temporary external fixation followed by delayed plating is indicated for forearm injuries. Both nonreamed nailing and definitive external fixation are effective in humeral fractures.

Temporary External Fixation

The "In-Board" Traction Concept

Severe wound contamination or fracture comminution can make primary definitive fixation either imprudent or impractical. Accordingly, traction may be entertained as an interim measure. However, with multiple injuries, traction interferes with mobilization, compro-

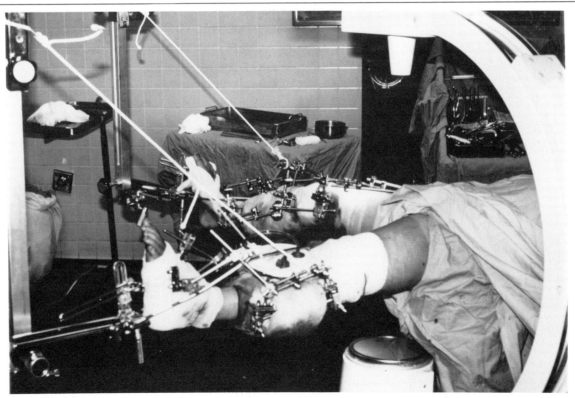

Fig. 32–4   Treatment of floating knee with external fixation for grade III open tibia and primary closed unreamed nailing for ipsilateral grade II femoral fracture.

mises pulmonary function, and often fails to provide sufficient fracture stability. In such cases, in-board traction using external fixation is a practical alternative.[74] Pin groups are placed on either side of the injured portion of the extremity and distracted with adjustable rods. This restores limb length and neutralizes the compressive force from surrounding muscles. The resulting localized traction pulls displaced fragments attached to surrounding soft tissues into relative alignment; this concept is known as "ligamentotaxis."[75]

In-board traction with external fixation permits unrestricted patient mobilization while stabilizing the injured tissues. Definitive open reduction and fixation can be accomplished subsequently. My associates and I regularly use in-board traction as a temporary means of fixation in the following clinical situations:

Wounds Precluding Open Reduction and Internal Fixation Several fracture patterns are best treated with open reduction and plate fixation. However, primary plating of open fractures can expose the patient to undue risk of deep infection when wounds are complicated by contamination or soft-tissue crush. This is a good indication for temporary in-board traction with external fixation followed by delayed open reduction and internal fixation (ORIF). For example, in a patient who had open and contaminated fractures of the humerus and forearm, temporary stability for the injured arm was achieved with external fixation after debridement. A standard lateral humeral half-frame was applied first. Pins were placed in the metacarpals. Adjustable rods were used to connect the humeral frame to the distal pins. The rods were distracted to restore length and alignment of the forearm. The patient underwent two additional debridements. During the interim, his arm was kept elevated and free from contamination by tying the fixator to an overhead frame. When the forearm wound was clean and ready for closure, a compression plating was performed. The distal extension of the fixator was then removed. The humeral frame was left in place for definitive treatment of the open humeral fracture (Fig. 32–5).

The Extremity With Multiple Fractures Temporary in-board traction for multiple comminuted fractures is particularly valuable in cases in which survival is doubtful or long extremity surgery at the time of admission would be intolerable. External fixation pin groups are placed to span fractured segments, including joints when necessary. This permits unrestricted patient mobilization during the first critical days after injury. It achieves rapid fixation of the injured soft tissues and fractures. It maintains length and alignment until the patient is sufficiently stable for delayed primary ORIF and/or definitive external fixation.

For example, we encountered a patient with head, chest, and abdominal injuries who also had an open ankle fracture-dislocation, open tibial fracture, and a comminuted distal femur. After debridement, pin groups were placed in her proximal femur, tibia, and calcaneus. Adjustable rods were placed between the pin groups and distracted to align and stabilize the fractures via soft-tissue traction. This made it possible to stabilize these multiple and complex fractures expeditiously without compromising subsequent mobility. Further debridement and definitive fracture fixation were accomplished several days later when the patient's overall condition had improved.

Reconstruction of Periarticular Injuries

Periarticular injuries usually result from high-energy vehicular accidents and are, therefore, frequently associated with other major injuries. We have encountered three general patterns of open periarticular injury: (1) large displaced articular fragments, (2) extensive articular comminution, and (3) major soft-tissue loss with or without fracture.

Major Articular Fragments

Open periarticular injuries with major displaced articular fragments obtain the best clinical results with primary intra-articular anatomic reduction using the minimum amount of metal. Edwards and Browner[76] evaluated 30 patients whose injuries included displaced intra-articular fractures. Approximately one half were treated with primary and one half with delayed fixation of articular fragments. Patients with primary restoration of articular congruity had considerably better late radiographic and clinical results. Primary, rather than delayed, fixation is important because the patient with multiple injuries is often unable to return to the operating room in a few days because of pulmonary, septic, or metabolic problems. If surgery is delayed a couple of weeks or more until the patient is stable, granulation tissue can invade the immobile articular cartilage, greatly compromising the ultimate result.

Primary fixation of displaced articular fragments with Kirschner wires and/or lag screws has not been associated with infection in our experience with over 30 open intra-articular fractures. A small amount of metal fully encased within cancellous bone appears to be well tolerated. In contrast, my colleagues and I have frequently observed infection after primary plating of periarticular open fractures.

Accordingly, when displaced articular fractures are associated with open metaphyseal fractures, my colleagues and I recommend primary wire or lag screw fixation of the articular fragments. External fixation can be used to stabilize associated epiphyseal or metaphyseal fractures (Fig. 32–6). Transfixion pins are placed transversely and parallel to the joint surface af-

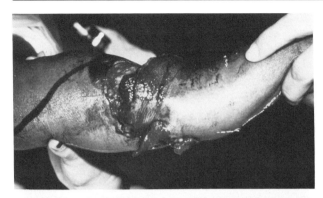
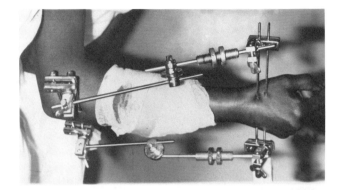
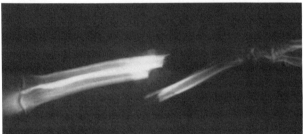
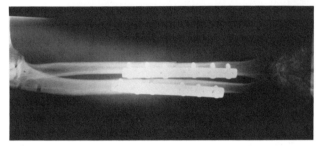

Fig. 32–5   In-board traction with fixator to maintain length and stability of grade III forearm fracture until delayed compression plating.

ter fixing the articular fragments with lag screws. The percutaneous pins can be placed as close as 1 or 2 cm from the subchondral plate to provide epiphyseal fixation without crossing the joint for the great majority of periarticular injuries.

Articular Comminution

When it is not possible to achieve stable fixation of major articular fragments, a temporary neutralization frame must be constructed across the joint. The frame should then be distracted somewhat to negate the compressive force of muscles crossing the joint and unload the articular surfaces so as to promote cartilage nutrition.[77]

When articular comminution is too extensive for interfragmentary fixation, external fixation across the joint can provide a definitive means of treatment. With distraction across the joint with the fixator, ligamentotaxis can achieve a reasonable reduction in many cases. After several weeks, callus between the cancellous fragments usually provides enough stability to begin joint motion within the fixator. The adjustable rods are replaced by hinges for the knee joint. This maintains axial alignment and distraction while permitting daily passive motion to help mold fragments and prevent joint adhesions. This technique is particularly useful in two situations. First, nonweightbearing joints such as the elbow, and particularly the wrist, do surprisingly well after treatment with an external fixator held in distraction. Unless there are discrete fragments that can be internally fixed to restore anatomic congruity, the wrist and

elbow will often do better with external fixation than with open articular surgery. Secondly, definitive treatment with ligamentotaxis for acetabular, knee, ankle, or foot comminuted articular fractures may be necessary by default in patients with multiple injuries who are not able to return to the operating room for ORIF within a couple weeks of injury. Although the results are generally not as good as those following meticulous restoration of articular congruity, my colleagues and I have had patients with functional hip, knee, ankle, and foot joints after treatment with external fixation and distraction alone.

Tissue Loss Crossing Joints

Major soft-tissue loss and/or arterial injury crossing the knee or other major joints is best treated with some form of stabilization. Even when there are no fractures, motion through the joint compromises soft-tissue healing and natural defenses against infection. In the case of arterial repairs, success is claimed with only relative traction immobilization,[78] but this greatly compromises patient mobility and makes adequate wound care very difficult. My colleagues and I have found external fixation to be the most effective method for stabilizing major soft-tissue injury crossing joints. Pin groups are placed proximal and distal to the joint. Mild distraction is applied to protect articular cartilage nutrition. Wounds are then covered with a combination of delayed closure, split-thickness skin grafting, and/or myocutaneous flaps within one or two weeks of injury when there is no remaining necrotic tissue or infection. Once the graft incorporates securely, it is possible to begin progressive motion across the injured joint with a hinged fixator or by temporarily loosening the fixator couplings on a daily basis.

External fixation is particularly effective in severe periarticular burns, soft-tissue avulsion from about the ankle or knee joint, and after saphenous vein arterial reconstructions.[79] Wound stability reduces pain, facilitates sterile wound care, and prevents contractures. Despite several weeks of semirigid joint fixation, these patients have surprisingly little loss of ultimate joint range of motion when there has been no concomitant intra-articular injury or surgery.

Wrist Fixation

Fixation across the wrist is one of the simplest and most effective transarticular external fixation constructs. Distraction across the wrist for an average of six weeks improves articular congruity by ligamento-taxis and maintains full radial length.[31] A simple wrist fixator is constructed by placing two or three 4-mm half-pins on the radial side of the distal radius and connecting these to 3-mm half-pins placed into the dorsoradial surface of the first metacarpal. For injuries with ulnar instability, an additional pin group can be placed into the fifth metacarpal. Several studies have found this technique to be easier, more adjustable, and better tolerated than formerly used pins-in-plaster techniques.[31,80] My colleagues and I noted pin loosening or drainage in less than 4% of pins about the wrist.

The wrist joint appears to tolerate six to eight weeks of external fixation in distraction very well. The standard radial half-pin frame is quite flexible and permits a small amount of motion across the carpal joints. This facilitates cartilage nourishment and helps prevent adhesions. Clinical results suggest that this approach is not associated with much greater loss of motion than observed after other forms of treatment for comparable wrist fractures. Schuind and associates[81] noted a 33% loss of wrist motion at six-month follow-up in 126 cases. Cooney[80] (100 cases) and D'Anca and associates[82] (87 cases) both reported that almost two thirds of their patients had no significant (less than 10%) late loss of wrist motion. Cooney also noted that patients treated with a fixator crossing the wrist had the same average range of motion as those treated with a special mini-fixator that did not cross the wrist.[80]

Elbow Fixation

The elbow has less tolerance for both external fixation and intra-articular fractures than other major joints. The simplest construct connects posterior distal humeral half-pins to proximal olecranon half-pins. However, if there is instability about the elbow, it is usually necessary to counteract the weight of the forearm with an additional pin group in the metacarpals. In lieu of pins in the proximal forearm, adequate elbow control

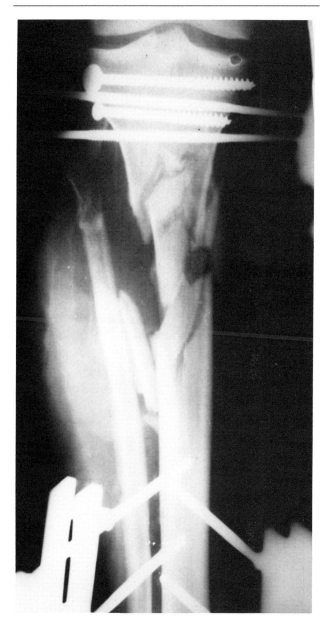

Fig. 32-6   Primary lag screw reduction of displaced articular fragments with external fixation of open metaphyseal fractures.

can usually be obtained by combining metacarpal pins with a plaster cuff about the forearm.[74] Rods then triangulate the metacarpal pins, humeral frame, and forearm cuff or pins.

Ankle Fixation

Both the tibiometatarsal and triangular frames are useful in the treatment of open or unstable injuries about the ankle. The tibiometatarsal frame consists of 3-mm half-pins placed across the base of the first and second metatarsals connected to 4-mm half-pins placed in the anteromedial aspect of the distal tibia with a single rod. Fifth metatarsal fixation with a second rod can be added for particularly unstable injuries. The tibiometatarsal frame makes the intervening joints stable by means of a biologic tension-band phenomenon. The foot is held in slight dorsiflexion, making the Achilles tendon and plantar fascia taut. The resulting balanced anterior and posterior compression stabilizes the intervening joints, yet permits enough micromotion for cartilage survival and maintenance of a reasonably supple foot.[11,54]

The tibiometatarsal frame is used to maintain reduction of open dislocations between the ankle and mid-foot. The frame also provides stability for injured soft tissues in degloving injuries about the hind-foot. On the other hand, this construct requires an intact plantar fascia and Achilles tendon posteriorly and a noncomminuted bony column anteriorly to maintain stability.[34]

When comminution precludes axial loading, the triangular frame is used. The original triangular frame, described by Connes[59] in 1977, consisted of transfixion pin groups placed across the metatarsals, tibia, and calcaneus. The calcaneal and metatarsal pin groups are connected by a simple rod. Adjustable rods connect the anterior tibial pins to the rod attached to both lower pin groups. Good stability with less tissue trauma is also achieved with half-pin fixation to the metatarsals and distal tibia connected to transfixion pins crossing the calcaneus. The triangular frame maintains length and foot position in cases with bone loss or comminution about the ankle or hind-foot (Fig. 32–7). It is also indicated after open disruption of the plantar fascia or Achilles tendon or in multiple open fracture-dislocations in which a stable reduction cannot be maintained with the simple tibiometatarsal frame.

In a study of 50 severe open foot and ankle injuries, Edwards and associates[47] found fixation about the ankle to be an effective and low-risk method for preserving functional foot position and bony alignment when treating severe periarticular injuries. Less than 2% of the metatarsal or distal tibial half-pins and calcaneal transfixion pins developed noticeable drainage or loosening. Clinical results were good for open dislocations and injuries with tissue loss, although patients with extensively comminuted fractures about the ankle and hind-foot did poorly despite these fixation methods.

Knee Fixation

External fixation across the knee joint is occasionally needed to stabilize open injuries with periarticular comminution, soft-tissue loss, or popliteal artery repair. It is difficult to stabilize the knee effectively without the use of transfixion pins across the distal femoral and proximal tibial metaphyses. Although transfixion pins should be avoided in both the femoral and tibial shaft, my colleagues and I found no greater incidence of pin-tract problems when we used transfixion rather than half-pins near the epiphyseal-metaphyseal junction. This

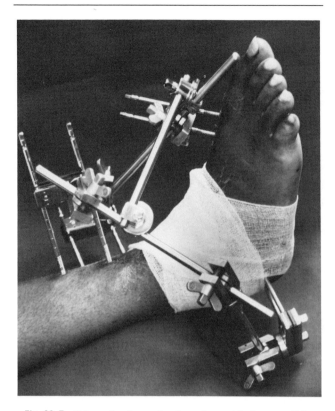

Fig. 32–7 Triangular frame fixation of unstable fracture dislocation with bone loss about the ankle.

was probably because the bone was largely cancellous with very little overlying muscle.

Most cases requiring fixation across the knee have open tibial and/or open femoral fractures requiring an independent tibial or femoral external fixation frame. When definitive external fixation is used for both tibial and femoral fractures, half-pins are used in the proximal femur and distal tibia with transfixion pins across the femoral and tibial epiphyses. The pin clamps on either side of the knee joint are initially attached with a medial rod and a lateral rod.

Hip Fixation

Fixation across the hip joint may be required to stabilize major groin wounds associated with open pelvic fractures or to stabilize open high subtrochanteric fractures or hip fracture-dislocations until ORIF can be performed. The pelvifemoral frame (Fig. 32–8) consists of proximal fixation to the pelvis with distal fixation to the femoral shaft.[79] Widely spaced 5-mm half-pins are placed in the ilia just posterior to the anterior iliac spines. The right and left iliac pin groups are connected with a bar. If there is pelvic disruption, a Slätis A-frame or Pittsburgh frame may be required. Proximal femoral fixation is achieved with widely spaced 5-mm half-pins directed anterior-to-posterior at the level of the lesser trochanter and a second set of half-pins is directed

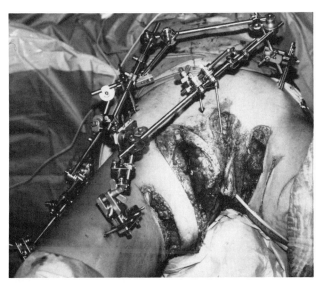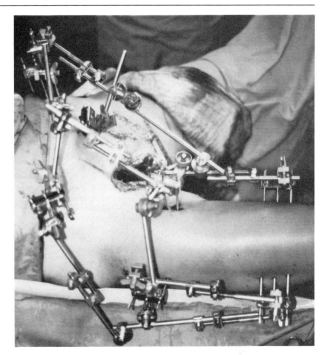

Fig. 32–8 Pelvifemoral fixator to stabilize open pelvic or proximal femoral injuries and mobilize the polytrauma patient.

lateral-to-medial at approximately the same level. The proximal pin groups are then connected to triangulate the proximal femoral fixation. When it is necessary to fix an open femoral shaft fracture, distal femoral fixation is obtained with medial-lateral transfixion pins. Stable fixation across the hip joint is achieved by connecting the ipsilateral iliac pin group to the lateral femoral half-pin group with an adjustable rod and the contralateral iliac pin group to the anterior proximal femoral half-pin group with a second adjustable rod. If pins are placed across the distal femur as well, a third adjustable rod can be connected from the medial side of these pins to the contralateral anterior ilium for particularly stable hip fixation.[83] Very effective distraction can be provided across the hip joint by extending the adjustable rods between the ilium and femoral pins. The diagonal direction of the rods directly opposes the muscle forces crossing the hip. Accordingly, it is possible to maintain reduction of central acetabular fractures.[74] My colleagues and I used this construct successfully to treat comminuted subtrochanteric fractures[79] and open pelvic disruptions combined with major groin wounds. The pelvifemoral fixator holds the leg in abduction to stabilize the injured tissues, facilitates groin wound care, and protects skin grafts without compromising the ability to turn and transfer these patients with multiple injuries.

The pelvifemoral frame permits enough hip joint micromotion to prevent clinically significant stiffness after as much as ten weeks of fixation. Although the pelvifemoral frame is somewhat complex and indicated for only the most severe injuries, it may well be the most important factor contributing to the 90% survival rate for the ten open injuries in one prospective study of pelvic disruptions.[63]

Joint Remobilization

The wrist, ankle, and hip tolerate relatively flexible external fixation and distraction for two to three months without clinically significant loss of ultimate joint motion. This may result, in part, from the relative laxity of the joint capsule in the case of the hip and the fact that the pelvifemoral, wrist, and tibiometatarsal frames do not block all motion at their respective joints. The knee and elbow, on the other hand, respond poorly to prolonged external fixation. An external fixator is able to block motion more completely than at the hip, and the elbow and knee joint capsules lie more closely opposed to synovium and cartilage.

Cartilage nutrition for synovial fluid perfusion depends on the movement of synovial fluid over the cartilage surface and intermittent loading. When joint surfaces are fixed, particularly in compression, nutrition is impaired, causing cartilage necrosis. Necrotic cartilage is often replaced by fibrocartilage, which may then form thick bands connecting both sides of the joint. Simultaneously, motionless synovium can fibrose and form adhesions between the joint capsule and periarticular bone.[77]

To minimize cartilage damage, mild distraction should be placed across any immobilized joint. More importantly, external fixation should be used to limit joint motion only as a temporary measure. As soon as debridements and needed internal fixation of articular fragments are accomplished, rods crossing the knee joint should be replaced by hinges.[54,61] Standard polycentric hinges designed for cast braces can be used to replace the rods connecting the distal femoral and proximal tibial frames. The flat metal pieces on each side of the hinges fit within standard Hoffmann pin clamps. The clamps are then attached to the femoral and tibial frames with couplings. The hinges should be centered over the joint's center of rotation. The resulting hinged fixator can maintain joint alignment and distraction while permitting flexion and extension. Hinges with adjustable nuts are preferable so that larger increments of knee motion can be permitted as healing progresses.

In articular fractures, it is particularly important to begin leg or knee motion early so as to minimize adhesions. This can be accomplished with continued passive motion in conjunction with the hinged fixator (Fig. 32-9). Once bone and/or soft-tissue healing has advanced to the point that control over the joint position or motion is required, the hinges are removed, with the independent femoral and/or tibial fixator(s) left in place.[11]

Soft-Tissue Reconstruction

Serial Debridement

High-energy open fractures are followed by several days of progressive ischemia. Energy dissipated within the soft tissues at the time of injury disrupts lymphatics, capillaries, and control of vascular permeability. Edema,

with increased tissue pressure, and further muscle necrosis follow. Accordingly, Gustilo and Mendoza[84] stated that "in open fractures with extensive soft tissue injury, one cannot expect to do a complete debridement initially, since inspection of the wound on the following day almost always reveals more dead tissue requiring a repeat debridement." Thus, patients with major open injuries should return to the operating room every two to four days for repeat debridement until evolving tissue necrosis ceases. Between debridements, the wounds should be loosely packed in an open fashion with moist gauze. To prevent contamination, the extremity can be suspended from an external fixator to the overhead frame.

It is important to remove all necrotic tissues, including bone. Remember, dead bone appears to be clean regardless of its bacterial content. Pus does not appear unless there is a blood supply to the area. Clinical experience and recent laboratory studies[85] document that live bone with an adequate blood supply survives under a moist dressing. Thus, it makes no sense to cover "exposed bone" hastily before adequate serial debridements, unnecessarily risking deep infection. Live bone forms bleeding points when abraded and grows granulation tissue. If this does not occur, cortical fragments are best removed. This is particularly true in the tibia where open fractures are most susceptible to deep infection. Bone defects can always be reconstructed in a well-vascularized and sterile environment. Indeed, fresh cancellous graft heals and unites faster than retained dead cortical fragments.

In a study of 202 grade III tibial fractures, Edwards and associates[12] occasionally attempted flap coverage

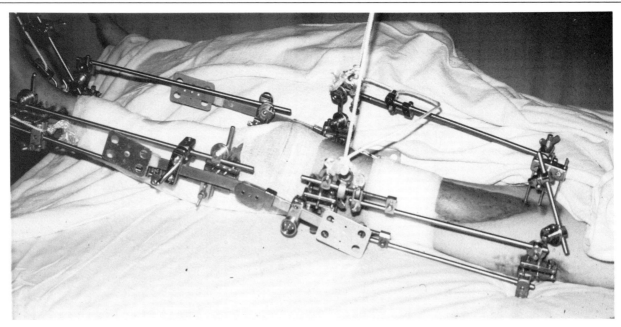

Fig. 32-9 Hinged fixator to restore knee joint motion while maintaining length and alignment of open periarticular fractures.

before removal of all nonviable bone in the first half of the series and experienced an infection rate of 21%. In the second half, my colleagues and I continued debridements until all nonviable tissues, including bone, were removed before we attempted coverage. This reduced our infection rate to 9%.

Soft-Tissue Reconstruction

When all wound surfaces are clean and viable, the simplest closure or plastic procedure that provides reliable coverage is performed. Before closure of major wounds, it is important to wait at least five days after injury when edema has resolved and the local circulation has recovered sufficiently to counteract residual bacteria. Prompt coverage thereafter helps prevent secondary wound infection.

Where there is little soft-tissue loss, delayed primary closure suffices. If there is any question about the wound or tissue tension on closure, retention wires can be placed and gradually tightened during dressing changes.

The balance of the wound is then covered with a split-thickness skin graft. Mesh grafting techniques, in particular, can speed physiologic coverage without completely blocking observation of the wound or natural drainage. Split-thickness skin grafting also provides adequate coverage over the granulation tissue that gradually forms on debrided living bone. If more durable coverage is needed or major bone reconstruction is necessary, elective flap coverage can be performed later.

Muscle and myocutaneous flaps are frequently needed in the reconstruction of open fractures. In my open fracture studies, flap coverage was used in 32% of tibias,[12] 21% of femoral injuries (usually about the knee),[62] and 9% of upper extremity injuries (usually about the elbow).[31] Flaps are indicated to cover an exposed fracture site, joint, or major tendons. Muscle flaps also bring a needed blood supply and osteoprogenitor cells to the fracture site in cases with extensive injury to the surrounding muscles.[86]

Two classes of flaps are useful in the reconstruction of open fracture wounds: muscle flaps and myocutaneous flaps. Muscle flaps are placed in the soft-tissue defect and subsequently covered with a split-thickness skin graft. Myocutaneous flaps include muscle together with its overlying subcutaneous tissue and skin. Myocutaneous flaps provide more cosmetic and durable soft-tissue coverage. However, they cause more disfigurement at the donor area.

A muscle can be rotated on its vascular pedicle or transferred to another location as a "free flap." Like Weiland and associates,[87] Edwards and associates[9] found the gastrosoleus rotational flap to be the most reliable source for reconstruction of anterior tibial wounds (Fig. 32–10). The medial head of the gastrocnemius, together with its overlying skin, is raised on its vascular pedicle and rotated to cover an anterior tibial defect. The donor site is covered by split-thickness skin. If the

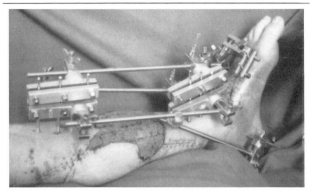

Fig. 32–10 Gastrosoleus rotational flap: muscle is detached distally, rotated on its proximal pedicle into the anterior tibial defect, and covered with split-thickness skin.

ipsilateral gastrocnemius is injured, the same flap can be raised from the opposite leg and is known as a cross-leg flap. The two legs are temporarily held together with external fixation until the base of the flap can be divided.[79] My colleagues and I achieved a 92% success rate with gastrosoleus rotational flaps in our open tibial series in contrast with a 66% success rate with free flaps.[12]

Free myocutaneous flaps can be obtained from several donor sites, but the latissimus dorsi is the most frequently used. Free flaps offer two major advantages. They can cover areas beyond the reach of conventional rotational flaps, such as the elbow, anterior knee, or foot and distal tibia. Secondly, they are able to cover larger wound areas than local pedicle flaps.[9] Despite these advantages, free flaps have some draw backs. Flap anastomosis to a posttraumatic one-vessel leg can jeopardize the injured extremity; hence, an arteriogram should be performed to evaluate leg vasculature before surgery. Moreover, severely injured extremities may not have healthy, unscarred vessels for anastomosis immediately proximal to the area for coverage; if the flap is anastomosed to a vessel within the zone of injury, the likelihood of flap failure is high.

Bony Union

When a major open fracture occurs in a patient with multiple injuries, delayed union is likely. High-energy open fractures are characterized by soft-tissue injury. Since fracture healing depends on these tissues for blood supply and osteoprogenitor cells, union will be slow without major reconstructive efforts. The problem is compounded in patients with multiple injuries by metabolic disturbances and negative nitrogen balance during the period when early callus formation normally occurs.

Average time to union varies among extremities according to their vascular and muscular anatomy. For grade III open fractures average time to full union is four months in the upper extremity,[31] 6.4 months in the femur,[62] and nine months in open tibial fracture.[12] Indeed, 33% of tibial injuries require more than one year of treatment to achieve sufficient union for full weightbearing without protection.

For open fractures with extensive tissue injury and bone loss, early myocutaneous flap coverage provides a healthy environment for bone repair. Cancellous grafting should be performed shortly thereafter if no callus is evident within eight to ten weeks of injury. My colleagues and I found grafting to be necessary in 28% of our open tibial cases.[12] Initial cancellous grafting is best performed through either the posterolateral approach described by Harmon[88] and Reckling and Waters[89] or by placing the cancellous bone directly into the fracture gap by detaching one edge of a mature myocutaneous flap.[11] Open cancellous Papineau grafting[90,91] is less successful than these closed grafting procedures for tibial shaft fractures. Papineau grafting is indicated only for partial metaphyseal bony defects, primarily in the femur.

When bone loss exceeds 6 cm, even muscle flap coverage with posterolateral and direct anterior grafting, combined with some shortening, may be inadequate. Two techniques offer promise for such large bony defects after soft-tissue coverage. These include vascularized bone grafts and bone transport procedures.

Three vascularized bone graft techniques should be considered. The ipsilateral fibula can be transposed along with the peroneal artery to fill a gap in the mid or distal tibia.[11] If the ipsilateral fibula or its vascular pedicle is not amenable to transposition, the contralateral fibula can be used to fill the defect by microvascular anastomosis of its pedicle to the peroneal artery.[92] Success rates of up to 89% have been reported with vascularized fibular grafts in carefully selected patients.[93]

The osseocutaneous graft described by Taylor and associates[94,95] can be helpful when there is segmental loss of bone, muscle, and skin (Fig. 32–11). Full-thickness iliac cortex based on a medial circumflex iliac artery pedicle is transferred along with its surrounding muscle and overlying skin. The composite graft is affixed to the fractured shaft by sagittal half-pins attached to an external fixator.[74] In my experience with this procedure, subsequent cancellous grafting is usually required as well.[12]

Ilizarov and associates[96] and several European surgeons[97,98] have described bone transport procedures for reconstructing major bone loss after shaft fractures. An osteotomy is performed across the uninjured metaphysis adjacent to the diaphyseal bone defect. The proximal metaphysis, intercolated bony segment, and distal shaft are fixed with external pins. The intercolated segment is gradually moved away from the metaphysis and into the bony defect. This is made possible

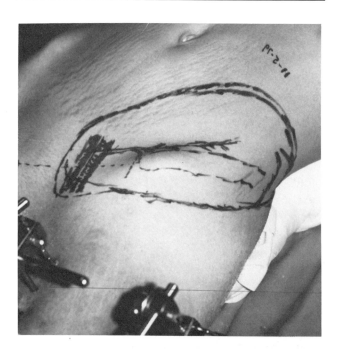

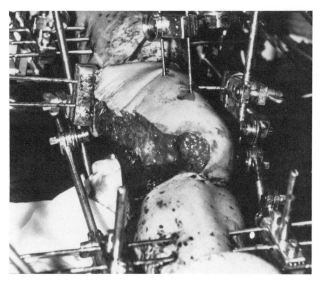

Fig. 32–11   Osseocutaneous groin flap for reconstruction of bone, muscle, and skin loss requires microvascular anastomosis and fixation for graft.

by the gradual lengthening of the callus that forms within the metaphyseal osteotomy as the intercolated fragment is moved away from the metaphysis and into the bony defect. Controlled studies of consecutive case series are required to determine the indications for this interesting reconstructive alternative in the treatment of open fractures.

Early use of electrical stimulation has also been suggested to accelerate union in severe open tibial fractures.[96,99,100] Clinical reports to date remain controversial for this approach as well. The Orthopaedic Trauma

Association has recently launched a double-masked multicenter study to determine the effect of electrical stimulation on delayed unions.

Union can also be accelerated by progressively loading the fracture once reconstruction of bony defects has been accomplished and callus is present. In stable fracture patterns with end-to-end apposition, an external fixator can be removed shortly after soft-tissue coverage is mature to permit physiologic loading in a cast.

On the other hand, early fixator removal can be a mistake in the treatment of high-energy fractures with bone loss or major comminution. Peripheral callus resists fracture bending. In these cases with extensive soft-tissue destruction, peripheral callus formation is depressed and premature removal of the fixator commonly results in angulation.[12,61] Functional union for these injuries is prompted not by early fixator removal but, rather, by maintenance of a stable milieu for the fracture and early bone grafting to build callus volume.[61]

Once bone grafting has stimulated callus formation, union can be accelerated by progressively loading the fracture. This can be accomplished to some extent by decreasing the rigidity of an external frame as fracture healing progresses. For example, the medial pin groups can be removed from a delta frame to convert it to an anterior half-pin frame. Similarly, transfixion pins can be cut laterally to convert a quadrilateral Vidal-type frame to a medial half-pin frame. Axial loading can also be increased by adding sliding elements to the external fixation frame.[11,101-103] Unfortunately, data are not available to determine how much axial displacement is desirable or at what stage of callus maturation it should be permitted. If the fibula unites before tibial union, a fibulectomy should be performed to restore axial loads across the healing tibial fracture.

Successful orthopaedic management of the patient whose multiple injuries include open fractures requires an organized clinical regimen incorporating the early stabilization and subsequent staged reconstruction of injured tissues. Although this therapeutic approach is often technically challenging and time-consuming, it helps minimize major complications and helps maximize both patient survival and restoration of normal extremity function.

References

1. Bone L, Bucholz R: The management of fractures in the patient with multiple trauma. *J Bone Joint Surg* 1986;68A:945–949.
2. Chapman MW: Early fracture stabilization in patients with multiple system trauma. Presented at the 12th International Conference on Hoffman External Fixation, Garmisch, 1986.
3. Johnson KD, Cadambi A, Seibert GB: Incidence of adult respiratory distress syndrome in patients with multiple musculos-

keletal injuries: Effect of early operative stabilization of fractures. *J Trauma* 1985;25:375–384.
4. Riska EB, Myllynen P: Fat embolism in patients with multiple injuries. *J Trauma* 1982;22:891–894.
5. Riska EB, von Bonsdorff H, Hakkinen S, et al: Prevention of fat embolism by early internal fixation of fractures in patients with multiple injuries. *Injury* 1976;8:110–116.
6. Patzakis MJ: Management of open fracture wounds, in American Academy of Orthopaedic Surgeons *Instructional Course Lectures, XXXVI*. Park Ridge, IL, American Academy of Orthopaedic Surgeons, 1987, pp 367–369.
7. Blick SS, Brumback RJ, Poka A, et al: Compartment syndrome in open tibial fractures. *J Bone Joint Surg* 1986;68A:1348–1353.
8. DeLee JC, Stiehl JB: Open tibia fracture with compartment syndrome. *Orthop Trans* 1981;5:430.
9. Edwards CC, Jaworski MF, Solana J, et al: Management of compound tibial fractures using external fixation. *Am Surg* 1979;45:190–203.
10. Edwards CC: Complications of external fixation, in Epps CH Jr (ed): *Complications in Orthopaedic Surgery*, ed 2. Philadelphia, JB Lippincott, vol 1, pp 103–125.
11. Edwards CC: Staged reconstruction of complex open tibial fractures using Hoffmann external fixation: Clinical decisions and dilemmas. *Clin Orthop* 1983;178:130–161.
12. Edwards CC, Simmons SC, Browner BD, et al: Severe open tibial fractures: Results treating 202 injuries with external fixation. *Clin Orthop*, in press.
13. Clancy GJ, Hansen ST Jr: Open fractures of the tibia: A review of one hundred and two cases. *J Bone Joint Surg* 1978;60A:118–122.
14. Karlström G, Olerud S: Fractures of the tibial shaft; a critical evaluation of treatment alternatives. *Clin Orthop* 1974;105:82–115.
15. Mears DC: Fracture healing: Pathophysiology and biomechanics, in Mears DC (ed): *External Skeletal Fixation*. Baltimore, Williams & Wilkins, 1983, pp 42–92.
16. Lazarides E, Revel JP: The molecular basis of cell movement. *Sci Am* 1979;240:100–113.
17. Meyer S, Weiland AJ, Willenegger H: The treatment of infected non-union of fractures of long bones. *J Bone Joint Surg* 1975;57A:836–842.
18. Ramsey WS: Analysis of individual leucocyte behavior during chemotaxis. *Exp Cell Res* 1972;70:129–139.
19. Rittmann WW, Perren SM: *Cortical Bone Healing after Internal Fixation and Infection*. New York, Springer-Verlag, 1974.
20. Wolff J: *Das Gasetz der Transformation der Knochen*. Berlin, August Hirschwald, 1892.
21. Perren SM, Cordey J: The concept of interfragmentary strain, in Uhthoff HK (ed): *Current Concepts of Internal Fixation of Fractures*. Berlin, Springer-Verlag, 1980, pp 63–77.
22. Müller ME, Allgöwer M, Schneider R, et al: *Manual of Internal Fixation*, ed 2. Berlin, Springer-Verlag, 1979.
23. Gustilo RB, Anderson JT: Prevention of infection in the treatment of one thousand and twenty-five open fractures of long bones: Retrospective and prospective analyses. *J Bone Joint Surg* 1976;58A:453–458.
24. Chapman MW: The use of immediate internal fixation in open fractures. *Orthop Clin North Am* 1980;11:579–591.
25. Chapman MW: The role of intramedullary fixation in open fractures. *Clin Orthop* 1986;212:26.
26. Rogers JF, Bennet JB, Tullos HS: Management of concomitant ipsilateral fractures of the humerus and forearm. *J Bone Joint Surg* 1984;66A:552–556.
27. Brumback RJ, Bosse MJ, Poka A, et al: Intramedullary stabilization of humeral shaft fractures in patients with multiple trauma. *J Bone Joint Surg* 1986;68A:960–970.
28. Dobozi WR, Hall RF: Flexible intramedullary nailing of humeral shaft fractures, in Browner BD, Edwards CC (eds): *The Science

and Practice of Intramedullary Nailing. Philadelphia, Lea & Febiger, 1987.

29. Stern PJ, Mattingly DA, Pomeroy DL, et al: Intramedullary fixation of humeral shaft fractures. *J Bone Joint Surg* 1984;66A:639–646.

30. Vander Griend R, Tomasin J, Ward EF: Open reduction and internal fixation of humeral shaft fractures. *J Bone Joint Surg* 1986;68A:430–433.

31. Edwards CC, Robertson RJ, Browner BD, et al: The use of external fixation in the upper extremity. *Orthop Trans* 1982;6:403.

32. Burny F, Hinsenkamp M, Donkerwolcke M: External fixation of the humerus: Analysis of 100 cases. Presented at the Seventh International Conference on Hoffmann External Fixation, Geneva, 1979.

33. Kenzora JE, Edwards CC, Browner BD, et al: Acute management of trauma involving the foot and ankle with Hoffmann external fixation. *Foot Ankle* 1981;1:348.

34. Edwards CC: External fixation about the foot and ankle, in Uhthoff HK (ed): *Current Concepts of External Fixation of Fractures.* Berlin, Springer-Verlag, 1982, pp 185–201.

35. Byers R, Day L, Trafton P, et al: Tibial fractures: Indications for internal and external fixation. *Orthop Trans* 1985;9:431.

36. Lottes JO, Hill LJ, Key JA: Closed reduction, plate fixation, and medullary nailing of fractures of both bones of the leg. *J Bone Joint Surg* 1952;34A:861.

37. Velazco A, Whitesides TE Jr, Fleming LL: Open fractures of the tibia treated with the Lottes nail. *J Bone Joint Surg* 1983;65A:879–885.

38. Wiss DA: Flexible medullary nailing of acute tibial shaft fractures. *Clin Orthop* 1986;212:122–132.

39. Bone LB, Johnson KD: Treatment of tibial fractures by reaming and intramedullary nailing. *J Bone Joint Surg* 1986;68A:877–887.

40. Hansen ST, Veith RG: Closed Kuntscher nailing of the tibia, in Browner BD, Edwards CC (eds): *The Science and Practice of Intramedullary Nailing.* Philadelphia, Lea & Febiger, 1987.

41. Bach AW, Hansen ST, Slovik S: Severe open tibial fractures: A prospective study of internal and external fixation for immediate stabilization. *Orthop Trans* 1985;9:430.

42. Schöntag H, Schottle H, Jungbluth KH: External fixation as an alternative when treating 2nd and 3rd degree open lower leg fractures. *Arch Orthop Trauma Surg* 1980;97:13.

43. Veliskakis KP: Primary internal fixation in open fractures of the tibial shaft. The problem of wound healing. *J Bone Joint Surg* 1959;41B:342–354.

44. Brown SA, Mayor MB, Merrittik M: Leukocyte migration inhibition test for metal sensitivity. Presented at the Second Conference on Materials for Use in Medicine and Biology, London, 1976.

45. Schurman DJ, Johnson BL Jr, Amstutz HC: Knee joint infections: A study of the influence of antibiotics, metal debris, hemorrhage, and steroids in a rabbit model. *J Bone Joint Surg* 1974;56A:850.

46. Green SA: *Complications of External Skeletal Fixation: Causes, Prevention, and Treatment.* Springfield, Charles C Thomas, 1981.

47. Edwards CC, Griffith PH, Kenzora JE, et al: Treatment of 50 severe injuries about the ankle. *Orthop Trans* 1982;6:415.

48. Behrens F, Searls K: External fixation of the tibia: Basic concepts and prospective evaluation. *J Bone Joint Surg* 1986;68B:246–254.

49. Finlay JB, Moroz TK, Rorabeck CH, et al: Stability of ten configurations of the Hoffmann external fixation frame. *J Bone Joint Surg* 1987;69A:734.

50. Oonishi H, Tatsumi M, Hasgawa T: Biomechanical studies on framework and insertion of pins of external fixation. *Orthopedics* 1984;7:658.

51. Vidal J, Nakach G, Orst G: New biomechanical study of Hoffmann external fixation. *Orthopedics* 1984;7:653.

52. Hein TJ, Chao EYS: Biomechanical analysis of the Orthofix axial external fixator. Presented at the meeting on Recent Advances in External Fixation, Riva del Garda, Italy, 1986.

53. Omer GE Jr, Pomerantz GM: Initial management of severe open injuries and traumatic amputations of the foot. *Arch Surg* 1972;104:696–698.

54. Edwards CC: New directions in Hoffmann external fixation: The Maryland experience with major trauma. Presented at the Seventh International Conference on Hoffmann External Fixation, Geneva, 1979.

55. Chapman MW, Pugh GA, Wood J, et al: Closed intramedullary nailing of femoral fractures. *Orthop Trans* 1982;6:326.

56. Browner BD, Blundon M, Brillhart AT, et al: Closed antegrade Ender nailing of femoral fractures. *Orthop Trans* 1982;6:325.

57. Pankovich AM, Goldflies ML, Pearson RL: Closed Ender nailing of femoral-shaft fractures. *J Bone Joint Surg* 1979;61A:222–232.

58. Winquist RA, Hansen ST Jr, Clawson DK: Closed intramedullary nailing of femoral fractures: A report of five hundred and twenty cases. *J Bone Joint Surg* 1984;66A:529–539.

59. Connes H: *Hoffmann's External Anchorage Techniques: Indications and Results,* ed 4. Paris, Edition Gead, 1977.

60. Coppola AJ Jr, Anzel SH: Use of the Hoffmann external fixator in the treatment of femoral fractures. *Clin Orthop* 1983;180:78–82.

61. Edwards CC: The timing of external fixation, in Uhthoff HK (ed): *Current Concepts of External Fixation of Fractures.* Berlin, Springer-Verlag, 1982, pp 27–42.

62. Edwards CC, Browner BD, Lewis CG, et al: Reconstruction of 44 severely injured open femurs using Hoffmann external fixation. *Orthop Trans* 1983;7:522.

63. Edwards CC, Meier PJ, Browner BD, et al: Results treating 50 unstable pelvic injuries with primary external fixation. *Orthop Trans* 1985;9:434.

64. Mears DC, Fu FH: External fixation in pelvic fractures. *Orthop Clin North Am* 1980;11:465–479.

65. Perry JF Jr: Pelvic open fractures. *Clin Orthop* 1980;151:41–45.

66. Rothenberger D, Velasco R, Strate R, et al: Open pelvic fracture: A lethal injury. *J Trauma* 1978;18:184–187.

67. Mucha P, Farnell MB: Analysis of pelvic fracture management. *J Trauma* 1984;24:379–386.

68. Fraser RD, Hunter GA, Waddell JP: Ipsilateral fracture of the femur and tibia. *J Bone Joint Surg* 1978;60B:510–515.

69. Gillquist J, Reiger Å, Sjödahl R, et al: Multiple fractures of a single leg: A therapeutic problem. *Acta Chir Scand* 1973;139:167–172.

70. McBryde AM, Blake R: The floating knee: Ipsilateral fractures of the femur and tibia. *J Bone Joint Surg* 1974;56A:1309.

71. Omer GE Jr, Moll JH, Bacon WL: Combined fractures of the femur and tibia in a single extremity: Analytical study of cases at Brooke General Hospital from 1961 to 1967. *J Trauma* 1968;8:1026–1041.

72. Ratliff AHC: Fractures of the shaft of the femur and tibia in the same limb. *Proc R Soc Med* 1968;61:906–908.

73. Karlström G, Olerud S: Ipsilateral fracture of the femur and tibia. *J Bone Joint Surg* 1977;59A:240–243.

74. Edwards CC, Browner BD: Indications for the Hoffmann fixator in severely injured patients, in Uhthoff HK (ed): *Current Concepts of External Fixation of Fractures.* Berlin, Springer-Verlag, 1982, pp 395–413.

75. Vidal J, Buscayret C, Connes H: Treatment of articular fractures by "ligamentotaxis" with external fixation, in Brooker AF Jr, Edwards CC (eds): *External Fixation: The Current State of the Art.* Baltimore, Williams & Wilkins, 1979, pp 75–81.

76. Edwards CC, Browner BD: Early management of open periarticular fractures with Hoffmann fixation. Presented at the S.I.C.O.T. Semi-Annual International Meeting, Rio de Janiero, Aug 21, 1981.

77. Fulkerson JP, Edwards CC, Chrisman OD: Articular cartilage, in Albright JA, Brand RA (eds): *The Scientific Basis of Orthopaedics,* ed 2. Norwalk, Appleton & Lange, 1987, pp 347–371.

78. Connolly J: Management of fractures associated with arterial injuries. *Am J Surg* 1970;120:331.

79. Edwards CC: Management of multisegment injuries in the poly-trauma patient, in Johnston RM (ed): *Advances in External Fixation*. Miami, Symposia Specialists, 1980, pp 43–60.

80. Cooney WP: External fixation of distal radial fractures. *Clin Orthop* 1983;180:44–49.

81. Schuind F, Donkerwolcke M, Burny F: External fixation of wrist fractures. *Orthopedics* 1984;7:841.

82. D'Anca AF, Steinlieb SB, Byron TW, et al: External fixator management of unstable Colles' fractures: An alternative method. *Orthopedics* 1984;7:853.

83. Edwards CC: The role of Hoffmann fixation in major trauma management. *Med Hygiene* 1983;41:1597.

84. Gustilo RB, Mendoza RM: Results of treatment of 1400 open fractures: 24 years of experience at Hennepin County Medical Center—Minneapolis, Minnesota, in Gustilo RB (ed): *Management of Open Fractures and Their Complications*. Philadelphia, WB Saunders, 1982, pp 202–208.

85. Zych G, DeLorenzi R, Latta L, et al: The effect of skeletal stability on healing of open wounds and viability of exposed bone. Presented at the 12th International Conference on Hoffmann External Fixation, Garmisch, 1986.

86. Ger R: Muscle transposition for the treatment and prevention of chronic post-traumatic osteomyelitis of the tibia. *J Bone Joint Surg* 1977;59A:784–791.

87. Weiland AJ, Moore JR, Hotchkiss RN: Soft tissue procedures for reconstruction of tibial shaft fractures. *Clin Orthop* 1983;178:42–53.

88. Harmon PH: A simplified surgical approach to the posterior tibia for bone-grafting and fibular transference. *J Bone Joint Surg* 1945;27:496–498.

89. Reckling FW, Waters CH III: Treatment of non-unions of fractures of the tibial diaphysis by posterolateral cortical cancellous bone-grafting. *J Bone Joint Surg* 1980;62A:936–941.

90. Papineau LJ: L'excision-greffe avec fermeture retardée délibérée dans l'ostéomyélite chronique. *Nouv Presse Med* 1973;2:2753–2755.

91. Vidal J, Buscayret C, Connes H, et al: Treatment of open frac-tures with a loss of osseous substance: Examples from clinical cases, in Brooker AF Jr, Edwards CC (eds): *External Fixation: The Current State of the Art*. Baltimore, Williams & Wilkins, 1979, pp 215–224.

92. Taylor GI: Microvascular free bone transfer: A clinical technique. *Orthop Clin North Am* 1977;8:425–447.

93. Weiland AJ: Vascularized bone transfers. *Orthop Trans* 1985; 9:399.

94. Taylor GI, Townsend P, Corlett R: Superiority of the deep circumflex iliac vessels as the supply for free groin flaps: Clinical work. *Plast Reconstr Surg* 1979;64:745–759.

95. Taylor GI, Watson N: One-stage repair of compound leg defects with free, revascularized flaps of groin, skin, and iliac bone. *Plast Reconstr Surg* 1978;61:494–506.

96. Ilizarov GA, Makushin VD, Kuftiryer LM, et al: *Recovery of Post-traumatic Bony Defects of the Tibia by the Lengthening of a Bony Fragment*, thesis, 1973.

97. Gallinaro M, Rossi P, Dettoni A, et al: Open fractures with loss of bone substance and soft tissue: Remarks on compression-distraction osteosynthesis. Presented at the meeting on Recent Advances in External Fixation, Riva del Garda, Italy, 1986.

98. Paley D: The treatment of nonunions of the tibia with bony defects by the Ilizarov technique. *Clin Orthop*, in press.

99. Barker AT, Dixon RA, Sharrard WJ, et al: Pulsed magnetic field therapy for tibial non-union. *Lancet* 1984;1:994–996.

100. Bassett CAL: The development and application of pulsed electromagnetic fields (PEMFs) for ununited fractures and arthrodeses. *Orthop Clin North Am* 1984;15:61–87.

101. De Bastiani G, Aldegheri R, Renzi Brivio L: The treatment of fractures with a dynamic axial fixator. *J Bone Joint Surg* 1984;66B:538–545.

102. Fischer DA: Skeletal stabilization with a multiplane external fixation device. *Clin Orthop* 1983;180:50–62.

103. Zbikowski JL: Biocompression. Presented at the Seventh International Conference of Hoffmann External Fixation, Geneva, 1979.

Injuries to the Muscle-Tendon Unit

William E. Garrett, Jr., MD, PhD

Introduction

Muscle-tendon unit injuries are among the most common injuries treated by orthopaedic surgeons and others involved with sports medicine. These injuries can take many forms, including contusions, lacerations, and muscle strains. We know much about injuries to bone, articular cartilage, and ligaments, but there is relatively little information from basic science and clinical studies to guide our treatment of muscle injuries.

Basic Anatomy and Physiology

The muscle-tendon unit usually reaches from one bone to another and crosses a joint. Muscle can produce force and motion by actively shortening. Muscle can also act to decelerate joint motion by resisting lengthening. Muscle fibers usually run from bone or tendon to attach to bone or tendon distally. Muscle fibers are arranged within muscle in many ways. Muscle fibers are syncytial cells, that is, they have many nuclei and result from the fusion of many mononuclear cells. The fibers are usually considerably shorter than the muscle belly. In some muscles the fibers are parallel to the muscle axis, but most often the fibers are arranged obliquely to the muscle axis.

Muscle fibers are grouped together in fascicles. These fascicles are surrounded by a connective-tissue network. There is also a connective-tissue framework between individual fibers. Each muscle-fiber cell membrane is associated with a connective-tissue basement membrane called the sarcolemma. These connective-tissue elements in muscle greatly influence the passive resistance of muscle to stretch. Within the muscle fiber the contractile proteins are arranged in parallel smaller units called myofibrils. The myofibrils are arranged as a series of repeating units called sarcomeres, which are 2 to 3 μ long. Within the sarcomeres are contractile proteins arranged as sliding filaments in a highly ordered array. This ultrastructure has been reviewed in more detail elsewhere.[1]

The motor nerve to the muscle enters at the motor point. The nerve fibers branch many times within the muscle. One motor nerve innervates many muscle fibers. A motor nerve and the muscle fibers it innervates is called a motor unit. Muscle fibers and motor units are different histochemically, physiologically, and biochemically.[1] Whole muscles consist of mixtures of motor units of different types.[2] The distribution of fiber type within the muscle influences its physiologic characteristics. Type 1 fibers have a slower contraction time, rely on aerobic energy sources, are fatigue-resistant, and have a highly developed mitochondrial energy system. Type 2 fibers have a faster contraction time and are less resistant to fatigue. Type 2 fibers are further subdivided into types 2A and 2B. Type 2A fibers are slower to contract but more fatigue-resistant than type 2B fibers.[2] Studies in humans have shown that a muscle's contractile speed and fatigability are related to the composition of its fiber types.[3,4]

Muscle fibers are not recruited randomly by the central nervous system for the production of muscle force. Rather, the recruitment of motor units is determined by the intensity and duration of the muscle contraction. In low-intensity contractions, type 1 motor units are involved. In more intense contractions, type 1 and type 2 motor units are involved. The preferential involvement of type 1 fibers in low-intensity, high-repetition exercise and the involvement of type 2 motor units in high-intensity exercise may well be related to the order of recruitment by the central nervous system.[5]

Muscle fibers are activated by the motor nerve. An activated muscle fiber shortens if its innate contractile force is greater than the applied resistance. This is termed a concentric contraction. An activated muscle may also lengthen if the applied resistance is greater than the force generated by the muscle. This is called an eccentric contraction. If the muscle is not allowed to change length at all during activation, an isometric contraction results. Muscle can generate significantly more tension during eccentric contractions than during concentric contractions. In laboratory testing, isometric contractions are often used to measure muscle force. Many studies in humans now measure muscle contractile ability by using concentric contractions at a controlled angular velocity. These are called isokinetic contractions. Muscle output is measured as torque throughout the range of motion for a given angular velocity.

There are many mechanisms of injury of skeletal muscle. Muscle may be sharply lacerated and completely or partially divided. The injury may involve a blunt contusion without skin disruption. Muscle may also be injured indirectly by excessive stretch with or without activation, as happens in a muscle strain. For the purposes of this discussion, muscle injuries are classified as sharp injuries (lacerations), blunt injuries (contusions), and indirect injuries (strains).

Muscle Lacerations

Sharp injury to the muscle is common in cases of trauma to an extremity. If the muscle is to recover from a sharp injury, the vascular supply must be adequate to allow healing. Suture or appositional repair must result in successful connection of the muscle segments. In addition, muscle fibers isolated from the motor point and nerve supply must be successfully reconnected to the nervous system. Clinical experience with muscle injuries shows that muscle repair may be associated with successful but not total recovery of function.

In laboratory studies evaluating the recovery of rabbit muscle after laceration,[6] suture repair resulted in successful healing of the laceration even without immobilization. The site of the laceration was histologically quite different from normal muscle. A dense connective-tissue scar was the predominant tissue in the laceration site (Fig. 33–1). Muscle regeneration across the scar site was patchy at best, with some myotubes present in the connective-tissue scar. The muscle segment isolated from the motor point did not show good evidence of reinnervation. Rather, the fibers showed the histologic characteristics of denervated muscle (Fig. 33–2). Although the repair process successfully reunited the two segments, the segment isolated from the nerve did not appear to be completely reinnervated.

Muscle function was also evaluated. Rabbit muscle did recover good function after total laceration and repair although it did not recover to normal. Approximately one half the muscle's ability to generate tension and two thirds of its ability to shorten were recovered (Fig. 33–3). Partial lacerations recovered significantly better function.

There have been few clinical studies of the recovery of muscle function after laceration. One recent study showed relatively good recovery of muscle if the functioning segment of muscle was connected to the distal tendon.[7] A tendon graft was used to connect the functioning proximal muscle segment to the tendon. After a follow-up of more than one year, approximately 40%

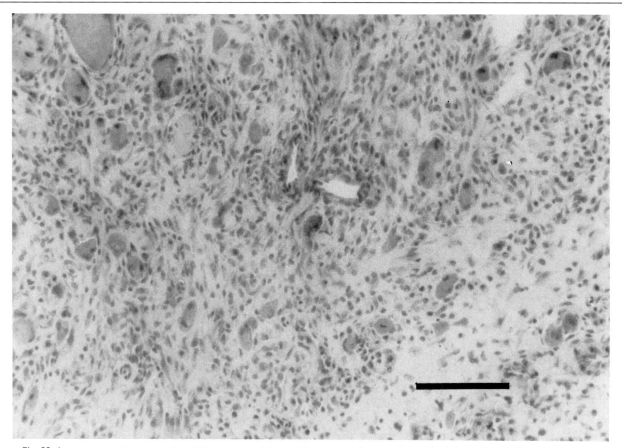

Fig. 33-1 A repaired laceration in rabbit extensor digitorum longus muscle seven days after injury. Some inflammatory cells and an intense fibroblastic reaction are present. Some myotubes are present but there is clearly poor regeneration of muscle tissue (bar gauge = 50 μ). (Reproduced with permission from Garrett WE Jr, Seaber AV, Boswick J, et al: Recovery of skeletal muscle after laceration and repair. *J Hand Surg* 1984;9:683–692.)

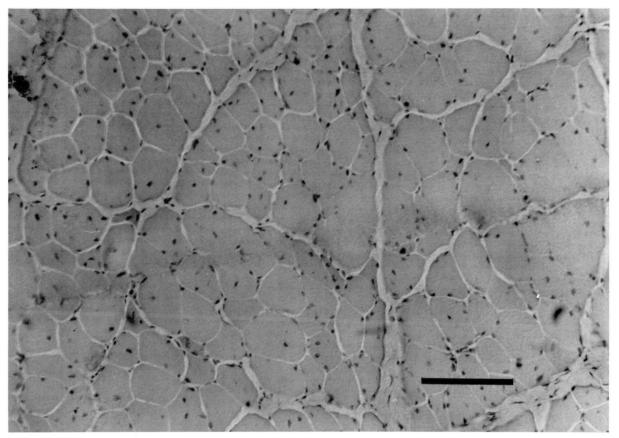

Fig. 33-2 Muscle 12 weeks after laceration. The distal muscle segment shown here was isolated from the motor nerve by the laceration. The histologic features of denervated muscle include variable fiber size, central nuclei, and increased connective tissue (bar gauge = 20 µ). (Reproduced with permission from Garrett WE Jr, Seaber AV, Boswick J, et al: Recovery of skeletal muscle after laceration and repair. *J Hand Surg* 1984;9:683–692.)

of the muscle strength was recovered. This represents useful function, of course, but is far from normal.

Recent experimental studies have shown that the recovery of muscle depends on the orientation of the laceration with respect to the axis of the muscle fibers and the location of the motor point.[8] Lacerations that transect muscle fibers or separate portions of the muscle from the nerve supply result in poorer recovery of muscle function.

Muscle Contusions

Direct injury to muscle by a blunt object is common, particularly in contact sports. The injury causes considerable pain and disability and recovery is often prolonged. In addition, a complicating condition called myositis ossificans occurs in a few of these injuries. Myositis ossificans involves the deposition of bone within the space normally occupied by muscle.[9] The new bone may be isolated within the muscle or it may have direct contact with the deeper bone and periosteum. In the laboratory, some animals show a proclivity toward per-

iosteal deposition of new bone whereas others demonstrate both periosteal and heterotopic deposition.[10,11]

Muscle contusion injuries have been described in several animals and studied by several techniques. Järvinen and Sorvari[12] contused the calf muscle of rats with a special apparatus and demonstrated its injury and recovery. The initial histologic pattern was one of hematoma formation and an inflammatory process. Eventually, the healing resulted in a dense connective-tissue scar without large areas of muscle regeneration. Mobilization led to less scar tissue and faster recovery of tensile strength.[13,14] Younger rats demonstrated a more intense healing response than did older rats.[15] These studies have several clinical implications.

Strict immobilization of contused muscle does not appear to be necessary for proper treatment. Early mobilization should be encouraged.[16] The initial reaction involves hematoma formation and an inflammatory reaction. Initial measures should be directed toward controlling the hematoma and subsequent measures should treat the inflammation.

Newer studies are defining the cellular and molecular events associated with injury and repair. In one study,

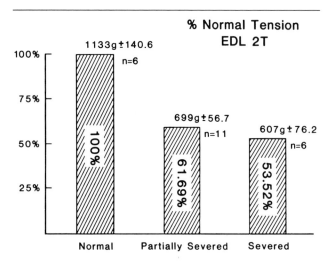

% Normal Tension
EDL 2T

Fig. 33-3 Recovery of muscle tension as a percentage of normal in totally severed and partially severed rabbit extensor digitorum longus muscle. The laceration was slightly distal to the middle of the muscle belly. The muscle was activated by motor nerve stimulation at twice the threshold voltage. (Reproduced with permission from Garrett WE Jr, Seaber AV, Boswick J, et al: Recovery of skeletal muscle after laceration and repair. *J Hand Surg* 1984;9:683–692.)

new protein synthesis occurred by day 2 with a peak in synthesis occurring five to 21 days after trauma.[17] Studies are needed to define the recovery of muscle function and the influence of various treatment regimens.

Muscle Strains

Muscle strain is defined as indirect injury to muscle caused by excessive stretch or tension and not associated with direct contact or trauma. These injuries have also been called muscle pulls, muscle tears, and muscle ruptures. They are very common in athletic and occupational situations. Relatively few clinical studies and fewer laboratory studies have addressed the pathophysiology of and recovery from these injuries.

Strain to Complete Disruption

Clinically, muscle strains involving complete muscle disruption are less common than incomplete muscle tears. They do, however, occur and serve as a good starting point for the investigation of muscle strains. An early study was done by McMaster more than 50 years ago.[18] He demonstrated that when muscle-tendon units were strained to failure, disruption never occurred in normal tendon. Previous tendon laceration or vascular disruption was necessary to create injury within tendon.

Almekinders and associates[19-21] created well-defined injuries in the muscle-tendon unit by grasping the distal tendon and applying stretch. Injury consistently occurred at the myotendinous junction. Muscle fibers usually tore within 1 mm of the true myotendinous

junction. In the rabbit, the muscle fibers insert into broad tendons of insertion. The visible tears began at the distal portion of the myotendinous junction. Histologically the muscle belly appeared essentially normal with all changes concentrated at the region of the distal myotendinous junction.

In more detailed later investigations,[22] different rabbit muscles with different architectural fiber arrangements were strained to failure. This was done in relaxed muscle without any nerve stimulation. In all the muscles tested, the failure occurred at the region of the myotendinous junction. Different rates of strain were also tested without change in the site of disruption. Finally, muscles were clamped and strained from the proximal or the distal tendon of the muscle. Failure still occurred at the distal myotendinous junction.

The structural and physiologic features of the myotendinous junction that make it more susceptible to injury are not understood in any detail, but a number of new studies have provided significant new information about the myotendinous junction. Extensive folding of the tendon surface greatly amplifies the area of contact between muscle and tendon at the junction. This allows a much greater surface for the transmission of force.[23] There are also a number of specialized structures at the junction. Force is transmitted through the myofibrils into thin terminal filaments that end beneath the sarcolemma in dense structures. The force is then transmitted across the plasma membrane and into the connective-tissue envelope of the basement membrane. From the basement membrane, force is next transmitted to the collagen fibrils of the tendon. Highly specialized structures allow for the efficient transmission of tension.[24]

The muscle fibers nearest the tendon do not stretch exactly as the midportions of the muscle fiber do in response to stress. The terminal sarcomeres are stiffer, particularly in the few millimeters of the fiber nearest the myotendinous junction.[25,26] The reason for this lack of homogeneity is not known. Complete disruption of muscle in response to stretch appears to occur within this region.

Muscle can be stretched passively or actively. The above studies pertain to passively stretched muscle. Clinically, many muscle injuries appear to occur when activated muscle is simultaneously stretched, thus producing an eccentric contraction. Injury to muscle produced during eccentric contractions has also been studied.[27] Muscle activation was accomplished by electrical stimulation of the motor nerve. The muscles were then stretched to failure. The site of disruption was unchanged, occurring near the myotendinous junction. Force and elongation to tear were also recorded. Electrically stimulated muscle disrupted at the same length increase as unstimulated muscle. A small increase in force to disruption was seen in the electrically stimulated muscle. The main difference in the biomechanical

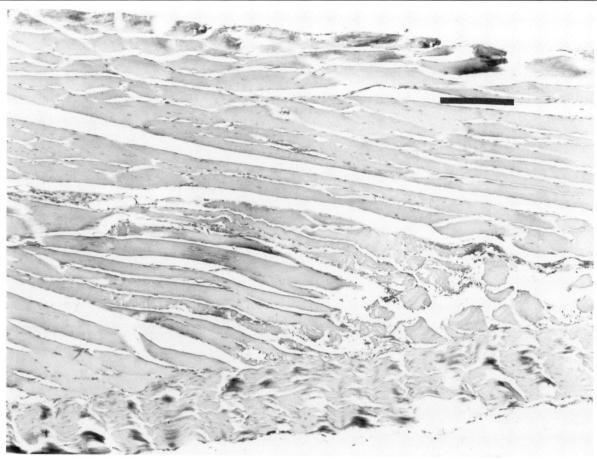

Fig. 33-4 Rabbit anterior tibial muscle immediately after nondisruptive strain injury. The tendon is at the lower margin of the micrograph. Some fibers are disrupted near the muscle-tendon junction while other fibers are not injured (bar gauge $= 300 \mu$).[30]

behavior between stimulated and passive muscle was the energy absorbed by the muscle before disruption. Stimulated muscle absorbed twice as much energy in response to stretch.

Muscle strains occur in a variety of situations. It has been postulated that the strength imbalance of antagonistic muscle may predispose the relatively weaker muscle to injury. Similarly, it has been clinically observed that fatigue increases the chance of muscle injury. These factors can be better understood if the capacity of muscle to absorb energy is considered. Both strength imbalance and fatigue make muscle less able to absorb energy before achieving a certain length increase. The length change necessary to create a strain should be no different in contracting muscle. However, the necessary energy may be absorbed by the strongly contracting muscle before it reaches a harmful length increase.

Partial Muscle Ruptures

The most common muscle strain injuries are not complete but partial disruptions of the muscle-tendon unit. Clinical studies have documented their impor-

tance and frequency but have not provided details regarding the pathophysiology of these injuries. A radiographic study of hamstring muscle strains has shown that acute muscle strains are characterized by an inflammatory reaction within the muscle. This was evidenced by a swollen and edematous muscle. A discrete intramuscular hematoma was not seen in indirect muscle injuries.[28,29] The pathologic lesion was located in the region near the myotendinous junction.

In experimental studies in the rabbit, incomplete tears of the muscle were produced by stretching the muscle into the elastic region of the load-deformation relationship.[30] The injury occurred near the myotendinous junction. Muscle fibers were disrupted near the tendon (Fig. 33-4). A small amount of hemorrhage was seen initially. During the next few days an inflammatory response occurred in the distal myotendinous junction (Fig. 33–5). Muscle fibers were disrupted near the tendon. This was followed by a significant fibroblastic response and scar tissue (Fig. 33–6). The mid-belly of the muscle appeared grossly normal at this stage.

These muscles were characterized physiologically during their recovery process. There was an initial decrease in contractile function as measured by the ability

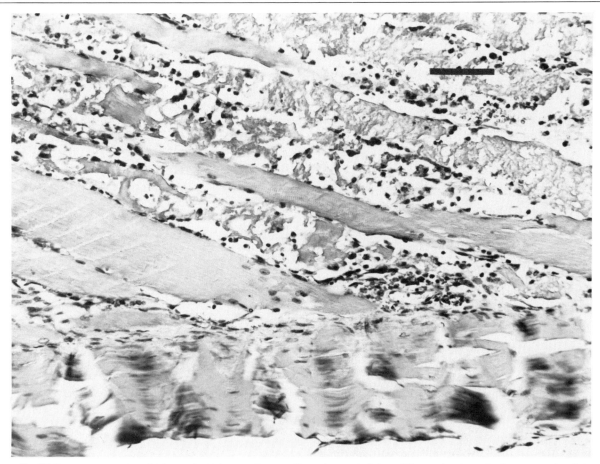

Fig. 33–5 Rabbit anterior tibial muscle 48 hours after nondisruptive strain injury. The tendon is at the lower margin of the micrograph. Some degenerating fibers are seen. There is an inflammatory reaction occurring around the degenerating fibers (bar gauge = 100 μ).[30]

to produce tension in response to nerve stimulation. By one week the muscle had almost completely recovered its ability to produce tension. In a study of the tensile strength of the muscle, Taylor and associates[31] found that the maximal force to disruption was considerably less in the recovery period, indicating a tendency to re-injury.

Prevention of muscle injury is of clinical importance. Studies in athletes have shown the effectiveness of an overall conditioning program on the prevention of injuries to muscle. However, the various components of the conditioning programs have not been evaluated individually to determine what precisely is necessary. A warm-up period of relatively light muscular exercise and a stretching routine are usually advocated as ways to prevent injury. Laboratory studies have shown that a warm-up period of muscle activation may indeed be beneficial in preventing strain injury. A single isometric contraction of rabbit muscle lasting ten to 15 seconds was effective in changing several of the biomechanical characteristics of this muscle. The preconditioned muscle required a greater length change before failure and developed more tension before failure.[32] Stretching

routines alone have also been investigated experimentally. Unactivated muscle showed characteristics of viscoelastic behavior and stress relaxation very similar to those in tendon.[33] Successive stretch-relaxation cycles during which the muscle was stretched to the same length showed a decrease in the tension developed during the first few cycles. Conversely, when the muscle was stretched to the same tension, the length increased significantly during the first four or five cycles. The stretching cycle, therefore, altered the stiffness of the muscle. It is uncertain at this point whether the muscle is less likely to suffer a strain injury after stretching.

Common Muscle Strain Injuries

Some muscles are much more susceptible to strain injury than others. Muscles that cross two joints are subject to stretch at both joints. These muscles are more likely to suffer a strain injury. In addition, muscles with a higher percentage of type 2 fibers are more likely to have injuries.[2] Sports requiring fast movement seem to be more likely to injure muscles.

The hamstrings are a frequently injured muscle group. They cross two joints and have a high proportion of

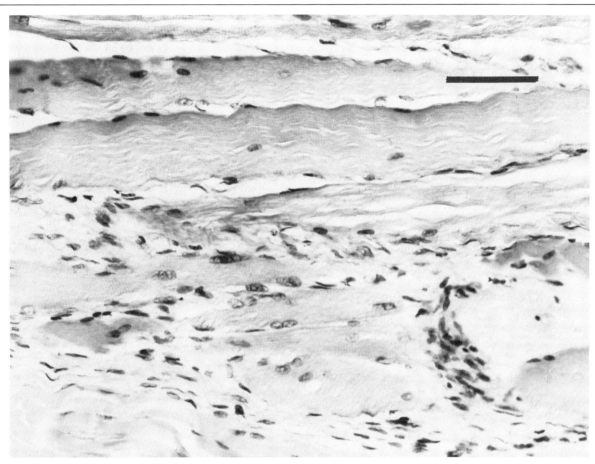

Fig. 33-6 Rabbit anterior tibial muscle seven days after nondisruptive strain injury. The tendon is at the lower margin of the micrograph. Near the myotendinous junction there is an increase in the number of fibroblasts and connective tissue between the muscle fibers (bar gauge = 100 μ).

type 2 fibers. They act largely as decelerators of the leg and work eccentrically. This muscle group is probably the one most subject to severe muscle strains.[34] The quadriceps muscle group is also subject to strain. The rectus femoris is the only quadriceps muscle that crosses two joints and it seems to be more susceptible to strain injury than the others. It also has a higher percentage of type 2 fibers.[2]

The gastrocnemius muscle is also susceptible to injury. Strains usually occur at the myotendinous junction of the medial head of the gastrocnemius.[35] This injury is often called a plantaris rupture although studies have repeatedly shown this injury occurs in the medial head of the gastrocnemius. This muscle crosses the knee and ankle joints. It also appears to be injured during eccentric loading. The adductor longus muscle, also frequently injured, probably avulses from its bony attachment and retracts proximally.[36]

In many respects injuries or strains in the low back region resemble muscle strains. These injuries occur during a period of increased loading and are usually not associated with any radiculopathy. The pain increases over several days as an inflammatory process might. Such injuries often occur in people performing physical activities to which they are unaccustomed. However, the exact nature of low back strains remains to be determined.

Summary

Injuries to muscles are very common in clinical practice. Our understanding of the pathophysiology lags far behind that of other orthopaedic injuries. The recent increase in research and emphasis on muscle injuries and sports medicine will, it is hoped, provide new data and a more scientific basis for treatment and prevention.

References

1. Garrett WE Jr: Basic science of musculotendinous injuries, in Nicholas JA, Hershmann EB (eds): *The Lower Extremity and Spine in Sports Medicine*. St. Louis, CV Mosby Co, 1986, pp 42–57.
2. Garrett WE Jr, Califf JC, Bassett FH III: Histochemical correlates of hamstring injuries. *Am J Sports Med* 1984;12:98–103.

3. Costill DL, Daniels JR, Evans W, et al: Skeletal muscle enzymes and fiber composition in male and female track athletes. *J Appl Physiol* 1976;40:149–154.

4. Tesch P, Karlsson J: Isometric strength performance and muscle fibre type distribution in man. *Acta Physiol Scand* 1978;103:47.

5. Thortenssen A: Muscle strength, fibre types and enzyme activities in man. *Acta Physiol Scand*, 1976, suppl, pp 439–444.

6. Garrett WE Jr, Seaber AV, Boswick J, et al: Recovery of skeletal muscle after laceration and repair. *J Hand Surg* 1984;9A:683–692.

7. Botte MJ, Gelberman RH, Smith DG, et al: Repair of severe muscle belly lacerations using a tendon graft. *J Hand Surg* 1987;12A:406–412.

8. Cheng MS, Seaber AV, Garrett WE Jr: Skeletal muscle function after different orientations of surgical laceration and repair. *Trans Orthop Res Soc* 1987;12:480.

9. Rothwell AG: Quadriceps hematoma: A prospective clinical study. *Clin Orthop* 1982;171:97–103.

10. Zaccalini PS, Urist MR: Traumatic periosteal proliferations in rabbits: The enigma of experimental myositis ossificans traumatica. *J Trauma* 1964;4:344–357.

11. Walton M, Rothwell AG: Reactions of thigh tissues of sheep to blunt trauma. *Clin Orthop* 1983;176:273–281.

12. Järvinen M, Sorvari T: Healing of a crush injury in rat striated muscle. *Acta Pathol Microbiol Scand* 1975;83:259–265.

13. Järvinen M: Healing of a crush injury in rat striated muscle. *Acta Pathol Microbiol Scand* 1975;83:269–282.

14. Järvinen M: Healing of a crush injury in rat striated muscle. *Acta Pathol Microbiol Scand* 1976;84:85–94.

15. Järvinen M, Aho AJ, Lehto M, et al: Age dependent repair of muscle rupture: A histological and microangiographical study in rats. *Acta Orthop Scand* 1983;54:64–74.

16. Jackson DW, Feagin JA: Quadriceps contusions in young athletes: Relation of severity of injury to treatment and prognosis. *J Bone Joint Surg* 1973;55A:95–105.

17. Lehto M, Järvinen M, Nelimarka O: Scar formation after skeletal muscle injury. *Arch Orthop Trauma Surg* 1986;104:366–370.

18. McMaster PE: Tendon and muscle ruptures: Clinical and experimental studies on the causes and location of subcutaneous ruptures. *J Bone Joint Surg* 1933;15:705–722.

19. Almekinders LC, Garrett WE Jr, Seaber AV: Pathophysiologic response to muscle tears in stretching injuries. *Trans Orthop Res Soc* 1984;9:307.

20. Almekinders LC, Garrett WE Jr, Seaber AV: Histopathology of muscle tears in stretching injuries. *Trans Orthop Res Soc* 1984;9:306.

21. Garrett WE Jr, Almekinders LC, Seaber AV: Biomechanics of muscle tears in stretching injuries. *Trans Orthop Res Soc* 1984;9:384.

22. Garrett WE Jr, Nikolaou PK, Ribbeck BM, et al: The effect of muscle architecture on the biomechanical failure properties of skeletal muscle under passive extension. *Am J Sports Med*, in press.

23. Trotter JA, Hsi K, Samora A, et al: A morphometric analysis of the muscle-tendon junction. *Anat Rec* 1985;213:26–32.

24. Tidball JG, O'Halloran T, Burridge K: Talin at myotendinous junctions. *Cell Biol*, in press.

25. Huxley AF, Peachey LD: The maximum length for contraction in vertebrate striated muscle. *J Physiol* 1961;156:150–165.

26. Gordon AF, Huxley AF, Julian FJ: Tension development in highly stretched vertebrate muscle fibres. *J Physiol* 1966;184:143–169.

27. Garrett WE Jr, Safran MR, Seaber AV, et al: Biomechanical comparison of stimulated and nonstimulated skeletal muscle pulled to failure. *Am J Sports Med*, in press.

28. Garrett WE Jr, Korobin M: Investigation of hamstring injuries using computed tomography. Presented at the American College of Surgeons Meeting, San Diego, California, May 23–26, 1984.

29. Garrett WE Jr, Rich FR, Nikolaou PK, et al: Computed tomography of hamstring muscle strains. *Am J Sports Med*, in press.

30. Nikolaou PK, Macdonald BL, Glisson RR, et al: Biomechanical and histological evaluation of muscle after controlled strain injury. *Am J Sports Med* 1987;15:9–14.

31. Taylor DC, Seaber AV, Garrett WE Jr: Immediate response of muscle to traumatic stretching. *Surg Forum* 1986;37:547–549.

32. Safran MR, Garrett WE Jr, Seaber AV, et al: The role of warm-up in muscular injury prevention. *Am J Sports Med*, in press.

33. Taylor DC, Seaber AV, Garrett WE Jr: Repetitive stretching of muscles and tendons to a specific tension. *Trans Orthop Res Soc* 1985;10:41.

34. Krejci V, Koch P: *Muscle and Tendon Injuries in Athletes.* Chicago, Year Book Medical Publishers, 1970, pp 1–35.

35. Millar AP: Strains of the posterior calf musculature ("tennis leg"). *Am J Sports Med* 1979;7:172–174.

36. Symeonides PP: Isolated traumatic rupture of the adductor longus muscle of the thigh. *Clin Orthop* 1972;88:64–66.

Professional Liability

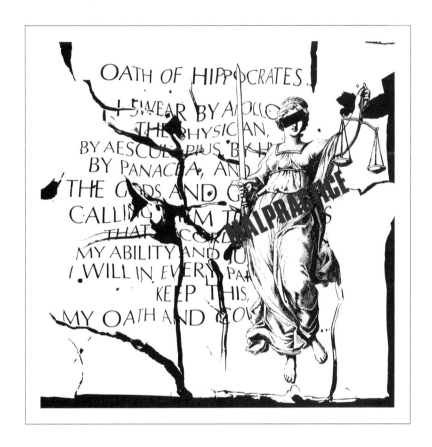

Handling Malpractice Stress:
Suggestions for Physicians and Their Families

Michael C. Reineck, MD

The malpractice issue has been with us for more than a decade, but it has slowly evolved from an issue of availability to one of affordability. A recent American Medical Association opinion poll of physicians showed that the cost of malpractice insurance has replaced previous concerns about governmental intervention and medical reimbursement systems.[1] Malpractice concern and stress has become part of the physician's personal and professional life. The malpractice issue is especially a topic of concern among surgeons.

Effects on Physicians' Families

An area that has received little attention is the effect that a malpractice suit has on physicians and their families. Such suits always produce significant stress that affects a physician immediately. The physician loses confidence and avoids further stress through patient referral or practice limitation.[1,2] Unfortunately, the physician may fail to recognize that the stress from a malpractice suit increases and accentuates stresses that are already occurring within the family.

The complex and extensive effects of a suit on the family are poorly understood and greatly underestimated by most physicians.[3] Many physicians fail to discuss the suit with their families in a mistaken attempt to protect them from the stress. This secrecy, rather than helping, actually compounds stress when family members sense there is a problem but do not know what it is. An uninformed spouse, aware of a change in the physician's behavior, may misinterpret this change. Communication helps the physician handle the stress and also provides the spouse with insight into the physician's mood changes. Through discussion, they can deal with their stress. Not surprisingly, the spouse's stress factors are very similar to those of the physician. The spouse's stress factors include (1) a deep sense of loss, (2) a feeling of marital isolation, (3) a fear of financial vulnerability, (4) social awkwardness, (5) a feeling of social isolation, and (6) a need to provide support for the family, especially the children.

At an appropriate time, the children should be informed and educated about the suit. As the suit becomes public knowledge, there may be a dramatic change in the children's relationship with their peers. The worst way for the children to learn of a suit is from friends whose sources of information are television, radio, newspapers, or hearsay. It is important that the children understand they are not the cause of the physician's anger. Children must be given the tools to handle possible taunting and questions from their peers. Children's stress factors will vary with their ages and personalities. Because they feel the loss of family mores, they have a need for reassurance and for verbalization at an appropriate level. Behavioral changes should be monitored carefully.

Coping With Stress

Dealing with the stresses caused by a malpractice suit requires a greater understanding of the problem. The AMA's Medical Auxiliary has prepared a booklet that explores the malpractice problem from the spouse's point of view.[4] It includes an excellent bibliography of additional publications. A number of booklets are available to give the physician and spouse a general overview of the malpractice and litigation process.[5-7] Audiotapes and videotapes may also be helpful.[8,9]

Reading about malpractice can provide physicians and their families with a foundation to cope with stress. Verbalization helps even more. To facilitate this verbalization, support groups of physicians and spouses are being formed throughout the country. The most successful programs combine the efforts of the medical societies and their auxiliaries. Most support groups have been formed at a local level to give personalized support that fits the specific needs of the physicians and spouses they serve. A number of state medical and specialty societies are active in coordinating the development of local support programs (see Appendix).

The AMA Auxiliary has responded to requests for support-group information by publishing a booklet that provides suggestions on how to form support groups.[10] In addition, this booklet contains a bibliography of further resources.

Wisconsin has established a support program that reaches out to physicians and spouses shortly after the allegation is filed. The contact letter informs the physician that a list of physicians willing to function in a support capacity will be sent on request. A separate letter from the Auxiliary sent to the spouse advises that a support group is available.

A third way to diffuse the anger and stress of a malpractice suit is to become active in solving the malpractice problem. Physicians and spouses can work for tort reform and join educational and support groups.

References

1. Harvey L: *AMA Surveys of Physicians and Public Opinion*. Chicago, American Medical Association, 1986.
2. *Professional Liability Insurance and Its Effects: Report of a Survey of ACOG's Membership*. Washington, DC, American College of Obstetricians and Gynecologists, 1985.
3. Bursztajn H, Feinbloom R, et al: *Medical Choices, Medical Chances: How Patients, Families, and Physicians Can Cope with Uncertainty*. New York, Dell Publishing Co, 1981.
4. *What Every Physician's Spouse Should Know...Professional Liability*. Chicago, American Medical Association Auxiliary, 1985.
5. *Understanding Malpractice Claims: A Guide for Physicians and Spouses*. Denver, Colorado Medical Auxiliary, 1983.
6. *Understanding Malpractice Claims*. Columbia, South Carolina Medical Association Auxiliary.
7. *Understanding Medical Liability Claims*. Pinehurst, North Carolina Medical Society Auxiliary.
8. Raines E: *Coping with Malpractice Problems*, audiocassette. Chicago, American Medical Association Auxiliary.
9. Illinois State Medical Society: *At the Heart of the Matter: The Role of the Expert Witness*, videotape. Chicago, Illinois State Medical InterInsurance Exchange.
10. *Professional Liability in the '80's: What Medical Auxiliaries Can Do*. Chicago, American Medical Association Auxiliary, 1985.

Appendix
Support Groups*

Alabama

Medical Association of Alabama
George Oetting
19 S Jackson
Montgomery, AL 36197
(205) 263–6441

Colorado

Medical Society and Auxiliary
Sandy Finney
PO Box 17550
Denver, CO 80217-0550
(303) 779–5455

Florida

Lee County Medical Society of Florida
Ann Wilke
PO Box 1704
Fort Meyers, FL 33902
(813) 936–1645

Georgia

Medical Association of Georgia
Stephen Davis, PhD
938 Peachtree St
Atlanta, GA 30309
(404) 876–7535

Indiana

Fort Wayne Medical Society
Larry Pickering
2414 E State Blvd, Suite 303
Fort Wayne, IN 46805
(219) 482–4589

Maryland

Medical and Chirurgical Faculty
Robert White
1211 Cathedral St
Baltimore, MD 21201
(301) 539-0872

Michigan

Michigan Academy of Family Physicians
H. F. Kendrick, MD
4036 S Shore Dr
Pontiac, MI 48054
(313) 685–6331

Mississippi

Mississippi Medical Association
Mrs. Ben (Linda) Martin
115 Sleepy Hollow Dr
Columbus, MS 39701
(601) 327–1471

New Jersey

Medical Society of New Jersey
Edward Reading
Two Princess Rd
Lawrenceville, NJ 08648
(609) 896–1766

North Carolina

North Carolina Medical Society and Auxiliary
Gail Clark, PhD
PO Box 1569
Pinehurst, NC 28374
(919) 295–1815

South Carolina

South Carolina Medical Society
Joy Drennen
PO Box 11188
Columbia, SC 29211
(803) 798–6207

Washington, DC

NCRI Medical Society of DC
Dorothy A. Starr, MD
2040 Belmont Rd, NW
Washington, DC 20009
(202) 462–7111

Washington

Washington State Medical Association Auxiliary
Listening Ear
Beryl Jean Kinny
PO Box 434
Ephrata, WA 98823
(509) 754–2572

Medical Society of Pierce County
George Tanbara, MD
1811 S K St
Tacoma, WA 98405
(206) 383–5777

Spokane County Medical Society
Tim Keller, MD
South 820 McCleaan, Suite 503
Spokane, WA 99204
(509) 747–3500

Wisconsin

LaCrosse County Medical Society and Auxiliary
Fe Albellera
1233 Lauderdale Pl
Onalaska, WI 54650
(608) 783–6141

State Medical Society of Wisconsin
Catherine Nimtz
330 E. Lakeside St
Madison, WI 53715
(608) 257–6781

---

*At the time of publication.

Psychological Reactions to Medical Malpractice Suits and the Development of Support Groups as a Response

Sara C. Charles, MD

Introduction

Although many people suggest that doctors should not take an allegation of malpractice "personally," most physicians experience it as a direct assault on their personal and professional integrity. As a result, doctors tend to perceive litigation as a stressful life event that results in considerable, albeit usually temporary, emotional disequilibrium. Such a response is normal and, to a large extent, unavoidable. It is, in fact, a function of their humanity.

Common Reactions to Being Sued

In studies of physicians in northern Illinois, 96% acknowledged some emotional reaction for at least a limited period.[1-4] These reactions were most commonly described as intense anger and "feelings of devastation." A variety of symptoms, often clustered into one of two groups, also developed (Table 35–1). The first cluster, associated with clinical depression and acknowledged by about 33% of doctors, included symptoms such as depressed mood, insomnia, loss of appetite, loss of energy, decreased libido, and, in some instances, suicidal ideation. The second cluster of symptoms, experienced by about 26% of doctors, was characterized by overwhelming anger accompanied by feelings such as frustration, irritability, headache, inner tension, gastrointestinal distress, insomnia, and depressed mood. In addition, some doctors acknowledged distractibility with lack of concentration, difficulties in making a decision, and general feelings of dissatisfaction and worry.

Approximately 16% of doctors experienced the onset of a physical illness or the exacerbation of a previously diagnosed one. These were usually stress-related illnesses such as coronary artery disease, hypertension, colitis, and duodenal ulcer.

A small percentage of doctors reacted to litigation by engaging in behaviors such as excessive use of alcohol (7% of study subjects), the abuse of drugs (less than 1%), and suicidal ideation (3% of study subjects).

The Emotional Course of a Malpractice Suit

Most physicians who are formally charged with malpractice immediately feel stunned and often deny or disavow the event. As the reality and degree of accusations are absorbed and the initial stunned reaction diminishes, the doctor generally begins to feel enormous anger. In many instances this translates into insomnia, depressed feelings, and the previously described symptom clusters. The development of these symptoms signals a period of emotional disequilibrium that may resolve within one to two weeks. Occasionally, these symptoms persist for a longer period, diminish and recur periodically, or last until the resolution of the suit or longer.

Litigation is by its very nature a lengthy and unpredictable process. Consequently, symptoms may recur whenever the lawsuit demands the doctor's attention. For example, a week or two after the delivery of the complaint and consultation with a lawyer and insurer, emotional equilibrium may return. A call many months later to schedule the first depositions may cause the whole spectrum of symptoms to re-emerge. This pattern may occur repeatedly over a number of years, depending on the degree of involvement with the case up to and including the time of the trial.

Deciding whether or not to go to trial or whether or not to settle is agonizing for many doctors. The unpredictable nature of a trial pits a doctor's wish to "clear his or her name" against the possibility of losing, creating a conflict. Losing may result in feelings of diminished self-confidence and increase the risk of financial loss to self and family. Doctors often feel very alone in these decisions despite well-intended advice from proponents on both sides. It is essential, of course, that doctors who go to trial are convinced of their competent performance in the situation in question and committed to active and persistent defense of their cases.

Many doctors who go to trial describe the experience as one of the most trying of their lives. It is a

Table 35–1
Self-reported symptoms of physicians after being sued

Symptoms	Study I[1] (1982)	Study II[2] (1983)	Study III[3] (1984)
Depression cluster	39.0%	35.0%	24%
Anger cluster	20.0%	31.0%	26%
Physical illness	16.0%	15.0%	18%
Alcohol misuse	2.0%	11.0%	8%
Drug misuse	0.7%	0.5%	0%
Suicidal ideation	2.2%	6.7%	0%

source of some support that over 70% of doctors who go to trial win, but it is a source of anxiety that a certain percentage do not. It is also of interest that for many doctors who win their trials there remains a sense of frustration and anger arising from a conviction that the whole process served no particular purpose and that they should not have been sued in the first place.

Many doctors are advised by legal counsel and insurance interests to settle the case, often for well-founded business or legal reasons. Some doctors who settled report lingering regrets and feelings of lack of vindication even though the settlements involved no admission or denial of guilt.

Irrespective of the final outcome of the suit, most doctors—especially those involved for lengthy periods—indicate that as a result of being sued, they will never be quite the same as before their involvement in litigation.

Why Doctors React to Malpractice Litigation

Litigation is an event that has certain inherently stressful characteristics.

Unpredictability After a suit is served, the doctor's name may be dropped from the complaint within six weeks or the doctor may still be waiting for trial five or six years later, often irrespective of the merits of the case. The manner by which lawyers proceed, the rules of law, the delays, the testimony of experts, the judge, and, if the case goes to trial, the jury, all contribute to the inherently unpredictable nature of the litigation process. This generates feelings of frustration and anxiety.

Loss of Control The average doctor, when faced with a stressful situation, tends to address the problem actively in order to regain control of the situation and reduce the feelings of discomfort engendered by the stress. Litigation, however, draws the doctor into the legal environment. The lawyer, offering reassurance, often tells the doctor not to worry, "just do what I tell you . . ." Few pieces of advice create more anxiety. Such advice tends to erode rather than support the doctor's characteristic mode of functioning, resulting in feelings of dependence and powerlessness, which in turn generate greater anxiety.

The Meaning of the Event Charges of negligence and incompetence are a direct assault on one's sense of self. They often engender feelings of shame and guilt. These must be evaluated in the context of the individual doctor's own feelings of competence, self-confidence, and idealism. In addition, each doctor has unique perceptions of the meaning of the event. My studies revealed that doctors generally experience the event in one of four ways. (1) When the plaintiff is a long-standing patient or relative of a friend, the result is often feelings of betrayal and anger. (2) When the lawsuit challenges feelings of competence, the doctor may feel greater anxiety about making decisions and overreact to ordinary practice stressors. (3) Often the doctor feels immense anger, believing that the medical malpractice situation is unmanageable or that the system works against the physician in some way. (4) Lastly, some doctors perceive litigation as time-consuming and bothersome and feel irritated and frustrated by the event.

Individual Coping Mechanisms Each doctor brings a unique life history, psychological characteristics, and pattern of dealing with stress to the litigation experience. The overall method of responding to the suit is highly variable.

Social Support Twenty-seven percent of the study subjects reported feeling alone and isolated from peers as a result of being sued.[1-4] Lawyers advise their clients not to "talk to anybody." Lawyers are correctly concerned that their clients not discuss details of their cases in a manner that would jeopardize their defense. There is a human need, however, to share the impact of any major life event with an understanding friend, associate, or spouse. There is a considerable body of research that supports the notion that the impact of a major stressor is modified by social support.

How To Cope With the Stress Produced by Litigation

Effective measures of coping can counteract the stressful characteristics of litigation.

Unpredictability (1) Recognize that the legal process is unpredictable in terms of its rules, the lawyers, the judge, the juries, the outcome. (2) Make active efforts to inform yourself about the process so that you can anticipate all the possibilities. (3) Ask your attorney to explain points of law and what you can anticipate throughout the process. (4) Familiarize yourself with the legal process by participation in mock depositions, trials, and other legal proceedings. (5) Participate in choosing your experts.

Degree of Control (1) Actively involve yourself in the defense of your case. (2) Review depositions. (3) Actively study the literature as it relates to your case. (4) Examine your ordinary office and practice procedures and make changes where indicated. (5) Examine your use of time and initiate changes that help you feel more in control. This may mean an increase or decrease in time with patients, more leisure, or change in office hours. (6) Do not practice in situations that demand compromising your professional standards. (7) Participate in loss prevention education, especially as it relates to keeping records, communication, and informed consent. (8) Work in professional groups that attempt to remedy the medical malpractice problem. (9) If particularly stressed by some aspect of the case, e.g., before a deposition or in preparation for trial, rearrange your office visits or cancel surgery or other clinical procedures, if necessary.

Meaning of the Event (1) Reflect on your own feelings of competence and take whatever measures necessary to solidify them. (2) Reflect on the meaning of your profession and your career and plan accordingly. (3) Examine how this event affects your relationships with patients, especially if the plaintiff is a long-term patient or friend. Work to neutralize negative feelings. (4) Consulting an expert on family finances and financial planning can often reduce anxiety.

Means of Coping (1) Your own life history may help you choose effective ways of coping. (2) Denial and suppression are useful mechanisms for most doctors. (3) Self-observation is essential. If somatic symptoms develop and do not soon diminish, consult your doctor. If persistent psychological symptoms, alcohol, or drug abuse develop, consult a specialist. (4) Re-examine your life and restructure it as necessary. Litigation is often a time to reorder priorities. (5) Arrange more or better use of leisure time. Active sports, "nonworking" vacations, and more family time are helpful diversions. (6) Make any changes in your practice necessary to make it less anxiety-provoking and more manageable.

Social Support (1) Recognize that most doctors need to share their reactions to the experience. (2) Identify those with whom you feel most comfortable about sharing your reactions. These may be another doctor, a spouse, a family member, a friend, office staff, or legal counsel. Most people are willing to hear you out. (3) If the above are unavailable, contact your local medical or specialty society for referral to a support group or available peer.

Physician Support Groups

A number of medical and specialty societies throughout the country have recognized that an increasing number of doctors have been affected by the stress engendered by malpractice litigation. One form of response is the development of a physician support group. The rationale for this particular response is the assumption that these physicians have experienced some disruption in their relationship to their role and to their interaction with others as a result of litigation. Support groups whose members share the same social environment and role are more likely to understand the nature of this disruption and, therefore, to provide

support. A number of models have been explored and developed. The Illinois State Medical Society has provided leadership in this regard, has served as a resource for interested groups, and has monitored information and progress in their development.[5] The following list represents efforts on the part of a variety of groups.

Informal Consultation This involves an informal conversation with a peer and is the most common model that doctors use. It provides a listening ear, is a humane response to an associate who is often sorely stressed, and it is not designed to focus or even discuss the legal merits of the case. The content of the conversation focuses on the physician's emotional reaction to being sued, and often just one session is sufficient to diminish the feelings of isolation, anger, shock, and dismay that result from being named in a suit.

Organized Physician Support Groups Models developed in different areas are based on confidential interactions among physicians, the focus of which is not the legal dimensions of the malpractice suit but rather the emotional reactions to it.

A group organized by the Illinois State Medical Society consists of a panel of physicians from various specialties, all of whom have been through the entire litigation process. They have volunteered to be available to any physicians who wish to talk about their experience. The stipulation that the participating panel members have experienced the entire process, including trial, is based on the knowledge that different physicians may need support at different stages of the litigation process. Physicians were informed of this group's existence by a notice in the *Illinois Medical Journal* and by communications from the Illinois Medical Inter-Insurance Exchange, particularly after notification of a suit.

The Wisconsin Medical Society has formed a panel of physicians similar to the above model but physicians on the referral panel, although they have been sued, have not necessarily experienced the entire litigation process. Also, support physicians may not be from the same specialty as the physician requesting consultation.

Joint Support Groups of Physicians and Spouses Spouses are encouraged to participate in the Wisconsin Medical Society panel with the physicians.

The Winnebago County Medical Society in Illinois has formed a panel of couples who have experienced the litigation process and who are available to provide support and confidential assistance to couples currently undergoing a malpractice suit.

The New Jersey Medical Society has formed a litigation stress support group that sponsors a monthly meeting open to all physicians and spouses. The group is open-ended and meets for approximately 90 minutes each time. The meeting is divided between an education program and a group discussion on principles of mutual self-help.

Ongoing Support Groups The support group model promoted by John-Henry Pfifferling, PhD, of the Center for Professional Well-Being, Durham, North Carolina, depends largely on a small group of interested individuals. The group is self-generated, confidential, and follows the principles outlined by Dr. Pfifferling. Its focus often extends beyond litigation to common stressors in medical practice. Because it is time-consuming and highly structured in terms of regular attendance and membership, and because the need for support in the litigation experience is sporadic, it has not proved to be a functional model at this time.

Professional Liability Support Groups The South Carolina Medical Association developed a steering committee of both medical society members and their auxiliary counterparts who provide support with general educational meetings two or three times a year. The committee also circulates educational materials. Although its primary goals are educational, a prominent side-effect of its efforts has been the emotional support it provides to sued physicians and their families.

In Maryland, physicians who have been sued receive an open invitation to a quarterly meeting aimed at enabling physicians to handle the stress of litigation better.

Publication of Information on Malpractice Litigation Many medical and specialty societies, as well as the American Medical Association and its auxiliary, have published booklets and media materials that provide information on medical malpractice litigation. The A.M.A. recently established a clearinghouse for such informational materials, making them available to all interested parties.

As the effects of litigation become more widely recognized, the need for an organized response may diminish because informal support mechanisms may be more readily available. In the meantime, the development of some kind of program that provides support is crucial for practicing physicians.

Summary

For doctors to cope with litigation effectively, it is critical that they obtain accurate information about the current climate of litigation. Despite the considerable evidence that the core issue is not one of gross physician negligence, there is still no substitute for the feelings of competence and self-confidence that derive from adherence to the highest standards of medical knowledge and care. When a suit occurs, these feelings are often the best antidote for the hurt and depressed feelings that almost always arise. It behooves the doctor to try to deal as effectively as possible with the symptoms and behavioral responses to litigation because of the subtle impact such changes have on doctor-patient relationships and patient care.

Acknowledgment

Material from this chapter was adapted and reprinted with permission from *The Physicians Support Group Brochure*. Chicago, Illinois State Medical Society, 1987.

References

1. Charles SC, Wilbert JR, Kennedy EC: Physicians' self-reports of reactions to malpractice litigation. *Am J Psychiatry* 1984;141:563–565.
2. Charles SC, Wilbert JR, Franke KJ: Sued and non-sued physicians' self-reported reactions to malpractice litigation. *Am J Psychiatry* 1985;142:437–440.
3. Charles SC, Warnecke RB, Wilbert JR, et al: Satisfactions, dissatisfactions, and new sources of stress among sued and non-sued physicians. *Psychosomatics*, in press.
4. Charles SC, Pyskoty CB, Nelson A: Physicians on trial: Self reported reactions to malpractice trials. *The Western Journal of Medicine*, in press.
5. Charles SC: Support group formed. *Ill Med J* 1985;167:6.

Index

Abrasion, in meniscus repair 209–221
Accessory navicular 79–80
Acetabular dysplasia 15–16
Acquired immune deficiency syndrome 13, 22
Afferent vascular system 29
AIDS 13, 22
Allograft (*see* Graft)
Amputation, for neoplasm 8
Anasplasia 3
Anatomy and structure,
    clubfoot 93–106
    femur 27–31, 59, 173–175
    hip 225–227
    muscle-tendon unit 275–276
    pelvic ring 119–121
    radiocarpal joint 189–190
Angiography,
    avascular necrosis 56–57
    neoplasm 4
    pelvic fracture 133–134, 139–141
Ankle (*see also* Foot and toes),
    fixation 265–266
    fracture classification 251–256
    remobilization 267–268
Anterior cruciate ligament,
    deficiency 209
    reconstruction 216
Apophysitis,
    calcaneal 78–79
    metatarsal 79
Artery 27–31
Arthritis,
    juvenile rheumatoid 83, 114
    osteoarthritis 69
    secondary 33
    septic 83–84
Arthrodesis,
    avascular necrosis 63, 67
    donor bone 15
    flatfoot 112
    skewfoot 114
    tarsal coalition 114
Arthroereisis 112
Arthrography, vs arthroscopy 191
Arthroplasty 45–47
Arthroscopic surgery 181–231,
    elbow 195–201
    hip 223–231
    meniscus 203–221
    wrist 183–194
Arthroscopy,
    portals 196–199, 212–213
    vs arthrography 191
Articular cartilage (*see* Soft tissue)
Aseptic necrosis 33–40
Avascular necrosis 25–73,

arthroplasty 45–47
bone,
    graft 42–43
    scan 53–54, 61–62
bracing 63
causes 41, 51, 59–60
decompression 42, 63
diagnosis 51–57, 61–62
electrical stimulation 44
epidemiology 41, 67
evaluation 41
femur,
    head 41–57
    proximal 27–31
fusion 47
hip 46–47, 67
history-taking 51
imaging 53–54
laboratory tests 51
metatarsal head 81–82
nonsurgical treatment 41–42, 63
osteotomy 43–44, 63
pediatric 59–65
physical findings 51
prophylactic surgery 42–44
prosthesis 46
staging 60–61
tarsal navicular 81
total hip replacement 46–47
treatment,
    electrical stimulation 44
    nonsurgical 41–42, 63
    surgical 42–44
types 59

Bennett's fracture 247–249
Biomechanics,
    femur 173–175
    flatfoot 111
    intoeing 107–108
    meniscus 209
    pelvic ring 119
Blood,
    clot, in meniscus repair 215–216
    group 13
    hemorrhage 129–134, 139–140
    supply,
        to bone 27–31
        to femoral head 30, 59
        to healing bone 30
        to meniscus 209–210, 213–214
        to proximal femur 27–31
Bone (*see also* individual listings),
    banks 11–24, 153,
        cost 14
        donor selection 13

medicolegal issues 22
procurement 13–14
retrieval 14
safety 14
storage 14
blood supply 27–31, 59
chronic disorders 77–80
cyst 78, 84–85
graft 11–24, 42–43, 63, 69, 153–154, 159, 164, 167–171, 176, 264, 269, 270
foot pain 77
necrosis (*see* Avascular necrosis)
nonunion 151–179,
femur 173–179
historical overview 153–154
humerus 161–165
radius 157–159
tibia 167–171
ulna 157–159
use of electricity 155–156
osteoporosis 69, 71, 80
scan 39–40, 53–54, 61–62
stock 11–24, 69, 175
trauma (*see* Fracture)
Bracing (*see also* Fixation), in avascular necrosis 63
Bucket-handle tear 205

Calcaneal apophysitis 78–79
Calcaneus (*see* Foot and toes)
Calcium,
malabsorption 69
with blood transfusion 130
Cerebral palsy 113
Children (*see* Pediatric orthopaedics)
Chilectomy 63
Classification (*see also* Staging),
ankle fracture 251–256
avascular necrosis 59–61
flatfoot 111
meniscal tears 203, 217–220
pelvic ring disruptions 124–126
Clotting factor 130
Clubfoot 87–106,
anatomy 93–106
computer modeling 99–100
criteria for surgery 87
postoperative care 92
resistant 93–106
surgical techniques 89–92, 101–104
Compartmentalization, of neoplasm 4–5
Complications, of surgery (*see* Surgery)
Compression plate 162, 167–171
Computed tomography,
clubfoot 99
flatfoot 114
neoplasm 4
pelvic ring 122–125, 133
Computer modeling, of clubfoot 99–100
Cyst,
bone 78, 84–85
metaphyseal 60

Decompression, in avascular necrosis 42, 63
Degenerative tears, of meniscus 206
Diagnosis,
avascular necrosis 51–57, 61–62

femoral anteversion 107
flatfoot 109
foot pain 77
nonunion, of forearm 158
pelvic injury 122–125, 133–134, 139–141
reflex sympathetic dystrophy 80
tarsal tunnel syndrome 80–81
wrist pain 80
Diagnostic techniques (*see also* individual listings),
angiography 4, 56–57, 133–134, 139–141
arthrography, vs arthroscopy 191
bone scan 39–40, 53–54, 61–62
computed tomography 4, 99, 114, 122–125, 133
isotope scan 4
magnetic resonance imaging 4, 39–40, 61–62
myelography 4
nuclear counting 4, 61–62
peritoneal lavage 131, 139
radiography 3–5, 33–40, 77, 78, 99, 111, 121–124, 133–136
Diaphysis,
femur, blood supply 27–31
radius, nonunion 157–159
ulna, nonunion 157–159
DNA concentration, in neoplasm staging 4
Double Cobra plate 143–150
Down's syndrome 109
Dysplasia,
acetabular 15–16
anaplasia 3
epiphyseal 59

Efferent vascular system 29
Ehlers-Danlos syndrome 109
Elbow,
arthroscopic surgery 195–201
complications 200
indications 195
portals 196–199
postoperative care 199–200
surgical technique 195–196
fixation 265
floating 262
stiffness 258
Electrical stimulation,
avascular necrosis 44
femur 176
humerus 164–165
nonunion 154, 155–156
tibia 270–271
Embolization, to control hemorrhage 140–141
Emergency care,
pelvic ring disruption 129–132
polytrauma 257
Epidemiology,
avascular necrosis 41, 67
factors affecting total hip replacement 68
Legg-Calvé-Perthes' disease 59
Epiphyseal arteries 28–29
Epiphysis (*see also* Femur),
blood supply 28–29, 59
deformity 59
Excision, vs resection 8
External fixation (*see also* Fixation) 257–273,
ankle 265–266
elbow 265

femur 260–261
foot 258–259
forearm 258
hip 266–267
humerus 163, 258
knee 266
metatarsal 258–259
pelvis 261
tibia 259
wrist 265

Femur,
    afferent vascular system 29
    anteversion 107–108
    avascular necrosis 41–65,
        early diagnosis 51–57
        in children 59–65
        overview 41–50
    blood supply 27–31, 59
    deficiency 16–18
    efferent vascular system 29
    electrical stimulation 176
    fixation 176–178, 260–261
    fracture 173–179, 260–261
        anatomy 173–175
        biomechanics 173–175
        salvage procedures 175–178
    intermediate vascular system 29–30
    intracortical circulation 27–28
    microcirculation 29
    nonunion 173–179,
        distal third 175
        proximal third 173–175
        salvage procedures 175–178
Fibroma, nonossifying 85
Fibrosarcoma 6
Finger (see Hand and fingers)
Fixation,
    ankle 265–266
    elbow 265
    external 257–273,
        bracing, in avascular necrosis 63
        in-board traction 262–263
        joint remobilization 267–268
        of isolated fractures 257–261
        of multiple fractures 261–263
        rigid 257–258
        temporary 262–263
        with muscle loss 259–260
    femur 176–178, 260–261
    flatfoot 113
    foot 258–259
    forearm 157–158, 258
    hip 266–267
    humerus 163, 258
    internal,
        compression plate 162, 167–171
        Double Cobra plate 143–150
        intramedullary nailing 162–163, 174–175
        wounds precluding 263
    knee 266
    metatarsal 258–259
    pelvis 135–136, 143–150, 261
    radius 157–159
    tibia 259
    ulna 157–159

wrist 265
Flap,
    muscle 269
    myocutaneous 264, 269, 270
    tears 204–205, 211
Flatfoot 109–115,
    differential diagnosis 109
    evaluation 111
    features of 109–110
    hypermobile 111–112
    prehallux syndrome 112–113
    skewfoot 114–115
    spastic 113
    tarsal coalition 113–114
    treatment 112
Floating elbow 262
Floating knee 261–262
Foot and toes (see also Ankle),
    apophysitis 78–79
    child's 75–115
    clubfoot (see Clubfoot)
    fixation 258–259
    flatfoot (see Flatfoot)
    Freiberg's infraction 81–82
    gait analysis 107–108
    heel bisector line 107–108
    infection 83–84
    intoeing 107–108
    Köhler's disease 81
    neoplasm 84–85
    pain 77–85
    reflex sympathetic dystrophy 80
    Sever's disease 79–80
    skewfoot 114–115
    spastic 113
    subtalar complex 82–83
    tarsal coalition 113–114
    tarsal tunnel syndrome 80–81
    trauma 77
Foot-progression angle 107–108
Fracture (see also anatomic locations),
    classification 251–256
    comminuted 164, 264
    fixation (see Fixation)
    fracture-dislocation 246–249
    isolated 257–261
    multiple 261–263
    nonunion (see Nonunion)
    oblique 241–243
    polytrauma 257–273
    problem 235–249
    spiral 241–243
    toddler's 77
Freiberg's infraction 81–82

Gage's sign 61
Gait analysis 107–108
Gaucher's disease 59
Genitourinary injuries 131
Giant-cell tumor 6
Graft,
    bone 11–24, 42–43, 63, 69, 153–154, 159, 164, 167–171, 176, 264, 269, 270
    medicolegal issues 22
    muscle flap 29
    myocutaneous flap 264, 269, 270

osseocutaneous 270
osteochondral 63
skin 164, 264

Hand and fingers (*see also* Wrist),
    fracture,
        distal phalanx 236–239
        metacarpal 243–244
        proximal phalanx 240–243
        sesamoid 246
    fracture-dislocation,
        Bennett's 247–249
        dorsal 246–247
        metacarpal 249
        volar 247
Heel bisector line 107–108
Hemorrhage 129–134, 139–140
Hepatitis B 13
Hip,
    arthroscopic surgery 223–231,
        anatomy 225–227
        complications 230–231
        surgical technique 223–225
    avascular necrosis 46–47, 67
    external rotation 107–108
    fixation 266–267
    fusion 47, 63
    remobilization 267–268
    total replacement 46–47, 67–73
Horizontal cleavage tear 205, 210–211
Humerus,
    fixation 163, 258
    floating elbow 262
    nonunion 161–166,
        distal third 163–164
        electrical stimulation 164–165
        middle third 162–163
        humoral sleeve 165
        proximal third 161–162
        radial nerve injury 164
        with infection 164
        with loss of substance 164
Hyperchromatism 3
Hyperthyroidism 69
Hypothermia 129–130
Hypothyroidism 59

Imaging (*see* Diagnostic techniques)
Implant (*see also* Graft),
    femur 46, 178
    total hip 67–73
In-board traction 262–263
Infections,
    foot 83–84
    nonunion 164
    polytrauma 257–258, 263
    septic arthritis 83–84
Instruments, arthroscopic 183–185, 204, 213
Intermediate vascular system 29–30
Internal fixation (*see also* Fixation),
    femur 174–178
    flatfoot 113
    forearm 157–158, 258
    humerus 258
    pelvis 135–136, 143–150
    radius 157–158

ulna 157–158
Intoeing 107–108
Intramedullary nailing 162–163, 174–175
Intramedullary pressure 30–31
Isotope scan 4

Joint (*see also* anatomic locations),
    distractor 213
    remobilization 267–268
Juvenile rheumatoid arthritis 83, 114

"Kissing patella sign" 107
Knee (*see also* Meniscus),
    fixation 266
    floating 261–262
    "kissing patella sign" 107
    remobilization 267–268

Laparotomy 132, 139
Legg-Calvé Perthes' disease 41, 59–65
Ligament (*see also* Soft tissue),
    anterior cruciate 209, 216
    laxity 109–110
    trauma, and foot pain 77
Limb-length discrepancy 51
Limb-salvage procedures,
    in neoplasm 8
    in nonunion 175–178

Magnetic resonance imaging,
    aseptic necrosis 39–40
    avascular necrosis 61–62
    neoplasm 4
Malpractice (*see* Medicolegal issues)
Marfan's syndrome 109
Méary's angle 110, 111
Medicolegal issues,
    bone banks 22
    professional liability 283–292
        common reactions 289–292
        coping with 285, 290–291
        effect on family 285
        stress 285–287
        support groups 286–287, 291–292
Meniscus 203–221,
    arthroscopic meniscectomy 203–208,
        classification of tears 203
        general principles 203–204
        instruments 204
        surgical techniques 204–208
    arthroscopic repair 209–221
        basic science 209–210
        blood clot preparation 215–216
        complications 220
        healing 217–220
        methods 210–212
        portals 212–213
        posterior incision 212
        postoperative care 216–217
        vascularity 213–214
        with anterior cruciate ligament surgery 216
Metacarpal (*see* Hand and fingers)
Metaphysis,
    blood supply 28–29
    cyst 60
Metastasis,

neoplasm 5–6
  reconstructive surgery 22
Metatarsal (*see also* Foot and toes),
  apophysitis 79
  fracture fixation 258–259
  Freiberg's infraction 81–82
  osteotomy 114–115
Morquio's syndrome 59
Multiple trauma (*see* Polytrauma)
Muscle (*see also* Soft tissue),
  anatomy 275–276
  contusion 277–278
  fiber types 275
  flap 269
  laceration 276–277
  mechanisms of injury 275–276
  muscle-tendon unit 275–282
  physiology 275–276
  rupture 279–280
  strain 278–281
Myelography 4
Myocutaneous flap 264, 269, 270

Navicular,
  accessory 79–80
  tarsal 81
Necrosis (*see also* Avascular necrosis), staging 33–40
Neoplasm 1–10,
  amputation 8
  anaplasia 3
  angiography 4
  articulation 6–8
  bone graft 18–22
  computed tomography 4
  excision, vs resection 8
  fibroma, nonossifying 85
  fibrosarcoma 6
  foot 24–25
  grade 3–4
  isotope scan 4
  limb-salvage procedures 8
  magnetic resonance imaging 4
  metastasis 5–6, 22
  myelography 4
  nuclear counting 4
  osteochrondroma 84
  osteoid osteoma 84
  osteosarcoma 6
  pleomorphism 3
  radiography 3–5
  sarcoma 6
  site 4–5
  staging 1–10
  surgery 6–10, 18–22
Nerve,
  radial 164
  reflex sympathetic dystrophy 80
  tarsal tunnel syndrome 80–81
  transcutaneous stimulation 80
Neuroblastoma 59
Nonunion,
  bone graft 153–154, 159
  electrical stimulation 154, 155–156, 164–165, 167–171, 176
  femur 173–179
  historical overview 153–154

humerus 161–166
  radius 157–159
  tibia 167–171
  ulna 157–159
  with infection 164
  with loss of substance 164
Nuclear counting 4, 61–62

Orthotics,
  clubfoot 104
  flatfoot 110, 112
  humeral sleeve 165
Osgood-Schlatter disease 79
Osteoarthritis 69
Osteochondroma 84
Osteoid osteoma 84
Osteomalacia 69, 71
Osteomyelitis 84
Osteonecrosis (*see also* Avascular necrosis) 67
Osteoporosis 69, 71, 80
Osteosarcoma 6

Pathoanatomy (*see* Anatomy and structure)
Pediatric orthopaedics,
  accessory navicular 79–80
  avascular necrosis 59–69
  bone trauma 77
  calcaneal apophysitis 78–79
  clubfoot 87–106
  flatfoot 109–115
  foot pain 77–85
  Freiberg's infraction 81–82
  gait analysis 107–108
  infection 83–84
  intoeing 107–108
  Köhler's disease 81
  ligament trauma 77
  metatarsal apophysitis 79
  neoplasm 84–85
  reflex sympathetic dystrophy 80
  Sever's disease 79–80
  subtalar complex 82–83
  tarsal tunnel syndrome 80–81
Pelvic ring disruptions 117–150,
  anatomy 119–121
  biomechanics 119
  classification of disruptions 124–126
  computed tomography 122–125, 133
  Double Cobra plate 143–150
  emergency care 129–132
  hemorrhage 129–134, 139–140
  initial management 129–137
  internal fixation 135–136
  laparotomy 132, 139
  mortality 139
  peritoneal lavage 131, 139
  posterior 143–150
  radiography 121–124, 133–136
  stability,
    assessment 119–127
    criteria 126–127
Periarticular injuries 263–268,
  ankle fixation 265–266
  articular fragments 263–264
  comminution 264
  elbow fixation 265

hip fixation 266–267
joint remobilization 267–268
knee fixation 266
with soft-tissue loss 264–265
wrist fixation 265
Periosteal arteries 128
Pleomorphism 3
Polytrauma,
bony union 269–271
in-board traction 262–263
initial care 257
isolated open fracture 257–261
multiple fractures 261–262
periarticular reconstruction 263–268
soft-tissue reconstruction 268–269
Prehallux syndrome 112–113
Professional liability (*see* Medicolegal issues)
Prosthesis (see *Implant*)
Protrusio 15, 46

Radial nerve injury 164
Radial tears 205–206
Radiation,
avascular necrosis 59
tumor transformation 6
Radiocarpal joint 191
Radiography,
aseptic necrosis 33–40
clubfoot 99, 11
foot pain 77, 78
neoplasms 3–5
pelvic ring 121–124, 133–136
Radius,
fracture fixation 258
nonunion 157–159
Reconstructive surgery (*see also* Graft),
metastatic defects 22
periarticular injuries 263–268
soft tissue 268–269
Reflex sympathetic dystrophy 80
Resection, vs excision 8
Rh-sensitization 13

Salvage procedures (*see* Limb-salvage procedures)
Sarcoma 6
Septic arthritis 83–84
Sesamoid fracture 246
Sever's disease 78–79
Shock 129–132
Sickle cell disease 59
Skewfoot 114–115
Soft tissue,
articular cartilage 30
ligament,
anterior cruciate 209, 216
laxity 109–110
trauma, and foot pain 77
loss, in periarticular injuries 264–265
muscle flap 269
muscle-tendon unit 275–282,
anatomy 275–276
contusion 277–278
fiber types 275
laceration 276–277
mechanisms of injury 275–276
physiology 275–276

rupture 279–280
strain 278–281
myocutaneous flap 264, 269, 270
osseocutaneous graft 270
reconstructive surgery 268–269
serial debridement 268–269
skin graft 164, 264
tendon, chronic disorders 77–80
Spasticity 113
Staging (*see also* Classification),
aseptic necrosis 33–40
avascular necrosis 60–61
neoplasm 1–10
Subtalar complex 82–83
Surgery (*see also* Fixation),
arthroscopic 181–231,
elbow 195–201
hip 223–231
meniscus 203–221
wrist 183–194
complications,
elbow 200
hip 230–231
meniscus 220
guidelines,
clubfoot 87
meniscus 203–204
reconstructive,
metastatic defects 22
periarticular injuries 263–268
soft tissue 268–269
techniques,
clubfoot 89–92, 101–104
elbow 195–199
hand 236–249
hip 223–225
meniscectomy 204–207
meniscus repair 210–217
pelvic ring disruption 135–136, 143–145
wrist 187–189
treatment,
avascular necrosis 42–47, 63
clubfoot 87
flatfoot 111–112
neoplasm 6–10, 18–22
nonunion (*see* Nonunion)
pelvic ring disruptions 134
Sutures 214–215
Syphilis 13

Tarsal,
coalition 113–114
tunnel syndrome 80–81
Tears,
fibrocartilage 191
meniscal 203–206
Tendon (*see also* Soft tissue),
chronic disorders 77–80
muscle-tendon unit 275–282
Thigh-foot angle 107–108
Tibia,
fixation 259
muscle loss 259–261
nonunion 167–171
torsion 108
Tinel's sign 80

Toddler's fracture 77
Toe (*see* Foot and toes)
Total hip replacement 46–47, 67–73
Treatment guidelines,
    clubfoot 87
    flatfoot 110
    intoeing 107–108
    meniscus 203–204
Tumor (*see* Neoplasm)

Ulna,
    fixation 258

nonunion 157–159
Uniform Anatomical Gift Act 22

VDRL test 13
Vitamin D 71

Wrist (*see also* Hand and fingers),
    arthroscopic surgery 183–194
    fixation 265
    remobilization 267–268